SKILLS FOR THE PATIENT CARE TECHNICIAN

SKILLS FOR THE PATIENT CARE TECHNICIAN

Susan King Strasinger, DA, MT(ASCP)
Visiting Assistant Professor
Medical Technology Program
The University of West Florida
Pensacola, Florida

Marjorie Schaub Di Lorenzo, MT(ASCP), SH
Adjunct Instructor
Division of Medical Technology
School of Allied Health Professions
University of Nebraska Medical Center
Omaha, Nebraska

Phlebotomy Program Coordinator
Continuing Education
Methodist College
Omaha, Nebraska

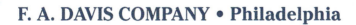

F. A. DAVIS COMPANY • Philadelphia

F. A. Davis Company
1915 Arch Street
Philadelphia, PA 19103

Printed in the United States of America

Last digit indicates print number: 10 9

Publisher, Health Professions: Jean-François Vilain
Senior Developmental Editor: Crystal Spraggins
Production Editor: Roberta Massey
Cover Designer: Louis J. Forgione

As new scientific information becomes available through basic and clinical research, recommended treatments and drug therapies undergo changes. The authors and publisher have done everything possible to make this book accurate, up to date, and in accord with accepted standards at the time of publication. The authors, editors, and publisher are not responsible for errors or omissions or for consequences from application of the book, and make no warranty, expressed or implied, in regard to the contents of the book. Any practice described in this book should be applied by the reader in accordance with professional standards of care used in regard to the unique circumstances that may apply in each situation. The reader is advised always to check product information (package inserts) for changes and new information regarding dose and contraindications before administering any drug. Caution is especially urged when using new or infrequently ordered drugs.

Library of Congress Cataloging-in-Publication Data

Strasinger, Susan King.
    Skills for the patient care technician / Susan King Strasinger,
Marjorie Schaub Di Lorenzo.
        p.   cm.
    Includes bibliographical references and index.
    ISBN 10: 0-8036-0355-X (alk. paper)   ISBN 13: 978-0-8036-0355-4
    1. Clinical medicine—Problems, exercises, etc.   2. Allied health personnel—Problems, exercises, etc.   3. Allied health personnel and patient—Problems, exercises, etc.
I. Di Lorenzo, Marjorie Schaub   II. Title.
    [DNLM: 1. Patient Care—methods—United States.   2. Allied Health Personnel—United States.   W 84 AA1 S88s 1999]
RC58.S77   1999
616–dc21
DNLM/DLC
for Library of Congress   98-44093
                                                                                                        CIP

PREFACE

Skills for the Patient Care Technician is a comprehensive text intended to meet the needs of the growing trend toward multiskilled healthcare workers. The self-contained units in the text are designed to provide flexibility in a variety of settings: structured educational programs, on-the-job training, cross-training of current healthcare personnel, continuing education, or home study.

Each unit begins with specific learning objectives followed by key terms that appear in bold italics when they are introduced in the text. Other technical terms appear in bold and are defined in a glossary at the end of the book. The basics of medical terminology are presented in Appendix I, followed by medical abbreviations related to the content of the text in Appendix II.

Included in the text are units covering safety precautions, anatomy and physiology, phlebotomy, specimen collection and handling procedures, electrocardiography, point-of-care-testing, respiratory care, nursing care, basic radiography, interpersonal skills, and quality assurance related to total quality management. The anatomy and physiology of body systems are integrated with the corresponding diagnostic tests and clinical procedures, disorders, and commonly administered medications. Phlebotomy theory and techniques are covered in-depth to provide eligible persons with the background necessary to sit for certification examinations.

Units are reinforced by study questions, practical exercises, and performance evaluation checklists for technical procedures. All procedures are written to comply with the standards set forth by the Occupational Safety and Health Administration, the Joint Commission on Accreditation of Healthcare Organizations, the National Committee for Clinical Laboratory Standards, the Commission of Office Laboratory Accreditation, and the American Academy of Radiology. Numerous illustrations, photographs, diagrams, charts, and tables are included to visually enhance the comprehension of complex information and technical procedures.

Multiskilled healthcare workers are designated by a variety of titles, including patient care technician, clinical medical assistant, and care team associate. In addition, persons using the text to learn additional skills may already have a primary title, such as radiographer, medical laboratory technician, certified nursing assistant, or phlebotomist. The authors have chosen the term *patient care technician* for this text, and we hope that our readers will understand the necessity of using one general term and will mentally substitute their particular designations while using the text.

The accompanying instructor's guide (available on a disk) will aid instructors by providing lecture outlines, answers to study questions and exercises, additional performance evaluation forms, objective unit tests, and a simulated phlebotomy certification examination. It should be particularly useful in maintaining continuity of instruction when the instruction must be provided by persons from varied healthcare specializations.

Susan King Strasinger
Marjorie Schaub Di Lorenzo

ACKNOWLEDGMENTS

Considering the multidisciplinary content of this text, the authors are indebted to many healthcare practitioners. Without our contributors—Mark L. Diana, MBA, RRT; Pamela B. DoCarmo, PhD, NREMT/P; Frankie Harris-Lyne, CLS(NCA); Marilyn Sinderbrand, BSRT(R); and Jonathan White, BSRT(R) (all from Northern Virginia Community College); and Marsha Cornell, MSN, from Armstrong College—this book would not have been possible. Additional appreciation is expressed to Marsha Cornell for her prompt assistance in completing and editing Unit 14. Also we extend our condolences to Bert Sulcer, RN, for his loss.

The artistic talents of Mary Butters Hukill and the photography skills of Frankie Harris-Lyne have provided the necessary visual enhancement to the text. We thank Sherman Bonomelli, Sara and Adam Mills, John Parker, Stephen Smith, Stephanie Tenny, and the radiology and respiratory students from NVCC for their patience during many photographic sessions.

We are most grateful for the technical assistance and photographic opportunities provided by Anita Sutherland, MT(ASCP), from Fauquier Hospital; Dee Wilkes, CMA, EMT II; John Yarwood, PA; paramedics Jonathan Wells and Ken Wilkes; and the staff of First Physicians of Orange Beach, Ruth Mills, MD; Doris Addison, LPN; Jerrie Holcombe; and Lisa Stowe.

CONTRIBUTORS

Marsha Cornell, MsN
Coordinator
PCT Program
Armstrong Atlantic State University
Savannah, Georgia

Mark L. Diana, MBA, RRT
Assistant Professor
Director, Respiratory Therapy and Pharmacy Technician Programs
Northern Virginia Community College
Annandale, Virginia

Pamela B. DoCarmo, PhD, NREMT/P
Program Head, Emergency Medical Services Technology
Northern Virginia Community College
Annandale, Virginia

Frankie Harris-Lyne, CLS (NCA)
Clinical Coordinator, Medical Laboratory Technician
Phlebotomy and Clinical Medical Assistant Programs
Northern Virginia Community College
Annandale, Virginia

Marilyn Sinderbrand, BSRT (R)
Program Head of Diagnostic Imaging
Northern Virginia Community College
Annandale, Virginia

Jonathan White, BSRT (R)
Clinical Coordinator of Radiography
Northern Virginia Community College
Annandale, Virginia

REVIEWERS

Barbara Ahern, RN, MSN, MEd, Coordinator Health Services, Shawsheen Valley Adult Technical Institute, School of Practical Nursing, Billerica, Massachusetts

Jean Bauer, BA, CLS(NCA), Laboratory Resource Center Coordinator, St. Paul Ramsey Medical Center, Department of Pathology, St. Paul, Minnesota

Laura B. Burcham, BS, RN, CMA, Education Coordinator, Shelby Baptist Medical Center, Alabaster, Alabama

David W. Chang, EdD, RRT, Professor/Director of Respiratory Therapy, Columbus State University, Columbus, Georgia

Michael Fugate, MEd, RT(R), Lead Didactic Faculty, Radiography Program, Santa Fe Community College, Gainesville, Florida

Linda R. Homa, BS, MT, Allied Health Advisor/Program Director/Consultant, Chattanooga State Technical Community College, Chattanooga, Tennessee

Linda S. Lahr, MS, MT(ASCP), Assistant Professor/Program Director, Department of Health Related Professions, East Tennessee State University, Elizabethon, Tennessee

Sally S. Lewis, MS, H.HTL(ASCP), Assistant Professor, Coordinator Health Care Competency Technology Program, Tarrant County Community College, Department of Health Sciences, Hurst, Texas

CONTENTS

UNIT 11

UNIT 12

UNIT **13**

UNIT **14**

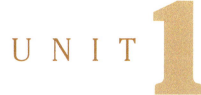

U N I T 1

INTRODUCTION TO THE HEALTHCARE FIELD

KEY TERMS

- *Accreditation* Process by which a program or institution documents meets established guidelines
- *Assault* Attempt or threat to touch or injure another person
- *Battery* Unauthorized physical contact
- *Civil lawsuit* Court action between individuals, corporations, government bodies, or other organizations (compensation is monetary)

■ **Continuous quality improvement**	Institutional program focusing on customer expectations
■ **Criminal lawsuit**	Court action brought by the state for committing a crime against public welfare (punishment is imprisonment and/or a fine)
■ **Ethics**	Principles of personal and professional conduct
■ **Informed consent**	Patient's right to know the method and risks before agreeing to treatment
■ **Invasion of privacy**	Unauthorized release of information
■ **Litigation**	Lawsuit
■ **Malpractice**	Medical care that does not meet a reasonable standard and results in harm
■ **Negligence**	Failure to perform duties according to accepted standards
■ **Patient's Bill of Rights**	Document written by the American Hospital Association stating the patient's rights during treatment
■ **Patient-focused care**	Centralization of patient care to the patient's location
■ **Quality assurance**	Methods used to guarantee quality patient care
■ **Quality control**	Methods used to monitor the quality of procedures
■ **Tort**	Wrongful act committed by one person against another person or property
■ **Total quality management**	Institutional policy to provide customer satisfaction

The healthcare delivery system is currently undergoing major changes in the manner in which patient care is provided. The rising cost of healthcare delivery has been a primary driving factor for these changes, which are designed to increase the efficiency of patient care and patient satisfaction. These changes have affected not only the manner and location in which patient care is performed but also the personnel providing patient services. Healthcare restructuring has resulted in the introduction of a new category of healthcare worker trained to perform a variety of basic patient-care procedures. Currently, these multiskilled healthcare workers are designated by a variety of titles, including patient care technician, clinical associate, clinical technician, healthcare technician, multiskilled practitioner, and care team associate. The authors of this text have chosen to use the term *patient care technician* (**PCT**).

This unit is designed to provide the PCT with an overview of the traditional structure of healthcare, the emerging concept of patient-focused care, the role of the PCT, and the legal aspects of healthcare and its regulation and management.

Healthcare Settings

PCTs are employed in a variety of healthcare settings, including acute-care hospitals, long-term care facilities, hospices, urgent care clinics, wellness centers, health maintenance organizations (**HMOs**), home healthcare, and physicians' office practices. Each facility has its own organizational structure based on the needs of its patients. All facilities have one goal in common, however: to provide quality care to the individual patient.

The skills used by the PCT vary, depending on the type of patient care provided by the facility. For example, a PCT working in an urgent care clinic or a physician's office will perform electrocardiograms (ECGs) much more frequently than will a PCT working in a long-term care facility.

The employment of PCTs in the hospital setting has occurred more recently than in other healthcare settings. This is a result of a new concept in the provision of healthcare, primarily referred to as ***patient-focused care***. The following sections provide a contrast between a traditional hospital structure and patient-focused care with regard to both infrastructure and the roles of healthcare providers.

Hospital Organization

A traditional hospital consists of a Board of Trustees, a Chief of Staff, a hospital administrator, and assistant administrators for service areas. The hospital is governed by the Board of Trustees, which is composed of private citizens. The board is ultimately responsible for the hospital operations and the medical staff. The Chief of Staff is the head of the medical team and acts as the liaison between the physicians, the Board of Trustees, and the hospital administrator. The Board of Trustees hires the hospital administrator to manage hospital operations. This person may be aided by assistant administrators who head each of the four main services of the hospital: professional service, nursing service, support service, and fiscal service. Figure 1–1 illustrates a traditional hospital structure.

PROFESSIONAL (ANCILLARY) SERVICE

Professional service consists of the departments of the hospital that assist the physician in the diagnosis (**Dx**) and treatment (**Rx**) of disease. Major departments in this service include, but are not limited to, radiology, radiation therapy, nuclear medicine, occupational therapy (**OT**), pharmacy, physical therapy (**PT**), respiratory therapy, and the clinical laboratory. The departments of electrocardiography (see Unit 13) and electroencephalography also provide professional services that aid in diagnosis.

NURSING SERVICE

Nursing service deals directly with patient care. Areas frequently included in this service are central supply; infection control; the cardiac care unit (**CCU**); emergency room (**ER**); intensive care unit (**ICU**); nursery; patient units; operating room (**OR**); and specialty areas such as cardiology, **endoscopy**, neurology, surgery, and urology. Healthcare team members associated with this service are registered nurses (**RNs**), licensed practical nurses (**LPNs**), certified nursing assistants (**CNAs**), and the unit secretary or ward clerk. The PCT is frequently a part of this service.

SUPPORT SERVICE

Support service is responsible for maintaining the hospital. Food service, grounds care, housekeeping, human resources, laundry, maintenance, purchasing, and security belong to this service.

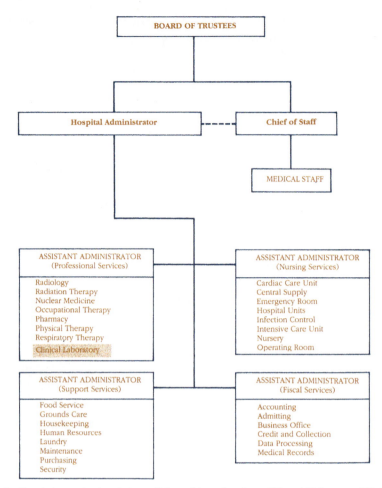

FIGURE 1–1 Hospital organizational chart. (Adapted from Strasinger, SK, and Di Lorenzo, MA: Phlebotomy Workbook for the Multiskilled Healthcare Professional. FA Davis, Philadelphia, 1996, p. 26, with permission.)

FISCAL SERVICE

Fiscal service manages the business aspect of a hospital. Included in this service are accounting, admitting, business office, credit and collection, data processing, and health information technology (medical records).

Professional Service Departments

In the traditional hospital structure the PCT interacts frequently with the professional service departments through scheduling patients for diagnostic procedures, preparing patients for procedures, transporting patients to the departments, and receiving test results. Under the concept of patient-focused care, the PCT is trained to perform some of the basic procedures associated with these departments on the nursing unit. This section provides a general description of the major professional service departments, the services performed, and the professional personnel working in these departments.

RADIOLOGY

The radiology department uses various forms of radiant energy to diagnose and treat disease. Some of the techniques include x-rays of teeth and bones, **computerized ax-**

ial tomography (CAT scan), contrast studies using barium sulfate, **cardiac catheterization**, **fluoroscopy**, **ultrasonography**, and **magnetic resonance imaging (MRI)**. A radiologist, who is a physician, administers diagnostic procedures and interprets radiographs. The allied healthcare professional in this department is a radiographer. The PCT may be trained to perform limited radiographic procedures, such as chest radiographs (see Unit 16).

RADIATION THERAPY

The radiation therapy department uses high-energy x-rays or ionizing radiation to stop the growth of cancer cells. Radiation therapy technologists perform these procedures. Because radiation therapy may affect the bone marrow, blood tests are often performed to monitor the immune status of patients.

NUCLEAR MEDICINE

The nuclear medicine department studies the characteristics of radioactive substances in the diagnosis and treatment of disease. Radioactive materials, called **radioisotopes**, emit rays as they disintegrate, and the rays are measured on specialized instruments. Two types of tests are used. In vitro (outside the body) tests analyze blood and urine specimens using radioactive materials to detect levels of hormones, drugs, and other substances. In vivo (inside the body) tests involve administering radioactive material to the patient by intravenous injection and measuring the emitted rays to examine organs and evaluate their function. Examples of these procedures are bone, brain, liver, and thyroid scans. Therapeutic doses of radioactive material also can be given to a patient to treat diseases. Nuclear medicine technologists perform these procedures under the supervision of a physician.

OCCUPATIONAL THERAPY

The OT department teaches techniques that enable patients with physical, mental, or emotional disabilities to function within their limitations in daily living. Occupational therapists provide this instruction and may be assisted by PCTs.

PHARMACY

The pharmacy department dispenses the medications prescribed by physicians. Persons trained to dispense medications are called pharmacists. The PCT associates with the pharmacy when requesting medications, picking up medications, collecting blood specimens to monitor medication levels, and monitoring patient responses to medications. PCTs do not administer medications without additional training and licensure in many states.

PHYSICAL THERAPY

The PT department provides treatment to patients who have been disabled through illness or injury by using procedures involving water, heat, massage, ultrasound, and exercise. Physical therapists are the professionals trained to provide this therapy. PCTs may be trained to assist patients receiving these treatments.

RESPIRATORY THERAPY

In the respiratory therapy department, patients with breathing disorders are treated by respiratory therapists. Respiratory therapists also perform arterial punctures to obtain blood to be analyzed for blood gases (oxygen and carbon dioxide). Much of the respiratory therapy department's work is performed at the patient's bedside. Therefore, PCTs are frequently trained to perform basic respiratory care procedures (see Unit 15).

CLINICAL LABORATORY

The clinical laboratory (**pathology**) provides data to the healthcare team to aid in determining a patient's diagnosis, treatment, and prognosis. The clinical laboratory is divided into specialized sections, including hematology/coagulation, chemistry, blood bank, serology (immunology), microbiology, urinalysis, and phlebotomy. Blood, bone marrow, culture, feces, urine, and other body fluid specimens are analyzed by medical technologists/clinical laboratory scientists (**MT/CLS**) and medical laboratory technicians/clinical laboratory technicians (**MLT/CLT**) in the clinical laboratory. Two additional sections of the clinical laboratory are histology and cytology. Histology technicians and technologists process and stain tissue obtained during surgery or autopsy for examination by the pathologist. Cytotechnologists process and examine tissue and body fluids for abnormal cells, such as cancer cells.

PCTs interact frequently with the clinical laboratory through the collection of specimens, delivery of specimens to the laboratory, preparation of patients prior to specimen collection, performance of basic laboratory tests at the patient's bedside (referred to as point-of-care testing; see Unit 12), and requisition and receipt of test results. The collection of blood specimens (**phlebotomy**) is usually performed by phlebotomists who are part of the clinical laboratory service or by PCTs. Proper specimen collection is essential for accurate test results, and many PCTs begin their careers as phlebotomists. Many phlebotomists are currently being trained to become PCTs.

Patient-Focused Care

As can be seen, a traditionally structured hospital consists of a large variety of highly specialized areas staffed by personnel trained to perform a limited number of specialized functions. During a typical hospital stay, a patient may be transported to several hospital departments and may see as many as 30 healthcare providers. Patient-focused care is designed to bring the care to the patient whenever possible and to have this care performed by a limited number of trained personnel. Providing this type of care requires some reorganization of the traditional hospital structure through decentralization of specialized departments. Equipment and personnel are relocated to patient-care units.

The degree of this decentralization varies greatly among institutions, and the process continues to evolve. At this time the most frequently adopted change is the cross-training of personnel to perform basic procedures from several departments. This cross-training began by teaching personnel already stationed on the nursing units to perform multiple procedures. The collection of blood specimens performed by clinical laboratory-based phlebotomists became a major part of this cross-training, resulting in the decentralization of phlebotomy and a decrease in the need for personnel trained only as phlebotomists. Therefore, phlebotomists became one of the first groups of healthcare workers not customarily stationed on the nursing units to be cross-trained and relocated to the patient-care areas. Respiratory therapists, who traditionally performed the majority of their functions in the nursing units, and emergency medical personnel, who consistently perform a variety of medical procedures, were other categories of healthcare personnel frequently selected for transfer to particular nursing units. Curricula are currently being developed to train persons without previous healthcare experience to perform these varied patient care functions. These programs are frequently called PCT programs.

The scope of patient-focused care currently ranges from the cross-training of persons already located in the nursing units to perform basic interdisciplinary bedside procedures to the actual relocation of the specialized radiology and clinical laboratory equipment, and personnel to the patient-care units. The type of equipment and personnel relocated is determined by the needs of the specific unit, such as **oncology**, cardiac care, and obstetrics (**OB**). Units also may perform their own admitting and discharging; maintain medical records; perform housekeeping and dietary functions; and have resident pharmacists, physical therapists, and other specialized healthcare personnel.

The advantages of patient-focused care include the reduction in time spent scheduling and transporting patients to specialized areas and the documentation associated with referring patients to various specialty areas, better infection control through minimized personnel contact, elimination of idle time for personnel trained to perform a small number of procedures, the familiarity between the patients and their healthcare givers, and the increased amount of time available for healthcare givers to provide direct patient care. The disadvantages of patient-focused care at this time appear to be temporary and include the time and expense of reorganizing hospital structure and cross-training personnel and the concern of employees about job security.

An increasing amount of medical equipment and testing procedures are being designed to meet the needs of patient-focused care. Therefore, healthcare workers can soon expect to experience some form of patient-focused care wherever they may be employed.

Duties of Patient Care Technicians

As discussed previously, the duties and technical skills required of PCTs will vary with the state and institution in which they are employed and also with the type of patient-care unit in which they work. Figure 1–2 shows a PCT working in a family practice center. In addition to needing technical, clerical, and interpersonal skills, the PCT must have strong organizational skills to efficiently handle a heavy workload and maintain accuracy, often under stressful conditions.

General duties and responsibilities of the PCT as related to the scope of this text include:

1 Caring for patients in a variety of healthcare settings
2 Correctly identifying patients or specimens prior to performing or ordering procedures
3 Collecting appropriate specimens for diagnostic tests by venipuncture and dermal puncture
4 Collecting nonblood specimens for diagnostic tests, using sterile technique when necessary
5 Performing point-of-care laboratory testing, including instrument calibration, quality control, and documentation
6 Performing and labeling a 12-lead ECG, identifying potentially dangerous readings
7 Assisting patients with activities of daily living, including hygiene and ambulation

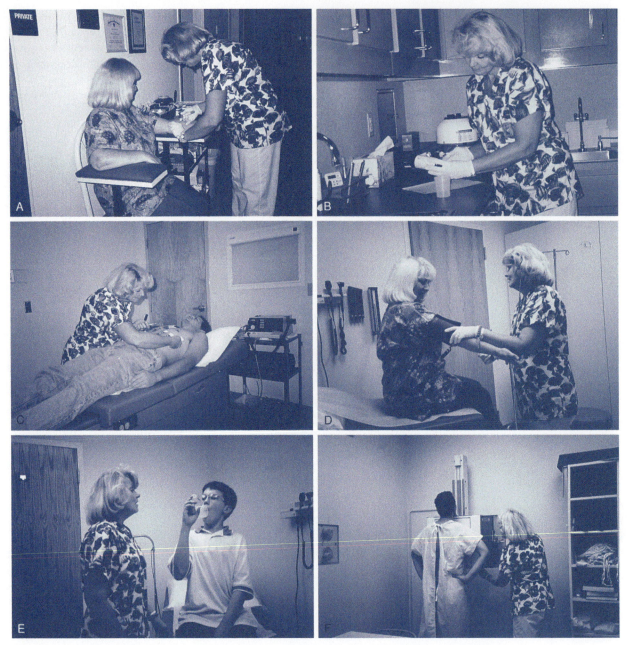

FIGURE 1–2   Examples of PCT duties. *A,* Performing phlebotomy. *B,* Performing chemical examination of urine. *C,* Performing an ECG. *D,* Taking a blood pressure. *E,* Instructing a patient in the use of a nebulizer. *F,* Performing a chest radiograph.

8 Performing and recording patient vital signs and reporting unusual observations or patient concerns to supervisors

9 Assisting with patient treatments

10 Performing and monitoring respiratory treatments, including spirometry, nebulization, pulse oximetry, and oxygen administration

11 Performing limited radiographic procedures

12 Maintaining patient documentation following healthcare setting requirements

13 Observing infection control guidelines and hospital policies

14 Interacting effectively with patients and healthcare personnel

15 Attending scheduled meetings and continuing education presentations

Desirable Personal Characteristics for Patient Care Technicians

PCTs are part of a service-oriented industry, and specific personal characteristics are necessary for success in this area.

DEPENDABILITY

Patient care is a team effort and relies on all members being present and on time when scheduled to work. Unnecessary delays in treatment result when not enough team members are present to perform necessary procedures such as early morning blood collection or the measuring of vital signs.

COMPASSION

PCTs deal with sick, anxious, and frightened patients every day. They must be sensitive to patient needs, understand a patient's concern about a possible diagnosis or fear of a needle when phlebotomy is being performed, and continually take the time to reassure each patient. A smile and a cheerful tone of voice are simple techniques that can put a patient more at ease.

FLEXIBILITY

The PCT, as well as other members of the patient-care team, is trained to perform a variety of unrelated tasks and will continue to expand this knowledge as new advances in medicine occur. Persons must be willing to adapt to these changes, accept additional responsibilities, and, above all, be team players.

HONESTY

The PCT should never hesitate to admit a mistake or to admit that he or she is unsure of the way to perform a procedure on a particular patient. A misidentified patient, mislabeled specimen, or improperly performed procedure can be critical to patient safety.

INTEGRITY

Patient confidentiality must be protected, and patient information should never be discussed with anyone who does not have a professional need to know it.

APPEARANCE

Each organization specifies the dress code it considers most appropriate, but common to all is a neat and clean appearance that portrays a professional attitude to the patient. Lab coats and smocks should be clean, pressed, and completely buttoned; shoes should be polished. Excessive jewelry, makeup, and perfume should not be worn, and long hair must be neatly pulled back. Personal hygiene is extremely important because of close patient contact, and special attention should be paid to bathing and use of deodorant and mouthwash. In general, a sloppy appearance indicates a tendency toward sloppy performance.

COMMUNICATION SKILLS

Good communication skills are critical for the PCT to function as the liaison between the nursing unit and the patients, their families and visitors, and other healthcare personnel. The three components of communication—verbal skills, listening skills, and nonverbal skills or body language—all contribute to effective communication by the PCT.

Verbal Skills

Verbal skills enable PCTs, who may be the primary contact with the patient and family, to introduce themselves, explain procedures, reassure the patient, and help to assure the patient that the procedure is being competently performed. Barriers to verbal communication that must be considered include physical handicaps such as deafness, patient emotions, level of patient education, age, and language proficiency. By recognizing these barriers, the PCT can be better equipped to communicate with the patient. When talking to a hearing-impaired patient, it is important to speak loudly and clearly, facing the patient to facilitate lipreading. Using a calm tone of voice may alleviate the fears of an emotional patient. To help the patient understand a procedure, the PCT must speak to the patient's age and educational level. Use age-appropriate phrases when communicating with children and, whenever possible, communicate at eye level. Avoid medical jargon and use terminology appropriate for laypersons. Every attempt should be made to locate someone who can translate for patients for whom English is not the first language. Most hospitals maintain a list of interpreters.

Listening Skills

Listening skills are a key component of communication. Allow the patient to express feelings and anxieties. Actively interact by providing appropriate feedback to let the patient know you understand and care. Active listening involves looking with complete attention directly at the patient.

Nonverbal Skills

Nonverbal skills or body language includes facial expressions, posture, and eye contact. It is estimated that these skills are responsible for 60% to 70% of face-to-face communication. Positive body language is demonstrated by a PCT who walks briskly into the room, displays a smile, and looks directly at the patient while talking. This makes patients feel that they are important and that you care about them and your work. Notice the PCT and patient in Figure 1–3.

Conversely, shuffling into the room, avoiding eye contact, and gazing out the window while talking are examples of negative body language and indicate boredom and disinterest in the patients and their tests.

Telephone Skills

Telephone skills are essential for all healthcare workers. PCTs should have a thorough understanding of the telephone system with regard to transferring calls, placing calls on hold, and paging personnel. Knowledge of emergency procedures such as reporting a fire (frequently called a Code Red) and requesting specialized personnel to assist in a cardiac arrest (Code Blue) is essential.

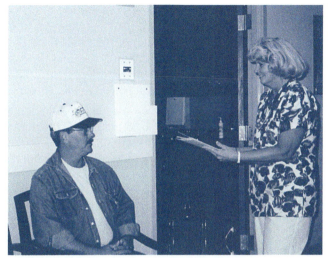

FIGURE 1–3 PCT communicating with a patient.

PCTs may frequently find themselves answering the telephone at the nursing station. The telephone in the nursing station is similar to a switchboard. Physicians call to check on patients and relay instructions to the staff, other hospital departments call regarding the scheduling of patients for specialized procedures or to report test results, and patients' family members call for information and reassurance. Unit personnel, including the PCT, call other hospital departments to schedule patient testing; check on test results; and order supplies, special meals, equipment, and services, such as housekeeping.

To observe the rules of proper telephone etiquette:

- Answer the phone promptly and politely, stating the name of the department and your name.
- Always check for an emergency before putting someone on hold, and return to calls that are on hold as soon as possible. This may require returning the telephone call after you have collected the required information.
- Keep writing materials beside the phone for recording information, such as patient test results, physician requests, test schedule changes, and phone numbers for returning calls. Test results should always be repeated to the caller to ensure accuracy, and the name of the caller should be recorded.
- Make every attempt to help callers and, if you cannot help, transfer them to another person or department that can. It is also helpful to give callers the number to which you are transferring them.
- Provide accurate and consistent information by keeping current with department policies, looking up information published in department manuals, or asking a supervisor.
- Speak clearly and make sure you understand the caller's question and that the caller understands the information you are providing.

Ethical and Legal Aspects of Patient Care

Principles of right and wrong (**ethics**) provide the personal and professional rules of performance and moral behavior as set by members of a profession. Medical ethics focus on the patient to ensure that all members of a healthcare team possess and exhibit the skill, knowledge, training, and professionalism necessary to serve the patient. PCTs are expected to follow these principles by performing only procedures for which they have been trained, adhering to established standards of performance, and continuing to improve their knowledge and skills.

PATIENT'S BILL OF RIGHTS

A document published by the American Hospital Association called the ***Patient's Bill of Rights*** specifies the essentials that a patient has the right to expect during medical treatment. A patient's rights and dignity must be protected during the process of providing quality care. The document addresses the following 12 areas:

1 Patients have the right to considerate and respectful care.
2 Patients have the right to obtain from their physician complete current information about their diagnosis, treatment, and **prognosis** in terms patients can reasonably be expected to understand.
3 Patients have the right to receive from a physician information necessary to give ***informed consent*** prior to a procedure. The information should include knowledge of the proposed procedure, with risks and probable duration of incapacitation. In addition, the patient has a right to information about medically significant alternatives.
4 Patients have the right to refuse treatment to the extent permitted by law and to be informed of the medical consequences of their action.
5 Patients have the right to privacy concerning their medical care. Case discussion, consultation, examination, and treatment should be conducted discreetly. Those not directly involved with a patient's care must have the patient's permission to be present.
6 Patients have the right to expect that all communication and records pertaining to their care will be treated as confidential.
7 Patients have the right to expect the hospital to make a reasonable response to their requests for services and to provide evaluation, service, and referral as indicated.
8 Patients have the right to obtain information regarding any relationship of their hospital to other healthcare and educational institutions, insofar as their care is concerned, and regarding the professional relationship among individuals who are treating them.
9 Patients have the right to be advised if the hospital proposes to engage in or perform human experimentation affecting their care or treatment. Patients have the right to refuse to participate in research projects.
10 Patients have the right to expect continuity of care, including future appointments and instructions on continuing healthcare requirements after discharge.
11 Patients have the right to examine and receive an explanation of their bill, regardless of the source of payment.
12 Patients have the right to know of hospital rules and regulations that apply to their conduct as a patient.

The PCT is directly involved with several sections of the Patient's Bill of Rights, including:

1 Patients may be difficult to deal with because they are afraid to be in the hospital or are angry because they have just received an unfavorable diagnosis. As the person with whom patients have the most contact, the PCT must develop a strong sensitivity to patients' feelings and treat all patients with respect and dignity.
2 Note that it is the physician, not the PCT, who must provide information concerning the purpose of test procedures. When questioned, PCTs should refer patients to their physicians. The PCT should only explain the procedure being performed on a patient. Also, test results are reported only to physicians or their designated representatives and are never given to patients or their family members.
3 Information necessary for a patient to provide informed consent must also come from a physician and not from the PCT. The PCT is frequently present when informed consent is being obtained from a patient and should be able to provide the appropriate signature forms and act as a witness.

4 The patient has the right to refuse a procedure, such as having blood drawn. If, after you have explained the procedure and stressed that it was requested by the physician to provide treatment, the patient still refuses, do not forcibly obtain a sample or perform a procedure. Notify the unit supervisor or the physician of the patient's refusal and note this information on the patient's chart.

5 PCTs will frequently be central to ensuring a patient's privacy, either when performing routine care procedures or when assisting with a physician's examination. Pulling the curtain around a patient's bed during procedures and knocking when entering a room are examples of privacy measures.

6 The patient's condition and test results are confidential and must not be discussed with anyone not directly involved with the patient's care or testing. Do not discuss patient information in elevators or in the cafeteria, where it may be overheard by bystanders.

LEGAL ISSUES

Failure to respect a patient's rights can result in legal action initiated by the patient or the patient's family. Medical law regulates the conduct of members of the healthcare profession. It differs from ethics, which are the principles of right and wrong conduct, by being legally required conduct. ***Litigation*** initiated as a result of illegal actions can be at the local, state, or national level and can result in criminal or civil prosecution. Penalties may include revocation of professional licenses, monetary fines, or imprisonment.

A ***criminal lawsuit*** is an action initiated by the state for the commission of an illegal act against the public welfare and can be punishable by imprisonment. A ***civil lawsuit*** is a court action between parties seeking monetary compensation for an offense. A wrongful act committed by one person against another is called a ***tort***. The threat to touch another person without his or her consent is termed ***assault***, and the actual touching is ***battery***. These are charges that could be initiated against a PCT who forcibly tries to collect a sample from a patient who refuses to have blood drawn. Release of confidential information is considered an ***invasion of privacy***.

Medical ***malpractice*** is misconduct or lack of skill by a healthcare professional that results in injury to a patient. ***Negligence***, which is defined as failure to give reasonable care by the healthcare provider, must be proven in medical malpractice. Examples of medical malpractice that could involve the PCT include:

1 Failure to raise a bed rail that has been lowered during a procedure, resulting in the patient's falling out of bed

2 Performing a procedure that the PCT is not trained to perform, resulting in complications for the patient

3 Misidentification of a patient or specimen, resulting in inappropriate treatment or possible death

All healthcare workers should carry malpractice insurance. Most institutions have policies covering all workers, and the PCT should confirm this coverage at the time of employment.

Regulation of Healthcare Providers

Healthcare agencies are governed by regulations that provide guidelines and rules for quality patient care. Accrediting agencies such as the Joint Commission on Accreditation of Healthcare Organizations (**JCAHO**) (Fig. 1–4) and individual state agencies exist to ensure a high standard of overall care for patients. To be eligible for reimbursement under Medicare and Medicaid, healthcare facilities must be accredited by an agency approved by the federal government.

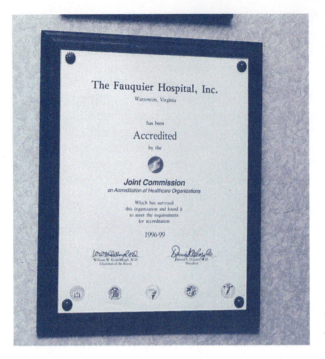

FIGURE 1–4 Certificate from the Joint Commission on Accreditation of Healthcare Organizations.

Accrediting agencies also exist for the regulation of healthcare specialty areas. Examples of these are the College of American Pathologists (**CAP**) and the Commission on Office Laboratory Accreditation (**COLA**) for clinical laboratories and the American College of Radiology (**ACR**) for radiology departments. Compliance with ***accreditation*** regulations is ensured by periodic on-site visits to facilities by inspection teams and through the performance of proficiency tests in areas such as laboratory testing. If deficiencies are present, the facility must correct them within a specified time and may be reinspected.

The qualifications of the personnel performing patient care are also regulated to ensure that procedures are performed only by persons with appropriate education and training. Healthcare personnel become certified and/or licensed in their particular fields through the completion of specified educational requirements and/or satisfactory performance on standardized proficiency examinations. At the present time there is no recognized route for **certification** or **licensure** of PCTs; however, this situation will most likely change in the near future. Many PCTs have already obtained certification in specialty areas of their field and are CNAs or certified phlebotomists. PCTs cannot perform procedures that require licensure or certification in a specialty area for which they do not have credentials. The educational requirements and scope of practice are ultimately determined by state regulations. Development of certification and licensure procedures for PCTs is currently under way.

Quality Assurance and Management

Quality assurance (**QA**) is the program through which healthcare facilities monitor and control processes designed to provide quality patient care at an established level. Performance of instrument and procedure *quality control* (**QC**), as discussed in Unit 12, is part of QA. Accrediting agencies require documentation of individual QC procedures, such as performance of instrument calibration and laboratory test controls, and documentation of the overall QA program.

Examples of the documentation required for a QA program are the following:

1 Written policies and procedures covering all aspects of service
2 Evidence of compliance with standards of good practice and achievement of expected results
3 Collection of data to monitor and evaluate the program
4 Actions taken to resolve problems

Departmental QC and QA programs are part of institutional ***total quality management* (TQM)** programs and ***continuous quality improvement* (CQI)** programs. Whereas QA is designed to maintain an established level of quality, TQM and CQI are designed to develop methods to continually improve the quality of healthcare. Standards from the JCAHO address this concept by requiring documentation showing that effective, appropriate patient care is being provided, as shown by patient outcomes. Areas addressed by the standards include availability of services, timeliness, continuity of care, effectiveness and efficiency of services, safety of services provided, and respect and care of the personnel providing services.

TQM is based on a team concept involving personnel at all levels working together to achieve a final outcome of customer satisfaction through implementation of policies and procedures identified by the CQI program. In the healthcare setting the patient is the ultimate customer; customers also include physicians, personnel in other departments, and the patient's family and friends.

Areas of concern in medical TQM are the infrastructure, including physical, personnel, and management structure; support services; and direct patient care. Although primarily associated with direct patient care, PCTs are involved in all of these areas. In fact, the concept of patient-focused care and the creation of the PCT are direct results of the response of TQM to address the concerns of the healthcare customers. Therefore, PCTs are in a unique position to contribute to the changing healthcare delivery system.

BIBLIOGRAPHY

Joint Commission on Accreditation of Healthcare Organizations: 1995 Comprehensive Accreditation Manual for Hospitals. JCAHO, Oakbrook Terrace, IL, 1995.
Lewis, MA, and Tamparo, CD: Medical Law, Ethics, and Bioethics in the Medical Office, ed 3. FA Davis, Philadelphia, 1993.
Strasinger, SK, and Di Lorenzo, MA: Phlebotomy Workbook for the Multiskilled Healthcare Professional. FA Davis, Philadelphia, 1996.
Vogel, DP: Patient Focused Care. Am J Hosp Pharmacol 50:2321–2329, 1993.

STUDY QUESTIONS

1. List eight healthcare settings in which PCTs may be employed.

   a. _____

   b. _____

   c. _____

   d. _____

   e. _____

   f. _____

   g. _____

   h. _____

2. Name the four services in a traditional hospital and a department of each.

   Service   *Department*

   a. _____   _____

   b. _____   _____

   c. _____   _____

   d. _____   _____

3. Match the following professional service departments and their functions:

   a. ____ Radiology   1. Teach daily living skills to disabled patients

   b. ____ Occupational therapy   2. Provide pulmonary therapy

   c. ____ Pharmacy   3. Perform CAT scans and MRIs

   d. ____ Physical therapy   4. Analyze blood and urine specimens

   e. ____ Clinical laboratory   5. Provide massage and exercise therapy

   f. ____ Respiratory therapy   6. Dispense medications

4. Define patient-focused care.

   _____

5. State two ways in which patient-focused care aids in controlling the cost of healthcare delivery.

   a. _____

   b. _____

6. State a way that failure of the PCT to demonstrate the following characteristics could affect the quality of patient care:

   a. Dependability _____

   _____

   _____

b. Compassion _____

_____

_____

c. Honesty _____

_____

_____

d. Integrity _____

_____

_____

7. Why is the appearance and personal hygiene of the PCT important to the patient?

_____

_____

_____

8. List four barriers to effective verbal communication and state a means to overcome each.

a. _____

_____

_____

b. _____

_____

_____

c. _____

_____

_____

d. _____

_____

_____

9. State two behaviors that represent negative body language.

a. _____

b. _____

10. How can a PCT demonstrate good telephone communication skills in the following situations?

a. Placing a call on hold

_____

_____

b. Providing instructions to a patient

_____

_____

   c. Responding to an inquiry from radiology concerning a patient's preparation

_____

_____

11. State an action by a PCT that would violate sections 1 through 6 of the Patient's Bill of Rights.

   a. Section 1: _____

_____

_____

   b. Section 2: _____

_____

_____

   c. Section 3: _____

_____

_____

   d. Section 4: _____

_____

_____

   e. Section 5: _____

_____

_____

   f. Section 6: _____

_____

_____

12. List two patient's rights that could result in a lawsuit if the PCT did not observe them.

   a. _____

   b. _____

13. The principles of right and wrong are called _____.

14. Differentiate between a criminal and a civil lawsuit.

_____

_____

_____

15. Describe two incidents that could cause a PCT to be charged with negligence.

   a. _____

_____

   b. _____

_____

16. A hometown professional football player was admitted to the hospital for blood work. Tests to rule out cancer of the prostate were ordered. The PCT obtained the blood specimens and delivered them to the lab. After work this PCT excitedly told friends about the famous person and the sad reason he was in the hospital. Is there anything ethically or legally wrong with this scenario?

_____

_____

_____

_____

17. List one agency that accredits healthcare facilities and two agencies that accredit specific healthcare departments.

a. Facilities _____

b. Department _____

c. Department _____

18. How does accreditation affect Medicare and Medicaid reimbursement?

_____

_____

_____

19. How do the roles of QA and TQM differ?

_____

_____

_____

20. List six areas relating to patient outcomes that are included in the JCAHO standards.

a. _____

b. _____

c. _____

d. _____

e. _____

f. _____

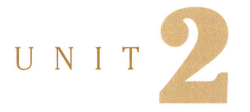
SAFETY

LEARNING OBJECTIVES

Upon completion of this unit, the reader will be able to:

1 Define the key terms associated with healthcare safety.
2 List the components of the chain of infection and the safety precautions that will break the chain.
3 Correctly perform routine handwashing.
4 Differentiate between category-specific isolation and transmission-based precautions.
5 Define universal precautions and discuss the Occupational Safety and Health Administration blood-borne pathogen policy.
6 State the precautions associated with body substance isolation.
7 Define standard precautions.
8 Correctly put on and remove protective apparel.
9 Safely dispose of sharp objects.
10 Describe safety precautions used when handling chemicals.
11 Discuss the purpose of Material Safety Data Sheets.
12 Identify the symbol for radiation.
13 Discuss the procedure to follow in cases of electrical shock.
14 List the basic steps to follow when a fire is discovered (RACE).
15 Correlate the classifications of fires to types of fire extinguishers.
16 Interpret the warnings of the National Fire Protection Association symbol.

KEY TERMS

- **Biohazardous** — Pertaining to a hazard caused by infectious organisms
- **Body substance isolation** — Guideline stating that all moist body substances are capable of transmitting disease
- **Category-specific isolation** — Isolation system grouping diseases into categories based on the mode of transmission
- **Disease-specific isolation** — Isolation system determining precautions for each individual disease
- **Nosocomial infection** — Infection acquired in the hospital
- **Personal protective equipment** — Apparel worn to prevent the transmission of pathogenic microorganisms

- ***Radioactivity***   Emission of radiant energy
- ***Standard precautions***   Guideline requiring the wearing of gloves when encountering moist body substances
- ***Transmission-based precautions***   Isolation procedures based on airborne, droplet, and contact disease transmission
- ***Universal precautions***   Guideline stating that all patients are capable of transmitting blood-borne disease

The healthcare setting contains a wide variety of safety hazards, many capable of producing serious injury or life-threatening disease. To work safely in this environment, the PCT must learn the existing hazards and the basic safety precautions associated with them and must learn to apply the basic rules of common sense required for everyday safety. As can be seen in Table 2–1, some hazards are unique to the healthcare environment and others are encountered routinely throughout life. These hazards affect not only the PCT but also the patient. Therefore, PCTs must be prepared to protect both themselves and their patients.

Biologic Hazards

BIOHAZARD

The healthcare setting provides an abundant source of potentially harmful microorganisms, including bacteria, fungi, parasites, and viruses. An understanding of the transmission (chain of infection) of microorganisms is necessary to prevent infection. The chain of infection requires a continuous link among three elements: a source, a method of transmission, and a susceptible host. The source refers to the location of the potentially harmful microorganisms and may be a person or a contaminated object. Microorganisms from the source must then be transferred to the host. This may occur through direct contact (host touches or is touched by the contaminated source), inhalation of infected material (**aerosol** droplets released by an infected patient or an uncapped tube in a centrifuge), ingestion of contaminated food or water (food poisoning), or a **vector** (malaria transmitted by mosquitoes). Although patients are considered the most logical susceptible host, anyone can serve as the host.

TABLE 2–1   **Types of Safety Hazards**

Type	Source	Possible Injury
Biologic	Infectious agents	Bacterial, fungal, viral, or parasitic infections
Sharp	Needles, lancets, and broken glass	Cuts, punctures, or blood-borne pathogen exposure
Chemical	Preservatives and reagents	Exposure to toxic, carcinogenic, or caustic agents
Radioactive	Equipment and radioisotopes	Radiation exposure
Electrical	Ungrounded or wet equipment and frayed cords	Burns or shock
Fire/explosive	Bunsen burners and organic chemicals	Burns or dismemberment
Physical	Wet floors, heavy boxes, and patients	Falls, sprains, or strains

Source: Strasinger, SK, and Di Lorenzo, MA: Phlebotomy Workbook for the Multiskilled Healthcare Professional. FA Davis, Philadelphia, 1996, p. 62, with permission.

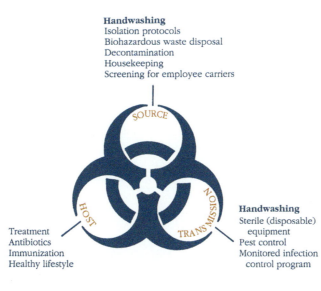

Handwashing
Isolation protocols
Biohazardous waste disposal
Decontamination
Housekeeping
Screening for employee carriers

Treatment
Antibiotics
Immunization
Healthy lifestyle

Handwashing
Sterile (disposable)
  equipment
Pest control
Monitored infection
  control program

FIGURE 2–1 Chain of infection and safety practices related to the biohazard symbol. (From Strasinger, SK, and Di Lorenzo, MA: Phlebotomy Workbook for the Multiskilled Healthcare Professional. FA Davis, Philadelphia, 1996, p. 63, with permission.)

Therefore, safety precautions are designed for both healthcare workers and patients. Once the chain of infection is completed, the susceptible host becomes the new source. The ultimate goal of biologic safety is to prevent completion of the chain. Figure 2–1 uses the universal symbol for **biohazardous** material to illustrate the chain of infection and demonstrates how it can be broken by following prescribed safety practices.

Previously uninfected patients who become infected during hospitalization represent approximately 5% of the patient population. The term **nosocomial infection** designates an infection contracted by a patient during a hospital stay. Although some of these **infections** may be caused by visitors, the majority are the result of personnel not following infection control practices.

HANDWASHING

Notice the emphasis on handwashing in Figure 2–1. Hand contact represents the number one method of infection transmission. PCTs circulate from one patient to another throughout their working hours, and without the observance of proper precautions such contact can provide an unlimited vehicle for the transmission of infection. It is essential to *change gloves and wash hands between patients.*

The importance of handwashing continues away from the patient setting for the purpose of protecting coworkers, family and friends, and the PCT. The PCT should always wash his or her hands before leaving the work area, at any time when the hands have been knowingly contaminated, and before going to designated break areas, as well as before and after using bathroom facilities.

The correct routine handwashing technique (Fig. 2–2) is as follows:

1 Wetting hands with warm water
2 Applying soap, preferably antimicrobial
3 Rubbing to form a lather, create friction, and loosen debris
4 Cleaning thoroughly between fingers and under fingernails and rings for at least 15 seconds and up to the wrist
5 Rinsing hands in a downward position
6 Drying with a paper towel
7 Turning off faucets with the used paper towel to prevent recontamination

More stringent procedures are used in surgery and in areas with highly susceptible patients, such as burn patients, immunocompromised patients, and newborns.

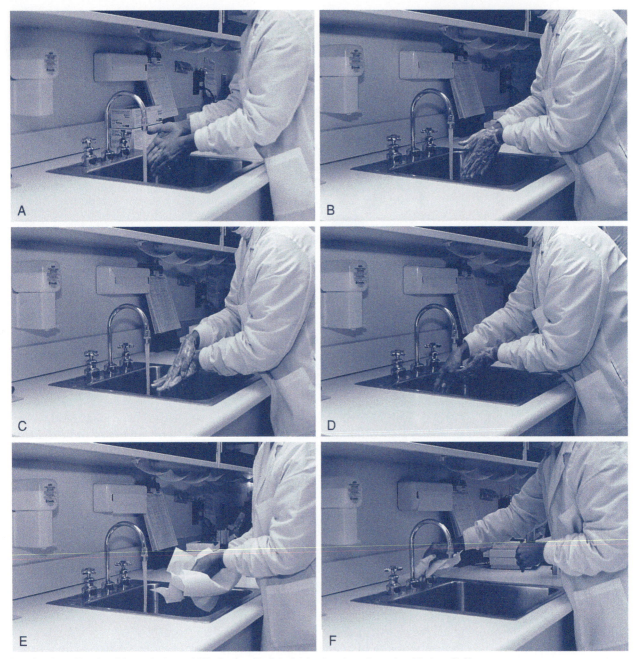

FIGURE 2–2   Handwashing technique. *A*, Wetting hands. *B*, Lathering hands and creating friction. *C*, Cleaning between fingers. *D*, Rinsing hands. *E*, Drying hands. *F*, Turning off water.

ISOLATION PRACTICES

Preventing the transmission of microorganisms from infected sources to susceptible hosts is critical in controlling the spread of infection. This is accomplished primarily through proper handwashing, wearing of ***personal protective equipment*** **(PPE)**, and placing particularly infective or highly susceptible patients in private rooms.

Guidelines for isolation practices are published by the Centers for Disease Control and Prevention (**CDC**) and are periodically revised to meet the changing needs of healthcare workers. A new guideline has recently been published, and it combines many of the previously used precautions. A brief review of past isolation guidelines will be helpful in understanding the new guideline.

Category-specific isolation grouped diseases together based on their mode of transmission. Table 2–2 presents some of the more commonly encountered categories. Modifications were made as new epidemiological information became available. For example, the designation "Blood Precautions" was changed to "Blood and Body Fluid Precautions" when acquired immunodeficiency syndrome (**AIDS**) appeared, "Tuberculosis Isolation" was separated from "Respiratory Isolation" when drug-resistant strains of the bacillus were identified, and "Protective Isolation" was found to be unnecessary, except in cases of severely immunocompromised patients.

Disease-specific isolation considered the mode of transmission of each individual disease. This procedure reduced the overuse of precautions caused by the grouping of all diseases into a small number of categories. It was more difficult for workers to follow this method.

Universal precautions were instituted to protect healthcare workers from exposure to blood-borne **pathogens,** primarily hepatitis B virus (**HBV**) and human immunodeficiency virus (**HIV**). Under universal precautions all patients are assumed to be possible carriers of blood-borne pathogens. Transmission may occur by skin puncture from a contaminated sharp object or by passive contact through open skin lesions or mucous membranes. The guideline recommends wearing gloves when collecting or handling blood and body fluids that are contaminated with blood, wearing face shields when there is danger of blood splashing on mucous membranes, and disposing of all needles and sharp objects in puncture-resistant containers without recapping.

The Occupational Exposure to Blood-Borne Pathogens Standard expanded universal precautions guidelines and was enacted into law to further protect workers. These regulations are monitored and enforced by the Occupational Safety and Health Administration (**OSHA**). Under the Occupational Exposure to Blood-Borne Pathogens Standard, all employers must have a written blood-borne pathogen exposure control plan available in the workplace and must provide necessary protection free of charge to employees. Specifics of the OSHA standard include:

1 Requiring all employees to practice universal precautions
2 Providing lab coats, gowns, face and respiratory protection, and gloves to employees and providing laundry facilities for nondisposable protective clothing

TABLE 2–2   **Category-Specific Isolation Classifications**

Type of Isolation	Conditions	Protective Apparel
Strict	Infectious diseases: chickenpox, measles, diphtheria, rabies, and staphylococcal and streptococcal pneumonia	Gown, mask, and gloves
Respiratory	Airborne infections: tuberculosis, mumps, whooping cough, and meningococcal meningitis	Mask and gloves for body substance contact
Enteric	Organisms causing disease through ingestion: *Salmonella, Shigella, Yersinia,* and intestinal parasites	Gown and gloves
Drainage/secretion	Skin, wound, and surgical infections	Gown and gloves
Blood/body fluid	Blood-borne pathogens: hepatitis and HIV	Gloves
Protective (reverse)	Immunocompromised patients: burns, nursery, and chemotherapy	Sterile gown, mask, gloves, and equipment

Source: Adapted from Strasinger, SK, and Di Lorenzo, MA: Phlebotomy Workbook for the Multiskilled Healthcare Professional. FA Davis, Philadelphia, 1996, p. 64, with permission.

3 Providing sharps disposal containers and prohibiting recapping of needles
4 Prohibiting eating, drinking, smoking, and applying cosmetics in the work area
5 Labeling all biohazardous material and containers
6 Providing immunization for HBV free of charge
7 Establishing a daily work surface disinfection protocol; the **disinfectant** of choice for blood-borne pathogens is sodium hypochlorite (household bleach diluted daily 1:10)
8 Providing medical follow-up to employees who have been accidentally exposed
9 Documenting regular training of employees in safety standards

Body substance isolation **(BSI)** is not limited to blood-borne pathogens but considers all body fluids and moist body substances to be potentially infectious. Personnel should wear gloves at all times when encountering moist body substances. A major disadvantage of the BSI guideline is that it does not recommend handwashing after removal of gloves unless visual contamination is present.

CURRENT ISOLATION CATEGORIES AND PRACTICES

New guidelines for preventing the transmission of infectious agents recognize that all body fluids, secretions, and excretions are capable of transmitting disease, and they contain provisions to prevent transmission of infection by airborne, droplet, and contact routes. The new guidelines have combined previous recommendations into a system that is much easier to follow.

The major features of universal precautions and body substance isolation have been combined and are called *standard precautions*. The old category-specific and disease-specific isolation practices have been condensed into *transmission-based precautions*.

Standard Precautions

Standard procedures should be used for the care of all patients and include the following:

1 Handwashing. Wash hands after touching blood, body fluids, secretions, excretions, and contaminated items, whether or not gloves are worn. Wash hands immediately after gloves are removed, between patient contacts, and when otherwise indicated to avoid transfer of microorganisms to other patients or environments. It may be necessary to wash hands between tasks and procedures on the same patient to prevent cross-contamination of different body sites.
2 Gloves. Wear gloves (clean, nonsterile gloves are adequate) when touching blood, body fluids, secretions, excretions, and contaminated items. Put on gloves just before touching mucous membranes and nonintact skin. Change gloves between tasks and procedures on the same patient after contact with material that may contain a high concentration of microorganisms. Remove gloves promptly after use, before touching noncontaminated items and environmental surfaces, and before going to another patient, and wash hands immediately to avoid transfer of microorganisms to other patients or environments.
3 Mask, Eye Protection, and Face Shield. Wear a mask and eye protection or a face shield to protect mucous membranes of the eyes, nose, and mouth during procedures and patient-care activities that are likely to generate splashes or sprays of blood, body fluids, secretions, and excretions.
4 Gown. Wear a gown (a clean, nonsterile gown is adequate) to protect skin and to prevent soiling of clothing during procedures and patient-care activities that are likely to generate splashes or sprays of blood, body fluids, secretions, or ex-

cretions. Select a gown that is appropriate for the activity and the amount of fluid likely to be encountered. Remove a soiled gown as promptly as possible, and wash hands to avoid transfer of microorganisms to other patients or environments.

5 Patient-Care Equipment. Handle patient-care equipment soiled with blood, body fluids, secretions, and excretions in a manner that prevents skin and mucous membrane exposures, contamination of clothing, and transfer of microorganisms to other patients and environments. Ensure that reusable equipment is not used for the care of another patient until it has been cleaned and reprocessed appropriately. Ensure that single-use items are discarded properly.

6 Environmental Control. Ensure that the hospital has adequate procedures for the routine care, cleaning, and disinfection of environmental surfaces, beds, bed rails, bedside equipment, and other frequently touched surfaces, and ensure that these procedures are being followed.

7 Linen. Handle, transport, and process linen soiled with blood, body fluids, secretions, and excretions in a manner that prevents skin and mucous membrane exposure and contamination of clothing and that avoids transfer of microorganisms to other patients and environments.

8 Occupational Health and Blood-Borne Pathogens. Take care to prevent injuries when using needles, scalpels, and other sharp instruments or devices; when handling sharp instruments after procedures; when cleaning used instruments; and when disposing of used needles. Never recap used needles, manipulate them using both hands, or use any other technique that involves directing the point of the needle toward any part of the body. Instead, use either a one-handed "scoop" technique or a mechanical device designed for holding the needle sheath. Do not remove used needles from disposable syringes by hand, and do not bend, break, or otherwise manipulate used needles by hand. Place used disposable syringes and needles, scalpel blades, and other sharp items in appropriate puncture-resistant containers that are located as close as practical to the area in which the items are used, and place reusable syringes and needles in a puncture-resistant container for transport to the reprocessing area. Use mouthpieces, resuscitation bags, or other ventilation devices as an alternative to mouth-to-mouth resuscitation methods in areas in which the need for resuscitation is predictable.

9 Patient Placement. Place a patient who contaminates the environment or who does not (or cannot be expected to) assist in maintaining appropriate hygiene or environmental control in a private room. If a private room is not available, consult with infection control professionals regarding patient placement or other alternatives.

Transmission-Based Precautions

Use of standard precautions with all patients effectively eliminates all but three of the traditional isolation categories. The remaining categories are airborne, droplet, and contact precautions. They are implemented in addition to the use of standard precautions for patients known to be infected with microorganisms that are transmitted by these routes.

Airborne precautions are necessary when microorganisms can remain infective while being carried through the air on the dried residue of a droplet or on a dust particle. PPE should include a mask or respirator. Filtration systems may be required in the patient's room. Examples of conditions requiring airborne precautions are tuberculosis, measles, and chickenpox.

Droplet precautions are required for persons infected with microorganisms transmitted on moist particles such as those produced during coughing and sneezing. Droplets are capable of traveling only short distances through the air (less than 3 ft); therefore, masks are worn when procedures requiring close patient contact are per-

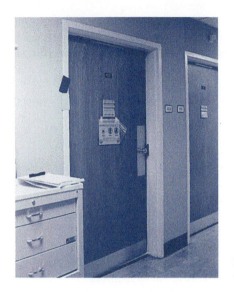

FIGURE 2–3 Isolation room with posted procedures and equipment stand.

formed. Examples of conditions requiring droplet precautions are diphtheria, pertussis, mumps, scarlet fever, and influenza.

Contact precautions are used when patients have an infection that can be transmitted by direct skin-to-skin contact or by indirect contact by touching objects in the patient's room. Gloves should be worn even if no contact with moist body substances is anticipated. Gowns are worn when entering the room and removed before leaving the room. After removing the gown and washing the hands, care must be taken to avoid touching objects in the room. Examples of conditions requiring contact precautions are impetigo, scabies, herpes simplex and herpes zoster, *Clostridium difficile*, and noncontained wounds and abscesses.

PCTs must be knowledgeable about hospital isolation practices. Warning signs for healthcare workers are posted on the doors of patient rooms (Fig. 2–3). They contain specific instructions for the type of protective apparel required, as shown in Figure 2–4.

PERSONAL PROTECTIVE EQUIPMENT

PPE encountered by the PCT includes gloves, gowns, masks, goggles, face shields, and respirators.

Gloves are worn to protect the healthcare worker's hands from contamination by patient body substances and to protect the patient from possible microorganisms on

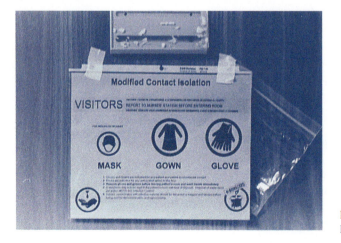

FIGURE 2–4 Transmission-based precautions sign.

the healthcare worker's hands. Wearing gloves is not a substitute for handwashing. Hands must always be washed when gloves are removed. A variety of gloves are available, including sterile and nonsterile, powdered and unpowdered, and latex and nonlatex. Allergy to latex is increasing among healthcare workers, and PCTs should be alert for any allergy symptoms, such as redness or rash, after removing gloves.

Gowns are worn to protect the clothing and skin of healthcare workers from contamination by patient body substances and to prevent the transfer of microorganisms between patient rooms. Gowns are removed and disposed of before leaving the patient's room when caring for patients under Contact Precautions. Fluid-resistant gowns should be worn when the possibility of encountering splashes or large amounts of body fluids is anticipated.

Masks are worn to protect against inhalation of infective microorganisms from patients on Droplet and Airborne Precautions. Masks and goggles are worn to protect the mucous membranes of the mouth, nose, and eyes from the splashing of body substances (Fig. 2–5). Face shields also protect the mucous membranes from splashes. They are most commonly worn when working with blood and body fluids outside of the patients' rooms. Respirators may be required when working with patients who have tuberculosis and are on Airborne Precautions.

Donning and Removing Personal Protective Equipment

Specific procedures must be followed when putting on and removing PPE. To prevent contact with or the spread of infectious microorganisms, apparel is put on before entering a room and is removed and disposed of before leaving the room. Care must be taken to avoid touching the outside contaminated areas of apparel when it is being removed.

Gowns are put on first. They usually tie in the back at the neck and waist and have tight-fitting cuffs. They should be large enough to provide full-body coverage, including closing at the back. Masks are tied first above the ears, securely molded to the face, and then tied at the neck. To provide maximum effectiveness, be sure the side labeled "outside" is facing outward. Gloves are put on last and stretched over the cuffs of the gown (Fig. 2–6).

PPE is removed in reverse order: gloves, mask, and gown, as shown in Figure 2–7. To avoid touching the outside of the gloves, one finger is slid under the glove, and the glove is removed by turning it inside out. Masks are untied by holding only the ends of the ties and are dropped into designated disposal bags. Gowns are untied at the waist before removing the gloves. For removal, the gown is untied at the neck and removed by turning it inside out. Hands are washed immediately after removing PPE.

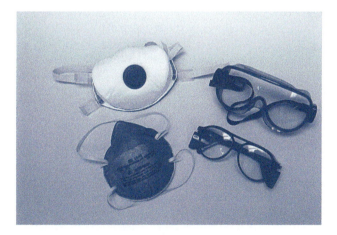

FIGURE 2–5 Face protective equipment.

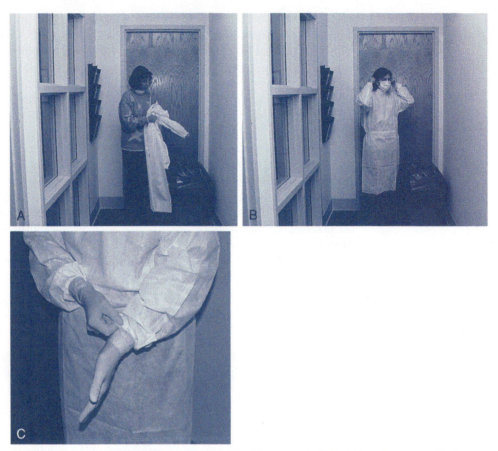

FIGURE 2–6   Donning PPE. *A*, Putting on gown. *B*, Putting on mask. *C*, Stretching glove over cuff of gown.

PATIENT-CARE EQUIPMENT

When dealing with isolation situations, special precautions must also be taken with equipment, such as phlebotomy and respiratory therapy materials brought into the room, and with specimens collected. Bring only necessary equipment into the room, but be sure to include duplicate phlebotomy collection tubes and enough supplies to perform a second venipuncture, should it be necessary. Tourniquets, gauze, alcohol pads, and pens may already be present in the room. All equipment taken into the room must be left in the room and, when appropriate, deposited in labeled waste containers. In the case of portable radiology equipment, the equipment is protected by plastic covering before being taken into the room. Upon completion of the x-ray procedures the plastic covering is removed and disposed of in the same manner as PPE. Specimens taken from the room should first be cleaned of any blood contamination and placed in plastic bags located at the door. Bags should be folded open to allow tubes to be added without touching the outside of the bag with contaminated gloves or tubes. Double bagging is required when contaminated waste is removed from isolation rooms, and a clean bag is required to be available immediately outside of the room.

Sharp Hazards

SHARP HAZARD

Exposure to sharp hazards is of particular concern to PCTs who perform phlebotomy, because needles and lancets are the primary pieces of equipment associated with blood collection. Needles may be part of vacuum tube blood collection equipment or may be attached to syringes used for blood collection or injection of medications. They can present a very serious hazard if proper safety precautions are not followed.

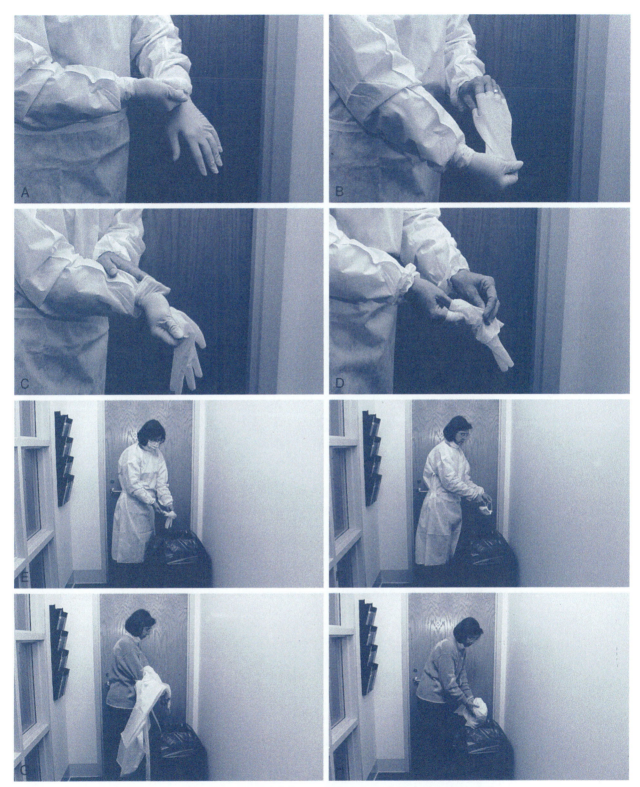

FIGURE 2–7   Removing PPE. *A*, Beginning glove removal. *B*, Removing first glove. *C*, Beginning removal of second glove. *D*, Removing second glove. *E*, Disposing of gloves. *F*, Disposing of mask. *G*, Removing gown. *H*, Disposing of gown.

The number one personal safety rule when using needles is to *never* manually re-cap a needle. Many safety devices are available for needle disposal, and they provide a variety of safeguards. Puncture-resistant containers are attached to the walls of patient rooms (Fig. 2–8*A*) for use when an entire assembly can be discarded. Do not reach into these containers when disposing of material, because accidental puncture may occur from a previously discarded needle. Containers must always be replaced when the safe-capacity mark is reached. Portable puncture-resistant containers that allow manual unscrewing or automatic removal of a needle from its holder (Fig. 2–8*B*) are located on phlebotomy trays and at specified blood collection stations. Needle holders that become a sheath, needles that automatically resheathe or become blunt, and needles with attached sheaths are also available (Fig. 2–9*A* and *B*). PCTs should be-

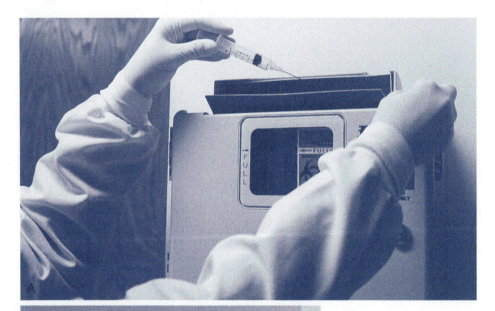

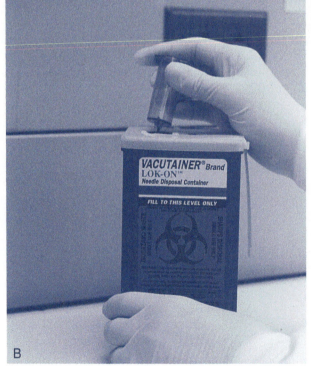

FIGURE 2–8   Sharps disposal containers. *A*, Wall unit. *B*, Portable unit.

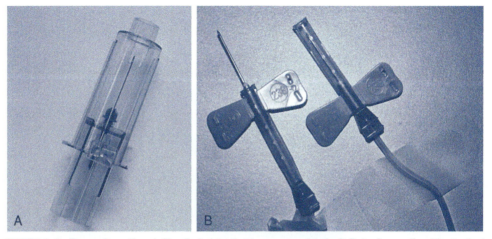

FIGURE 2–9   Types of needles. *A*, Needle holder that becomes a sheath. *B*, Butterfly needle with attached sheath.

come proficient with the disposal equipment in their area before performing puncture procedures on patients.

Lancets and butterfly apparatuses are equally, if not more, dangerous. They should be carefully disposed of in puncture-resistant containers immediately after use and never left lying on the work surface. Many lancets now have retractable points, and automatic needle covers have been developed for the butterfly apparatus.

Chemical Hazards

POISON

The same general rules for handling biohazardous materials apply to chemically hazardous materials to avoid getting these materials in or on your body, clothes, or work area. It should be assumed that every chemical in the workplace is hazardous. When skin contact occurs, the best first aid is to flush the area with large amounts of water.

Chemicals should never be mixed together, unless specific instructions are followed, and they must be added in the order specified. This is particularly important when combining acid and water because acid should always be added to water to avoid the possibility of sudden splashing.

All chemicals and reagents containing hazardous ingredients in a concentration greater than 1% are required to have a Material Safety Data Sheet (**MSDS**) on file in the work area. By law, vendors must provide these sheets to purchasers; it is the responsibility of the facility, however, to obtain and keep them available to employees. The MSDS contains information on physical and chemical characteristics, risk of fire or explosion, reactivity, health hazards, primary routes of entry, exposure limits and **carcinogenic** potential, precautions for safe handling, spill clean-up, and emergency first aid information. Containers of chemicals that pose a high risk must be labeled with a chemical hazard symbol.

OSHA requires all facilities that use hazardous chemicals to have a written Chemical Hygiene Plan. The purpose of the plan is to detail appropriate work practices, procedures, methods of control, protective equipment, and special precautions that must be taken when working with particularly hazardous chemicals. Employees must receive documented training in the procedures detailed in the plan. They must also have access to the plan at all times. Examples of required safety equipment and information are illustrated in Figure 2–10.

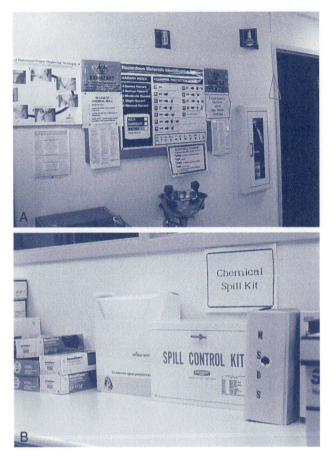

FIGURE 2–10 Chemical safety aids. *A*, Equipment. *B*, Information and supplies.

Radioactive Hazards

PCTs may come in contact with ***radioactivity*** while performing limited radiographic procedures, transporting patients to and from the radiology department, and caring for patients receiving radioactive treatments.

The amount of radioactivity present in most medical situations is very small and represents little danger. Exposure to radiation is dependent on the combination of time, distance, and shielding. Persons working in a radioactive environment are required to wear measuring devices to determine the amount of radiation they are accumulating.

PCTs should be familiar with the radioactive hazard symbol shown in the margin. This symbol must be displayed on the doors of all areas in which radioactive material is present. Exposure to radiation during pregnancy presents a danger to the fetus, and PCTs who are pregnant or think they may be should avoid areas with this symbol.

Electrical Hazards

The healthcare setting contains a large amount of electrical equipment with which PCTs have frequent contact. The same general rules of electrical safety observed outside the workplace apply. The danger of water or fluid coming in contact with equipment is greater in the hospital setting.

Electrical equipment is closely monitored by designated hospital personnel; PCTs should be observant for any dangerous conditions such as frayed cords and overloaded circuits and should report them to the appropriate persons. Equipment that has become wet should be unplugged and allowed to dry completely before reusing. Equipment should also be unplugged before cleaning. It is required that all electrical equipment be grounded with a three-pronged plug.

As an additional precaution, when drawing blood or performing other procedures, PCTs should avoid contact with electrical equipment in the room because current from improperly grounded equipment can pass through the PCT and metal instruments to the patient.

When a situation involving electrical **shock** occurs, it is important to remove the source of electricity immediately. This must be done without touching the person or the equipment because the current will pass on to you. Turning off the circuit breaker, unplugging the equipment, and moving the equipment using a nonconductive glass or wood object are safe procedures to follow.

Fire and Explosive Hazards

FIRE HAZARD

The JCAHO requires that all healthcare institutions have posted evacuation routes and detailed plans to follow when a fire occurs. PCTs should be familiar with these procedures and with the basic steps to follow when a fire is discovered. The following is a list of actions all employees are expected to follow:

1 *R*escue—anyone in immediate danger
2 *A*larm—activate the institutional fire alarm system
3 *C*ontain—close all doors to potentially affected areas
4 *E*xtinguish—attempt to extinguish the fire, if possible

The National Fire Protection Association (**NFPA**) classifies fires with regard to the type of burning material and also classifies the type of fire extinguisher that is used to control them. This information is summarized in Table 2–3. The multipurpose ABC fire extinguishers are the most common, but the label should always be checked before use.

The Standard System for the Identification of the Fire Hazards of Materials, NFPA 704, is a symbol system used to inform firefighters of the hazard they may encounter when fighting a fire in a particular area. The color-coded sections contain information relating to health, flammability, reactivity, use of water, and personal protection. These symbols are placed on doors, cabinets, and reagent bottles. An example of hazardous material symbols is shown in Figure 2–11.

TABLE 2–3   **Types of Fires and Fire Extinguishers**

Fire Type	Composition of Fire	Type of Fire Extinguisher	Extinguishing Material
Class A	Wood, paper, or clothing	Class A	Water
Class B	Flammable organic chemicals	Class B	Dry chemicals, carbon dioxide, foam, or halon
Class C	Electrical	Class C	Dry chemicals, carbon dioxide, or halon
Class D	Combustible metals	None	Sand or dry powder
		Class ABC	Dry chemicals

Source: Strasinger, SK, and Di Lorenzo, MA: Phlebotomy Workbook for the Multiskilled Healthcare Professional. FA Davis, Philadelphia, 1996, p. 70, with permission.

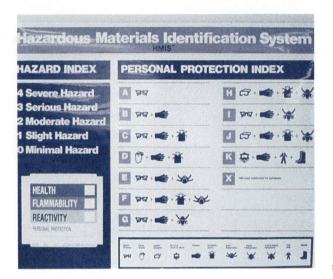

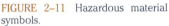

FIGURE 2–11 Hazardous material symbols.

Physical Hazards

These hazards are not unique to the healthcare setting, and routine precautions observed outside the workplace apply. General precautions to consider are to avoid running in rooms and hallways, watch for wet floors, bend the knees when lifting patients and boxes, keep long hair pulled back, avoid dangling jewelry, and maintain a clean, organized work area. PCTs should select comfortable, closed-toe shoes that provide maximum support.

BIBLIOGRAPHY

Baron, EJ, Peterson, LR, and Finegold, SM: Diagnostic Microbiology. CV Mosby, St. Louis, 1994.

Centers for Disease Control and Prevention: Guideline for Isolation Precautions in Hospitals, Parts I and II. Internet, Jan. 1, 1996.

National Fire Protection Association: Hazardous Chemical Data, No.49. NFPA, Boston, 1991.

Occupational Exposure to Blood-Borne Pathogens, Final Rule. Federal Register, 29 (Dec 6), 1991.

Occupational Exposure to Hazardous Chemicals in Laboratories, Final Rule. Federal Register, 55 (Jan 31), 1990.

Update, Universal Precautions for Prevention of Transmission of Human Immunodeficiency Virus, Hepatitis B Virus and Other Blood-Borne Pathogens in Health Care Settings MMWR (Morb Mortal Wkly Rep) 37:377, 1988.

STUDY QUESTIONS

1. List an example of each of the following healthcare hazards.

   a. Biologic _____

   b. Sharp _____

   c. Chemical _____

   d. Radioactive _____

   e. Electrical _____

   f. Fire or explosive _____

   g. Physical _____

2. List four methods by which infection can be transferred from the source to the host.

   a. _____

   b. _____

   c. _____

   d. _____

3. When drawing blood from five patients in ICU, how many pairs of gloves should be used? _____

4. A patient who develops staphylococcal pneumonia after entering the hospital has a _____ infection.

5. Define the following:

   a. Body substance isolation _____

   b. Universal precautions _____

   c. Standard precautions _____

6. List the three categories of transmission-based precautions.

   a. _____

   b. _____

   c. _____

7. The recommended disinfectant for blood and body fluid spills is

   _____ .

8. Name two viruses transmitted by blood and body fluids.

   a. _____

   b. _____

9. Indicate the correct order for putting on and removing protective apparel by placing a 1, 2, or 3 opposite the listed apparel.

	Putting On	*Removing*
a. Gown	_____	_____
b. Gloves	_____	_____
c. Mask	_____	_____

10. When a caustic solution such as phenol is spilled on the skin, what is the recommended first aid? _____

11. True or False. Water should always be added to acid. _____

12. Give an example of when a PCT should avoid areas with a radiation symbol.

_____

13. List three ways to remove the source of an electrical shock.

a. _____

b. _____

c. _____

14. The first things to do when a fire is discovered are to

a. *R* _____

b. *A* _____

c. *C* _____

d. *E* _____

15. What type of fire can be extinguished using water? _____

16. Match the following symbols with the numbered hazard they represent.

a. _____ 1. Biologic

b. _____ 2. Sharp

c. _____ 3. Chemical

d. _____ 4. Radioactive

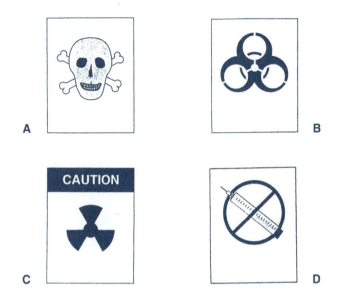

A   B

C   D

17. After reading the Blood-Borne Pathogen Exposure Control Plan for your training facility, state the name of the control officer responsible for the plan.

_____

EVALUATION OF HANDWASHING TECHNIQUE

RATING SYSTEM   2 = Satisfactory   1 = Needs improvement   0 = Incorrect/did not perform

_____ **1.** Turns on warm water

_____ **2.** Dispenses an adequate amount of soap onto palm

_____ **3.** Creates a lather

_____ **4.** Creates friction, rubbing both sides of hands

_____ **5.** Rubs between fingers and under nails

_____ **6.** Rinses hands in a downward position

_____ **7.** Obtains paper towel, touching only the towel

_____ **8.** Dries hands with paper towel

_____ **9.** Turns off water using paper towel

_____ **10.** Does not recontaminate hands

Total points _____

Maximum points = 20

COMMENTS

EVALUATION OF PERSONAL PROTECTIVE EQUIPMENT (GOWNING, MASKING, AND GLOVING)

RATING SYSTEM   2 = Satisfactory   1 = Needs improvement   0 = Incorrect/did not perform

_____   **1.** Correctly washes hands

_____   **2.** Picks up gown, touching only the inside

_____   **3.** Puts on gown with opening at the back

_____   **4.** Ensures that gown is large enough to close in the back

_____   **5.** Ties neck strings followed by waistband

_____   **6.** Positions mask with proper side facing outward and ties top string above the ears

_____   **7.** Securely positions mask over nose

_____   **8.** Ties bottom string at back of neck

_____   **9.** Puts on gloves

_____   **10.** Pulls gloves over cuffs of gown

_____   **11.** Unties gown at the waist

_____   **12.** Removes gloves, touching only the inside

_____   **13.** Deposits gloves in biohazard container

_____   **14.** Unties mask at neck and then head

_____   **15.** Touches only strings of mask

_____   **16.** Deposits mask in biohazard container

_____   **17.** Unties gown at neck

_____   **18.** Removes gown, touching only the inside

_____   **19.** Deposits gown in biohazard container

_____   **20.** Correctly washes hands

Total points _____

Maximum points = 40

COMMENTS

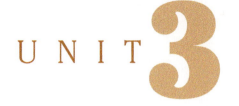

UNIT 3

BASIC ANATOMY AND PHYSIOLOGY

LEARNING OBJECTIVES

Upon completion of this unit, the reader will be able to:

1 Define the key terms associated with basic anatomy and physiology.
2 Explain the levels of organization of the human body.
3 Use directional terms to describe position and location of body structures.
4 List the body cavities and name the main organs contained in each cavity.
5 State the four quadrants and name the nine smaller regions of the abdominopelvic cavity.
6 List all the body systems and identify their functions and major components.
7 List the major disorders associated with each body system.
8 Recognize the major diagnostic tests and commonly used medications associated with each body system.

A basic knowledge of anatomy and physiology provides the basis for further study in the healthcare professions. Anatomy is the study of the structure of the body, and physiology is the study of how the body functions. Knowing the location and the function of each body part is essential to communicating effectively with coworkers in the medical setting. Understanding normal physiology will make disorders and diseases easier to understand.

Organizational Levels of the Body

The human body develops into a complex organism through different levels of structure and function from the simplest to the most complex. Each level includes the previous level to build on. These levels of organization are cells, tissues, organs, body systems, and the organism.

CELLS

The smallest functioning unit of the body is the cell. More than 30 trillion cells provide the basic building blocks for the structures that make up the human body. Size, shape, and composition of the cell determine cell function. There are several types of cells, each with a specialized function and the ability to carry out specialized chemical reactions to communicate with other cells throughout the body.

TISSUES

Groups of specific cells with similar structure and function form the types of body tissue and together perform specialized functions. There are four basic types of tissue:

- Epithelial tissue—flat cells in a sheetlike arrangement that cover and line body surfaces
- Connective tissue—blood, bone, and adipose cells that support and connect tissues and organs and provide a support network for the organs
- Muscle tissue—long, slender cells that provide the contractile tissue for movement of the body
- Nerve tissue—cells that are capable of transmitting electrical impulses to regulate body functions

ORGANS

Organs are body structures formed by the combination of two or more types of tissue. Each organ is a specialized component of the body (such as the heart, brain, skin, and kidneys) and accomplishes a specific function.

TABLE 3–1   **Summary of Body Systems**

System	Function	Organs
Integumentary	Protects against harmful pathogens and chemicals and regulates temperature	Skin, hair, nails, and glands
Skeletal	Supports and protects internal organs, stores minerals, and acts in blood cell formation	Bones, ligaments, joints, and cartilage
Muscular	Allows skeletal movement and heat production	Muscles and tendons
Nervous	Recognizes and interprets sensory stimuli and regulates responses to stimuli by coordinating other body systems	Brain, spinal cord, and nerves
Respiratory	Exchanges oxygen and carbon dioxide between the air and circulating blood	Nose, pharynx, larynx, trachea, bronchi, and lungs
Digestive	Breaks down food to usable molecules to be absorbed by the body and eliminates waste products	Mouth, pharynx, esophagus, stomach, small intestine, and large intestine
Urinary	Removes waste products and regulates water and salt balance	Kidneys, ureters, urinary bladder, and urethra
Endocrine	Produces and regulates hormones	Thyroid gland, parathyroid gland, adrenal gland, pancreas, pituitary gland, ovaries, testes, thymus, and pineal gland
Reproductive	Allows sexual reproduction and development of male and female sexual characteristics	Female: ovaries, fallopian tubes, uterus, vagina, and breasts Male: testes, epididymides, vas deferens, seminal vesicles, prostate gland, bulbourethral glands, and penis
Circulatory	Transports oxygen, nutrients, and waste products	Heart, arteries, veins, and capillaries
Lymphatic	Returns excess tissue fluid to the bloodstream and defends against disease	Lymph vessels, ducts, lymph nodes, spleen, tonsils, and thymus

BODY SYSTEMS

Groups of organs functioning together for a common purpose make up the body systems. The major body systems are the integumentary, skeletal, muscular, nervous, respiratory, digestive, urinary, endocrine, reproductive, circulatory, and lymphatic. Table 3–1 lists the organs and functions of each body system.

ORGANISM

Several body systems make up a complete living entity called an organism. The human body has attained the highest level of organization. The ability of these body systems to work together to sustain life and keep the body functioning normally, despite constantly changing internal and external conditions, is an essential function referred to as homeostasis.

Anatomic Description of the Body

KEY TERMS		
■ ***Anatomic position***	Body position used in anatomic descriptions (body is erect and facing forward with the arms at the side and the palms facing forward)
■ ***Frontal plane***	Vertical plane dividing the body into the anterior (front) and the posterior (back) portions
■ ***Midsagittal plane***	Vertical plane dividing the body into equal right and left portions
■ ***Sagittal plane***	Vertical plane dividing the body into right and left portions
■ ***Transverse plane***	Horizontal plane dividing the body into upper and lower portions

DIRECTIONAL TERMS

Healthcare providers effectively communicate with one another and the patient through universally adopted reference systems for the anatomic description of the body. These reference systems include directional terms, body planes, and body cavities. The ***anatomic position*** for the body is standing erect, the head facing forward, and the arms by the sides with the palms facing to the front. When studying anatomic illustrations, note that the right and left sides are opposite to your own.

Directional terms indicate the location and position of an area or body part, and Table 3–2 contains common directional terms.

BODY PLANES

An anatomic plane is an imaginary flat surface that divides portions of the body or an organ into front, back, right, left, upper, and lower sections. The ***frontal plane*** divides the body into **anterior** (front or **ventral**) and **posterior** (back or **dorsal**) portions. The ***sagittal plane*** divides the body vertically into right and left portions. A ***midsagittal plane*** vertically divides the body into equal right and left portions. The ***transverse plane*** is a cross-sectional division separating the body horizontally into upper (**superior**) and lower (**inferior**) portions. Figure 3–1 illustrates the body planes.

TABLE 3–2   **Common Directional Terms**

Term	Definition	Example
Anterior	In front of or before	The chest is anterior to the spine.
Posterior	Toward the back	The spine is posterior to the chest.
Superior	Above/in an upward direction	The head is superior to the chest.
Inferior	Below/in a downward direction	The chest is inferior to the head.
Proximal	Point of attachment near the body center	The knee is proximal to the foot.
Distal	Point of attachment further from center	The foot is distal to the knee.
Lateral	To the side	The shoulder is lateral to the chest.
Medial	Nearest the midline	The chest is medial to the shoulder.
Ventral	The front side	The chest is on the ventral side of the body.
Dorsal	The back side	The spine is on the dorsal side of the body.
Superficial	Toward the surface	The skin is a superficial organ.
Deep	Toward the interior	The artery is deep in the body.

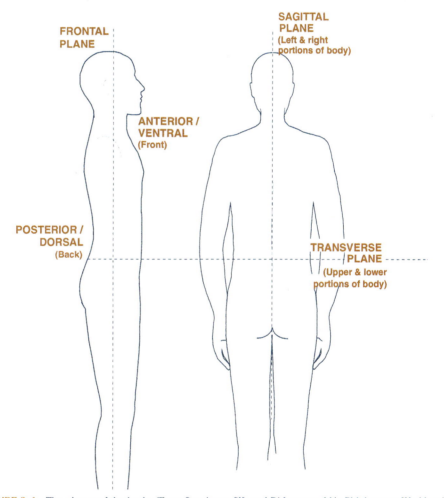

FIGURE 3–1   The planes of the body. (From Strasinger, SK, and Di Lorenzo, MA: Phlebotomy Workbook for the Multiskilled Healthcare Professional. FA Davis, Philadelphia, 1996, p. 81, with permission.)

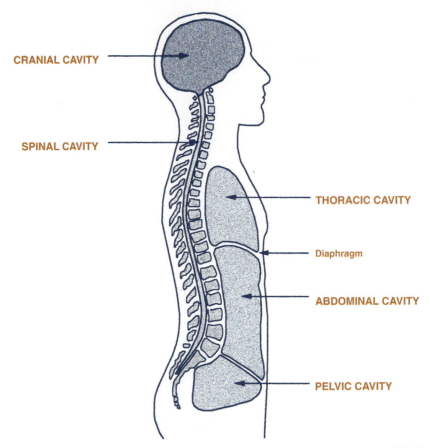

FIGURE 3–2   The cavities of the body. (From Strasinger, SK, and Di Lorenzo, MA: Phlebotomy Workbook for the Multiskilled Healthcare Professional. FA Davis, Philadelphia, 1996, p. 82, with permission.)

Computerized axial tomography (**CAT scan**) is a radiographic technique that produces an x-ray of the body in a transverse plane to detect soft body tissue diseases. Magnetic resonance imaging (**MRI**) uses a magnetic field rather than x-rays to produce images of the body in all three planes.

BODY CAVITIES

Body cavities are hollow spaces containing the internal organs. Classified into two major groups depending on their location, the anterior and posterior cavities enclose five subcavities (Fig. 3–2).

The ventral cavity (anterior) consists of the **thoracic** cavity, abdominal cavity, and pelvic cavity. Pleural membranes line the organs of the thoracic cavity. The parietal

TABLE 3–3   **Body Cavities and Their Organs**

Plane	Cavity	Organs
Anterior	Thoracic	Lungs and heart
	Abdominal	Stomach, small and large intestines, spleen, liver, gallbladder, pancreas, and kidneys
	Pelvic	Bladder, colon, ovaries, and testes
Posterior	Cranial	Brain
	Spinal	Spinal cord

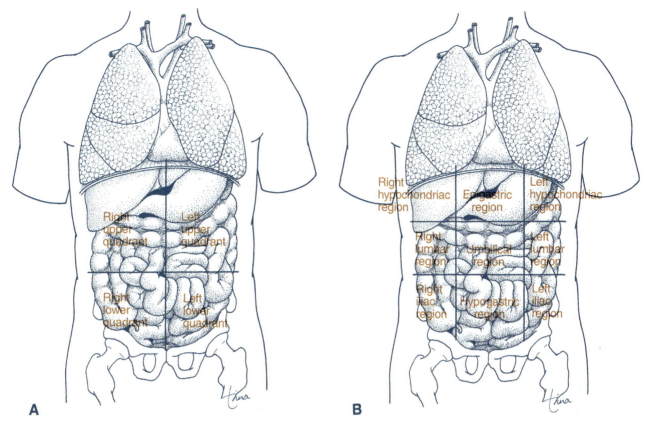

FIGURE 3–3 The abdominopelvic cavity. *A*, Four quadrants. *B*, Nine regions. (From Scanlon, VC, and Sanders, T: Essentials of Anatomy and Physiology, ed. 2. FA Davis, Philadelphia, 1995, p. 17, with permission.)

pleura lines the chest wall, and the visceral pleura covers the lungs. The **peritoneum** lines the abdominal cavity and the mesentery covers the outer surface of the abdominal organs. A muscular wall called the diaphragm separates the thoracic and abdominal cavities. The dorsal cavity (posterior) contains the cranial cavity and spinal cavity. Meninges are the membranes that line these cavities. Table 3–3 lists the main organs contained in these cavities.

Abdominopelvic Cavity

The abdominopelvic cavity combines the abdominal cavity and the pelvic cavity. An imaginary cross formed by a transverse plane and a midsagittal plane that cross at the **umbilicus** divides the abdominopelvic cavity into four quadrants for clinical evaluation and diagnostic purposes. The four divisions are right upper quadrant (**RUQ**), right lower quadrant (**RLQ**), left upper quadrant (**LUQ**), and left lower quadrant (**LLQ**). A patient with appendicitis might present with right lower quadrant pain (Figure 3–3*A*). Using an imaginary "tic-tac-toe" pattern across this large section, nine smaller regions are formed (Figure 3–3*B*). This pattern illustrates a point of reference to locate the internal organs to precisely identify the source of pain or to designate the exact location of tumors, ulcers, surgical incisions, skin lesions, and body structures.

The nine regions of the abdominopelvic cavity are:

- Upper section—the right hypochondriac, epigastric, and left hypochondriac
- Middle section—the right lumbar, umbilical, and left lumbar
- Lower section—the right iliac, hypogastric, and left iliac

Body Systems

INTEGUMENTARY SYSTEM

KEY TERMS

- ***Dermis*** — Inner layer of the skin
- ***Epidermis*** — Outer layer of the skin
- ***Erythema*** — Redness or inflammation of the skin
- ***Keratin*** — Tough protein found in the outer skin, hair, and nails
- ***Melanin*** — Black pigment in the outer skin
- ***Sebaceous gland*** — Oil-producing gland
- ***Subcutaneous*** — Layer of connective and fat tissues under the skin
- ***Sudoriferous gland*** — Sweat-producing gland

The integumentary system consists of the skin, hair, nails, ***sebaceous*** (oil) ***glands***, and ***sudoriferous*** (sweat) ***glands***. The skin is the body's largest organ. On the average adult, it weighs about 7 lb and when stretched out would cover about 18 sq ft.

Function

The skin covers the outer surface of the body and provides the functions of protection, regulation, sensation, and secretion.

Skin protects the body against invasion by microorganisms and environmental chemicals, minimizes the loss or entry of water, helps block the harmful effects of sunlight, and helps produce vitamin D.

Skin regulates temperature by insulating the body and raising or lowering body temperature in response to environmental changes. Blood vessels in the skin dilate to bring blood to the surface when the body needs to lose heat and constrict to allow blood to flow to the muscles and organs when the body needs to conserve heat.

Embedded in the skin are sensory receptors to receive the sensations of heat, cold, pain, touch, and pressure that provide information about the external environment.

Millions of glands under the skin produce secretions to lubricate the skin and produce sweat to keep the body cool.

Components

The outer ***epidermis*** and the inner ***dermis*** make up the two main layers of the skin. A layer of ***subcutaneous*** tissue connects the skin to the underlying muscles.

The epidermis is the thinnest layer of skin and contains no blood vessels or nerve endings. It depends on the blood supply in the capillaries of the dermis to provide oxygen and nutrients. Four or five layers of stratified (layered) squamous epithelial cells make up the epidermis. The two most important layers are the innermost layer (**stratum germinativum**) and the outermost layer (**stratum corneum**).

In the stratum germinativum, cells undergo division (**mitosis**) to continually produce new cells that push the older cells toward the outer skin surface. These cells produce the hard protein called ***keratin***. As the cells move up to the outermost layer of the epidermis, away from the nutrients in the dermis capillaries, they die. Older skin cells become dry and flake away. A layer of skin replaces itself about once a month.

Melanocytes, the cells that produce the skin pigment ***melanin***, are located in this layer. The amount of melanin produced determines the darkness of skin color. Exposure to the ultraviolet (**UV**) rays of the sun stimulates the melanocytes to produce increased amounts of melanin, which protects the skin by darkening the color.

The stratum corneum is the outermost layer of the epidermis, consisting of dead cells filled with keratin. Keratin acts as a waterproof coat that prevents the loss or entry of water and resists the entry of pathogens and harmful chemicals.

The dermis lies below the epidermis. Thicker than the epidermis, this irregular fibrous connective tissue contains capillaries, lymph vessels, nerve fibers, sudoriferous glands, sebaceous glands, and hair follicles. A layer of dermal papillae acts as peglike projections that help bind the dermis to the epidermis. The uneven ridges and grooves created by this junction form the fingerprints and footprints.

Connective tissue and fat tissue make up the subcutaneous layer directly beneath the dermis. This tissue connects the skin to the underlying organs, protects and cushions the deep tissues of the body, stores fat for energy, and acts as a heat insulator.

Hair consists of dead cells filled with keratin. Hair fibers grow in sheaths of epidermal tissue called hair follicles. Mitosis takes place in the hair root at the base of the follicle. The new cells produce keratin, obtain their color from melanin, and grow into the visible portion of the follicle, the hair shaft. Attached to each hair follicle are tiny smooth muscles called arrector pili or the pilomotor. These muscles pull the hair follicles upright to form "goosebumps" when stimulated by cold or fear.

Nails consist of hard keratin plates that cover and protect the fingers and toes. As with the hair fiber, new cells constantly form in the nail root of a nail follicle. The new cells produce keratin and then die to form the nail plate.

Sudoriferous glands are small coiled glands with ducts extending up through the epidermis to small pores on almost all body surfaces. The forehead, armpits, upper lip, palms, and soles are the areas of highest concentration. Activated by high external temperature and exercise, the perspiration (sweat) produced by these glands regulates body temperature by evaporation and eliminates waste products through the pores of the skin.

Sebaceous glands are the oil-secreting glands of the skin. Secreted through tiny ducts into hair follicles or directly to the skin surface to prevent drying of the hair and skin is an oily substance called **sebum**. Secretion of sebum varies with age. Adolescents have increased production and the elderly often have dry, fragile skin caused by decreased sebum production.

Disorders

The following are disorders of the integumentary system:

- Acne—an oversecretion of sebum by sebaceous glands that causes blockage of ducts and the formation of pustules; it is triggered by hormonal changes of puberty and is most common in adolescents and persons with oily skin.
- Eczema—an allergic reaction with an itchy rash that may blister and is aggravated by infection, emotional stress, food allergy, and sweating.
- Fever blisters (cold sores)—an area of inflammation caused by the herpes simplex virus. Usually presents at the edge of the lip; may become dormant and then may be triggered by stress or illness.
- Fungal infections—tinea infections such as ringworm, athlete's foot, and jock itch caused by the dermatophyte fungi that can produce itching, scaling, and ***erythema***.
- Impetigo—a highly contagious bacterial infection caused by *Staphylococcus* or *Streptococcus,* frequently seen in younger children; may present with erythema and progress into blisters that rupture, producing yellow crusts.
- Keloid—excess collagen scar formation in the area of surgical incisions or skin wounds.

TABLE 3–4 Diagnostic Tests Associated with the Integumentary System

Test	Clinical Correlation
Culture and sensitivity (**C & S**)	Bacterial infection
Fungal culture	Fungal infection
Gram stain	Microbial infection
Potassium hydroxide (**KOH**) prep	Fungal infection
Skin biopsy (**Bx**)	Malignancy

- Psoriasis—a chronic inflammatory skin condition characterized by itchy, scaly, red patches; the scales are on top of raised lesions called plaques.
- Skin cancer—squamous cell carcinoma, basal cell carcinoma, and **malignant** melanoma are the most common. (Kaposi's sarcoma is a form of skin cancer associated with AIDS.)
- Warts—raised, rounded, skin-colored, rough growths, usually on the hands and feet; caused by a virus.

Diagnostic Tests

The most frequently ordered diagnostic tests associated with the integumentary system and their clinical correlations are presented in Table 3–4.

Medications

Table 3–5 lists the names and purpose of the most commonly used medications for the integumentary system.

MUSCULOSKELETAL SYSTEM

Bones, joints, and muscles make up the musculoskeletal system. The framework and support for the body is provided by 206 bones, together with the joints, cartilage, and ligaments. More than 600 muscles attached to the bones of the skeleton by tendons move the skeleton and cause the movement of the organs.

TABLE 3–5 Commonly Used Medications for the Integumentary System

Type	Generic and Trade Names	Purpose
Anesthetics	Local: Dyclone, Solarcaine, and Xylocaine	Relieve itching and pain
Antibiotic agents	Bactroban, Mycitracin, Neosporin, and Polysporin	Eliminate infection
Antifungal agents	Desenex, Fungizone, Lotrimin, Micatin, and nystatin	Inhibit growth of fungi and yeast
Anti-inflammatory agents	Steroids: Aristocort, Decadron, hydrocortisone, and Temovate	Relieve redness, swelling, tenderness, and painful inflammation
Antipruritic agents	Atarax, Claritin, Benadryl, Topicort, and Zyrtec	Prevent itching
Antiseptic agents	Betadine, isopropyl alcohol, pHisoHex, and Zephiran	Inhibit growth of pathogens
Antiviral agents	Denavir, Famvir, and Zovirax	Inhibit viral diseases
Emollients	Dermassage, Desitin, and Neutroderm	Soothe dry skin
Keratolytics	Carmol, DuoFilm, Karalyt, and Saligel	Loosen and destroy outer layers

Skeletal System

KEY TERMS		
	▪ *Articulation*	Joint/connection
	▪ *Bursa*	Sac of synovial fluid located between a tendon and a bone to decrease friction
	▪ *Cartilage*	Flexible connective tissue surrounded by gel (located where bones come together)
	▪ *Hematopoiesis*	Formation of blood cells in the bone marrow
	▪ *Ligament*	Fibrous connective tissue that binds bones together at the joint
	▪ *Sarcoma*	Malignant tumor containing embryonic connective tissue
	▪ *Synovial*	Pertaining to lubricating fluid secreted by membranes in joint capsules
	▪ *Tendon*	Connective tissue that binds muscles to bones

Function

The five main functions of the skeletal system are support, protection, movement, mineral storage, and blood cell formation (***hematopoiesis***). As the framework of the body, the skeletal system provides support and protects vital organs. Movement is possible because bone is the anchor point for muscles, joints, ***tendons***, and ***ligaments***. Phosphorus and calcium are stored in the bones and are released to the blood as needed. The important function of hematopoiesis takes place in the center (marrow) of bones.

Components

The components of the skeletal system are the bones, joints, tendons, ***cartilage***, and ligaments.

Bone Composition

Bone-forming cells called **osteoblasts** and bone-reabsorbing cells called **osteoclasts** provide a process by which calcium phosphate deposits are laid down in specific patterns in a gel-like matrix. The osteoblasts produce an enzyme to combine calcium and phosphorus into calcium phosphate that makes the bones hard and rigid. The osteoclasts remove bone debris and smooth and shape the bones. Cartilage is the flexible part of the skeletal system and is found where bones come together. Cartilage fibers are embedded in a gel-like material versus the calcified substance found in bones and therefore provide greater flexibility.

Bone Types

There are four classes of bones, and this classification is usually based on shape. The *long bones* are found in the extremities. These are the bones of the leg (**femur, tibia,** and **fibula**) and the arm bones (**humerus, radius,** and **ulna**). *Short bones* are the wrists (**carpals**), hands (**metacarpals**), ankles (**tarsals**), and feet (**metatarsals**). *Flat bones* are for the protection of the inner organs, such as the heart and brain. They have a broad surface for the attachment of muscles. Examples of flat bones are the **cranium**, ribs, **scapula**, and **sternum**. *Irregular bones* have unusual shapes, such as the bones of the vertebrae, **sacrum**, and **coccyx**. Figure 3–4 shows the major bones of the body.

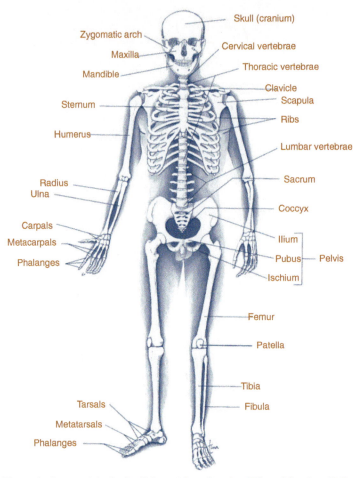

FIGURE 3–4   The major bones of the body. (Adapted from Scanlon, VC, and Sanders, T: Essentials of Anatomy and Physiology, ed. 2. FA Davis, Philadelphia, 1995, p. 109, with permission.)

Joints

Each bone connects (***articulates***) to another bone by forming an immovable (**synarthrosis**), partially movable (**amphiarthrosis**), or free-moving (**diarthrosis**) joint. The skull bones have immovable joints called cranial sutures, and vertebrae have partially movable joints; most joints in the body (knee, hip, elbow, wrist, and foot), however, are free moving.

All free-moving joints are ***synovial*** joints and consist of a synovial cavity, a joint capsule, and a layer of articular cartilage. Articular cartilage covers the ends of each bone, providing a smooth surface and acting as a cushion against jolts. The synovial cavity is the space between the bones at the joint and is separated by a joint capsule. The joint capsule fits over the ends of the two bones and secures the joint together tightly by ligaments (strong connective tissue). The synovial membrane lining the joint capsule secretes synovial fluid, a thick and slippery fluid, to prevent friction and allow easy movement of bones. Small sacs of synovial fluid called ***bursae*** located between the joint and tendons allow tendons to slide easily across joints. Figure 3–5 illustrates a synovial joint.

Disorders

The following are disorders of the musculoskeletal system:

- Ankylosing spondylitis—pain affecting the back and the joints of the lower back.
- Arthralgia—pain without swelling or redness in the joints that can be caused by tension, virus infections, unusual exertion, or accidents.

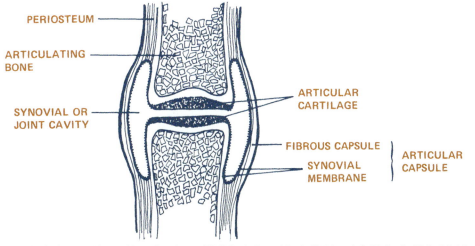

FIGURE 3–5   Synovial joint. (From Strasinger, SK: Urinalysis and Body Fluids, ed. 3. FA Davis, Philadelphia, 1994, p. 165, with permission.)

- Arthritis—inflammation of the joint causing swelling, redness, warmth, and pain upon movement. The four most common types are osteoarthritis, rheumatoid arthritis, gout, and ankylosing spondylitis.
- Bursitis—inflammation of the bursae (sacs of synovial fluid) located between the joints and the tendons, commonly causing swelling and pain in the shoulder, elbow, or heel.
- **Fractures** (Fx) (Figure 3–6)—breaking of bone caused by stress, cancer, or metabolic disease. The different types of fractures are:
  - *Comminuted (Fx)*—the bone has splintered into many pieces by two or more intersecting breaks.
  - *Compound (open)*—the bone is broken with fragments protruding through the skin.
  - *Greenstick*—the bone is partially bent and partially broken; often seen in children.
  - *Impacted*—the bone fragment is driven into another bone.
  - *Simple (closed)*—the bone is broken with no puncture through the skin.
- Gout—painful metabolic condition caused by uric acid crystals forming in the joints, frequently the big toe, the ankle or the knee; occurs mostly in men.
- Lyme disease—result of an infection caused by a spirochete bacterium carried by deer ticks; an oval rash, fever, headache, stiff neck, and backache can develop 3 to 20 days after the bite of an infected tick. The synovial membrane becomes infected, producing joint, neurologic, or cardiac problems.
- Osteoarthritis—occurs in later life and causes knobby swelling at the most distant joint of the fingers.
- Osteoma—a benign or malignant bone tumor. Malignant tumors, **sarcomas**, are named for the specific tissue affected:
  - *Fibrosarcoma*—fibrous connective tissue
  - *Lymphosarcoma*—lymphoid tissue
  - *Chondrosarcoma*—cartilage
  - *Osteosarcoma*—bone
  - *Ewing's sarcoma*—shaft of the long bones
- Osteomalacia—softening of the bones, resulting from the inability to absorb calcium because of a vitamin D deficiency; often called rickets. It is seen in infants and children and may result in bone deformity.
- Osteomyelitis—inflammation of the bones and bone marrow caused by a bacterial infection; often caused by local trauma to the bone such as improper microtechniques in phlebotomy.

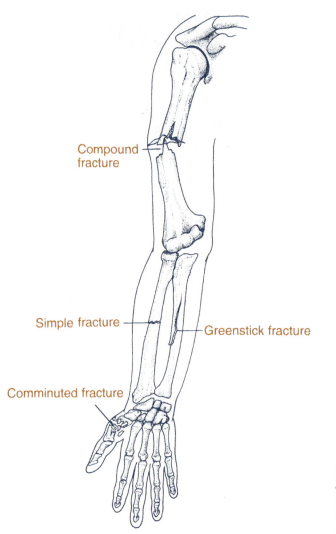

Compound fracture

Simple fracture

Greenstick fracture

Comminuted fracture

FIGURE 3–6 Types of fractures. (From Scanlon, VC, and Sanders, T: Essentials of Anatomy and Physiology, ed. 2. FA Davis, Philadelphia, 1995, p. 107, with permission.)

- Osteoporosis—bone disease involving decreased bone density producing porous bones that can become brittle and easily broken. Causes include a lack of protein, calcium, or Vitamin D; high doses of corticosteroids; or the lack of estrogen in postmenopausal women.
- Paget's disease—a metabolic disorder in which new abnormal bone replaces spongy bone, resulting in the deformity of flat bones and the bowing of the legs; usually affects adults over the age of 35.
- Rheumatoid arthritis (**RA**)—chronic inflammation of the joints due to an autoimmune reaction involving the joint connective tissue. The inflammation causes painful swelling and can produce crippling deformities as it spreads from the inflamed synovial membrane to the cartilage of a joint. RA usually starts in midlife and is diagnosed with a blood test to determine the presence of the autoantibody (rheumatoid factor [**RF**]).
- Scoliosis—a lateral curvature of the spine with deviation to either the right or left that gives the spine the shape of an "S." It can be **congenital** or can develop in early teen years because of poor posture.
- Spina bifida—congenital disorder characterized by an abnormal closure of the spinal canal, resulting in malformation of the spine.
- Systemic lupus erythematosus (**SLE**)—autoimmune disease affecting the connective tissue; cartilage, bones, ligaments, and tendons; usually seen in women of childbearing years. A hallmark of the disease is the classic butterfly rash that appears across the cheeks and the bridge of the nose.

Diagnostic Tests

The most frequently ordered diagnostic tests associated with the skeletal system and their clinical correlations are presented in Table 3–6.

Medications

Table 3–7 lists the names and purpose of the most commonly used medications for the skeletal system.

Muscular System

KEY TERMS

- *Cardiac muscle*   Striated muscle of the heart
- *Insertion*   Movable attachment point of a muscle to a bone
- *Origin*   Stationary attachment point of a muscle to a bone
- *Skeletal muscle*   Striated voluntary muscle that moves bones
- *Smooth muscle*   Unstriated involuntary muscle of the internal organs and blood vessels
- *Striated*   Marked with grooves or stripes

The muscular system works in conjunction with the skeletal and nervous systems to provide body movement. Composed of long, slender cells called fibers, muscles make up 42% of body weight. Each muscle consists of fibers held together by connective tissue enclosed in a fibrous sheath.

Function

Muscles attach to the bones of the skeleton by tendons. The ability of the muscle to contract provides the body with movement, posture, and heat production. A special type of contraction called **tonicity** maintains posture. It is a partial contraction of skeletal muscles that shortens only a few muscles and does not allow movement. Muscles held in position resist the pull of gravity. Heat produced through chemical changes

TABLE 3–6   **Diagnostic Tests Associated with the Skeletal System**

Test	Clinical Correlation
Alkaline phosphatase (**ALP**)	Bone disorders
Antinuclear antibody (**ANA**)	Systemic lupus erythematosus
Arthroscopy	Joint trauma
Calcium (**Ca**)	Bone disorders
Computerized axial tomography (CAT scan)	Body structure examination
Culture and sensitivity (C & S)	Microbial infection
Fluorescent antinuclear antibody (**FANA**)	Systemic lupus erythematosus
Gram stain	Microbial infection
Magnetic resonance imaging (MRI)	Body structure examination
Phosphorus (**P**)	Skeletal disorders
Rheumatoid arthritis (RA)	Rheumatoid arthritis
Synovial fluid analysis	Arthritis
Uric acid	Gout
X-ray	Bone structure

TABLE 3–7 **Commonly Used Medications for the Skeletal System**

Type	Generic and Trade Names	Purpose
Analgesics	Non-narcotic: Aleve, aspirin, Motrin, Nuprin, and Tylenol Narcotic: Demerol, morphine sulfate, Percocet, and Vicodin	Relieve swelling, fever, and pain
Anti-inflammatory agents	Nonsteroidal: Anaprox, aspirin, Motrin, and Naprosyn Steroids: Celestone, Decadron, and Kenalog	Relieve bone and joint pain
Antirheumatic agents	Gold therapy, Imuran, Plaquenil, and Rheumatrex	Treat rheumatoid arthritis

involved during muscle contraction maintains a constant body temperature. Muscles not only provide skeletal movement but also pass food through the digestive system, propel blood through blood vessels, and contract the bladder to expel urine.

Components

The three types of muscle found in the body are skeletal, smooth, and cardiac. They are classified by their function and appearance. The three types of muscle are shown in Figure 3–7.

Skeletal muscle is a *striated* voluntary muscle that attaches to bones and is responsible for movement of the body. It is called a voluntary muscle because a person has control over its activity. It is a striated muscle because of its cross-striped appearance when examined microscopically.

Smooth muscle is an unstriated involuntary (**visceral**) muscle that lacks the cross-striped appearance microscopically. It is controlled by the autonomic nervous

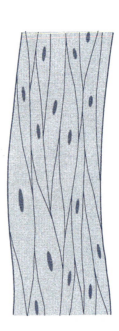
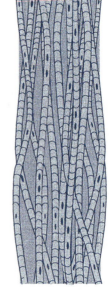

Skeletal / Striated   **Smooth / Unstriated**   **Cardiac**

FIGURE 3–7   The three types of muscle. (From Strasinger, SK, and Di Lorenzo, MA: Phlebotomy Workbook for the Multiskilled Healthcare Professional. FA Davis, Philadelphia, 1996, p. 121, with permission.)

system. Smooth muscle is found in the walls of veins and arteries and in the internal organs of the digestive, respiratory, and urinary systems; smooth muscle functions without any conscious control by the individual.

Cardiac muscle is the muscle of the heart wall. Like skeletal muscle, it is a striated muscle, but it is also an involuntary muscle. Controlled by the autonomic nervous system, cardiac muscle rhythmically contracts without any conscious control by the individual.

Movement

Tendons, cords of fibrous connective tissue, attach skeletal muscle to bones. A muscle attaches to a stationary bone, the *origin*, and to a movable bone, the *insertion*. As the muscle contracts and shortens, the insertion bone moves toward the stationary bone. A muscle pulls when it contracts, but it cannot push. An opposing muscle contracts to pull the bone in the other direction. A muscle that produces movement is the prime mover, and the opposing muscle is an antagonist. Table 3–8 lists the major muscle movements. The concept of muscular movement is illustrated in Figure 3–8.

Disorders

The following are disorders of the muscular system:

- Atrophy—wasting away of muscle, caused by inactivity.
- Carpal tunnel syndrome (**CTS**)—caused by pressure on the median nerve as it passes through the ligaments, bones, and tendons; characterized by pain and tingling in the fingers and hand that may radiate to the shoulder.
- Fibromyalgia syndrome (**FMS**)—a condition with muscle pain, chronic pain, fatigue, sleep problems, irritable bowel syndrome, morning stiffness, anxiety, and memory problems.
- Muscular dystrophy (**MD**)—an inherited disorder in which the muscles are replaced by fat and fibrous tissue and progressively weaken.
- Myalgia—muscle pain that can be caused by tension, viral infections, exertion, accidents, or, in rare cases, cancer or thyroid disease.
- Myasthenia gravis—a neuromuscular disorder of the skeletal muscle that affects the transmission of nerve impulses to the muscles of the eyes, face, and limbs.
- Poliomyelitis—viral infection of the nerves controlling skeletal movement resulting in muscle weakness and paralysis.
- Tendinitis—inflammation of the tendons caused by excess exertion; common locations are the rotator cuff around the shoulder, biceps, and Achilles tendon (large tendon that connects the calf muscles to the back of the heel).

TABLE 3–8 **Major Muscle Movements***

Motion	Action
Abduction	Moving away from the middle of the body
Adduction	Moving toward the middle of the body
Extension	Straightening of a limb
Flexion	Bending of a limb
Pronation	Turning the palm down
Supination	Turning the palm up
Dorsiflexion	Elevating the foot
Plantar flexion	Lowering the foot
Rotation	Moving a bone around its longitudinal axis

*Grouped in pairs of antagonistic function.

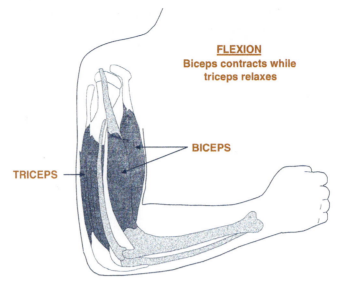

FIGURE 3–8 An example of muscular movement. (From Strasinger, SK, and Di Lorenzo, MA: Phlebotomy Workbook for the Multiskilled Healthcare Professional. FA Davis, Philadelphia, 1996, p. 120, with permission.)

Diagnostic Tests

The most frequently ordered diagnostic tests associated with the muscular system and their clinical correlations are presented in Table 3–9.

Medications

Table 3–10 lists the names and purpose of the most commonly used medications for the muscular system.

NERVOUS SYSTEM

KEY TERMS

- *Afferent neuron* Nerve cell carrying impulses to the brain and spinal cord (sensory neuron)

- *Autonomic nervous system* System regulating the body's involuntary functions by carrying impulses from the brain and spinal cord to the muscles, glands, and internal organs

TABLE 3–9 **Diagnostic Tests Associated with the Muscular System**

Test	Clinical Correlation
Computerized axial tomography (CAT scan)	Soft tissue examination
Creatine kinase (**CK[CPK]**)	Muscle damage
Creatine kinase isoenzymes (**CK-MM, MB**)	Muscle damage
Electromyogram (**EMG**)	Muscle function
Lactic acid	Muscle fatigue
Magnesium (**Mg**)	Musculoskeletal disorders
Magnetic resonance imaging (MRI)	Soft tissue examination
Myoglobin	Muscle damage
Potassium (**K**)	Muscle function

TABLE 3–10   **Commonly Used Medications for the Muscular System**

Type	Generic and Trade Names	Purpose
Analgesics	Non-narcotic: Aleve, aspirin, Motrin, Nuprin, and Tylenol	Relieve swelling, fever, and pain
Muscle relaxants	Flexeril, Paraflex, Parafon Forte, DSC, Robaxin, and Soma	Relax muscle spasms
Neuromuscular blocking agents	Flaxedil, Norcuron, and Tracrium	Relax muscles

- **Axon** — Fiber of nerve cells that carries impulses away from the cell body of the neuron
- **Central nervous system** — Brain and spinal cord
- **Dendrite** — Fiber of nerve cells that carries impulses to the cell body of the neuron
- **Efferent neuron** — Nerve cell carrying impulses away from the brain and spinal cord (motor neuron)
- **Meninges** — Protective membranes around the brain and spinal cord
- **Myelin sheath** — Tissue around the axon of the peripheral nerves
- **Neuroglia** — Connective tissue cells of the nervous system that do not carry impulses
- **Neuron** — Nerve cell
- **Peripheral nervous system** — All nerves outside the brain and spinal cord
- **Synapse** — Point at which an impulse is transmitted from one neuron to another

The nervous system is the communication system for the body. It controls and regulates all body systems to maintain homeostasis. Nerve impulses cause muscles to contract to move bones and enable one to hear, see, taste, think, and react.

Function

The primary functions of the nervous system are to recognize sensory stimuli, to interpret these sensations, and to initiate the appropriate response that provides the communication, integration, and control of all body functions. Electrical nerve impulses traveling by way of a nerve fiber and the release of a chemical substance called a neurotransmitter accomplish these functions. The specialized cell of the nervous system is the **neuron**; its type varies, depending on the function it performs.

Components

The nervous system is divided into the **central nervous system (CNS)** and the **peripheral nervous system** (PNS). The CNS lies in the center of the body and consists of the brain and the spinal cord. The PNS consists of nerves located outside the skull and spinal column; it extends out into the body and connects the brain and spinal cord to all parts of the body.

Cell body
Neuron

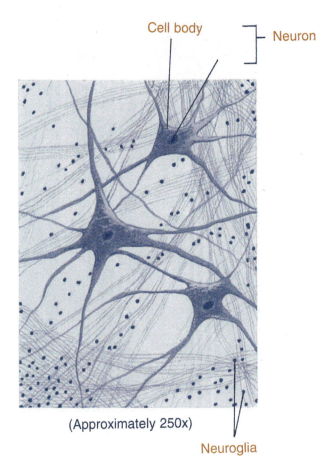

(Approximately 250x)

Neuroglia

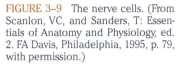

FIGURE 3–9   The nerve cells. (From Scanlon, VC, and Sanders, T: Essentials of Anatomy and Physiology, ed. 2. FA Davis, Philadelphia, 1995, p. 79, with permission.)

Two types of cells are present in the nervous system. The main functioning cell that conducts nerve impulses is the neuron. The second type of cell is the *neuroglia*, which acts as nerve glue or connective support for neurons and does not conduct nerve impulses. Figure 3–9 illustrates the nerve cells.

Different types of neurons are classified by the way they transmit impulses. Sensory neurons, also called *afferent neurons*, transmit impulses from the sensory organs to the brain and spinal cord. Motor or *efferent neurons* transmit impulses away from the brain and spinal cord to the muscles and glands to produce a response of either contraction or secretion. Central neurons or **interneurons** transmit impulses from sensory neurons to motor neurons.

A neuron consists of three main parts: *dendrites*, a cell body, and an *axon*. Several dendrites branch out to receive and carry impulses to the cell body. The axon, which is a single long projection, extends out and carries impulses away from the cell body. Axons are covered by a protective *myelin sheath* that acts as a special insulator and can accelerate electrical impulses. Because myelin is a white fatty substance, the axons have a white appearance and are therefore called the white matter. Gray matter consists of all the fibers, dendrites, and nerve cell bodies that are not covered with the myelin sheath and have a gray appearance.

The point at which the axon of one neuron and the dendrite of another neuron come together is called a *synapse*. Nerve impulses are transmitted at the synapse. The nerve impulse from an axon stops at the synapse; chemical signals are sent across the gap; and the impulse then continues along the dendrites, the cell body, and the axon of the next neuron.

The CNS, consisting of the brain and spinal cord, is the communication center of the nervous system. It receives impulses from all parts of the body, processes the information, and initiates a response. The brain and spinal cord are continuous through an opening in the base of the skull.

The brain is one of the largest organs in the body and is the center for regulating body functions. The major structures of the brain are the **cerebrum**, the **cerebellum**, the **diencephalon**, and the **brain stem**. The cerebrum is the largest part of the brain and consists of two hemispheres divided by a longitudinal fissure (groove). Each hemisphere is divided into lobes that have the same name as the cranial bone they are near (frontal, parietal, temporal, or occipital). The cerebrum governs all sensory and motor activity. The cerebellum is located in the posterior part of the brain and coordinates voluntary movement, equilibrium, and balance. The diencephalon consists of the **thalamus** and **hypothalamus**. The thalamus relays all sensory impulses except olfactory and emotional behavior. The hypothalamus regulates autonomic nerve impulses and endocrine activity. The brain stem consists of the midbrain, **medulla oblongata**, and the **pons**. It is the conduction pathway between the brain and the spinal cord.

The spinal cord has an ascending nerve tract to carry sensory impulses to the brain. A descending nerve tract carries motor impulses away from the brain to the muscles and organs.

The skull bones provide protection for the brain, and the vertebrae provide protection for the spinal cord. Three layers of connective tissue membranes called *meninges* cover the brain and spinal cord to provide additional shock-absorbing protection. The thick outermost layer is the **dura mater**, which lines the skull and vertebral canal. The middle layer is the **arachnoid membrane**. The innermost layer is the **pia mater**, which is a thin membrane covering the surface of the brain and spinal cord. The subarachnoid space located between the arachnoid and pia mater contains the **cerebrospinal fluid** (CSF). CSF circulates through the inner ventricles of the brain, the central canal of the spinal cord, and the subarachnoid space to cushion the brain and spinal cord from shocks that could cause injury; it supplies nutrients to the cells.

Normally CSF is clear and colorless, containing proteins, glucose, urea, salts, and a few white blood cells. Infection (meningitis) or cerebral hemorrhage can cause the fluid to become cloudy. To diagnose these conditions, the physician must extract some CSF for laboratory analysis. A **lumbar puncture** is performed by inserting a needle between the vertebrae of the lower spine and aspirating fluid into a syringe. Three or four tubes of fluid are collected, each with approximately 1 mL of fluid. The first tube is tested in the chemistry section for substances such as glucose and protein. The specimen in the second tube is cultured in the microbiology section for infectious agents. The third tube is analyzed in the hematology section, where cell counts and cell identification are performed.

The nerve network branching throughout the body from the brain and spinal cord is the PNS. The 12 pairs of cranial nerves connect to the brain by passing through openings to the skull. Cranial nerves distribute to the head and neck regions of the body, except for the tenth cranial nerve, called the vagus, which controls the structures of the neck, chest, and abdomen. The 31 pairs of spinal nerves pass through the openings in the vertebral column. Spinal nerves distribute in a bandlike fashion to the trunk and to the upper and lower extremities.

The PNS includes the *autonomic nervous system* (**ANS**). It consists of the motor neurons to control the involuntary bodily functions, such as heartbeat, stomach contractions, respiration, and gland secretions. The ANS has two divisions, the sympathetic and parasympathetic. They function opposite one another and are controlled by the hypothalamus to keep the body in a state of homeostasis. The sympathetic division controls stress situations such as anger or fear by increasing the heart rate and dilating vessels. The parasympathetic division controls relaxed situations by decreasing the heart rate and the other body activities to normal levels.

Disorders

The following are disorders of the nervous system:

- Alzheimer's disease—characterized by diminished mental capabilities, including memory loss, anxiety, and confusion.

- Amyotrophic lateral sclerosis (**ALS**)—a disorder of the motor neurons in the brain and spinal cord that causes skeletal and muscular weakness; also called Lou Gehrig's disease.
- Bell's palsy—inflammation of a facial nerve that causes paralysis and numbness of the face.
- Cerebral palsy—associated with birth defects, this condition is marked by partial paralysis and poor muscular coordination.
- Cerebrovascular accident (**CVA**)—stroke; can be caused by cerebral hemorrhage or arteriosclerosis, hardening of the arteries. A decrease in the flow of blood to the brain causes destruction of the brain tissue from a lack of oxygen.
- Encephalitis—inflammation of the brain caused by a virus; symptoms are lethargy, stiff neck, or convulsions. A lumbar puncture to analyze the CSF can confirm the diagnosis.
- Epilepsy—recurring seizure disorders resulting from abnormal electrical activity or malfunctioning of the chemical substances of the brain.
- Meningitis—inflammation of the membranes of the brain or spinal cord caused by a variety of microorganisms; severe headaches, fever, and stiff neck are common symptoms.
- Multiple neurofibromatosis—fibrous tumors throughout the body that cause crippling deformities.
- Multiple sclerosis (**MS**)—a chronic degenerative disease of the CNS that destroys the myelin sheath of the brain and spinal cord; the myelin sheath is replaced by hard, plaquelike lesions that interfere with the transmission of nerve impulses, resulting in diminished motor control. Muscle weakness, poor coordination, and paralysis may occur.
- Myelitis—inflammation of the spinal cord.
- Neuralgia—pain of the nerves.
- Neuritis—inflammation of nerves associated with a degenerative process.
- Parkinson's disease—chronic disease of the nervous system characterized by muscle tremors, muscle weakness, and loss of equilibrium; frequently a disease of the elderly, with stiffness of joints, unblinking eyes, and slowness of movement.
- Reye's syndrome—an acute disease that causes edema of the brain and fatty infiltration of the liver and other organs; viral in origin, seen in children following aspirin administration.

TABLE 3–11 **Diagnostic Tests Associated with the Nervous System**

Test	Clinical Correlation
Cerebrospinal fluid (**CSF**) analysis	
Cell count/Differential	Neurologic disorders or meningitis
Culture and Gram stain	Meningitis
Glucose and protein	Neurologic disorders or meningitis
Computerized axial tomography (CAT scan)	Soft tissue examination
Creatine kinase isoenzymes (**CK-BB**)	Brain damage
Culture and sensitivity (C & S)	Microbial infection
Drug screening	Therapeutic drug monitoring or drug abuse
Electroencephalogram (**EEG**)	Brain function
Gram stain	Microbial infection
Lead	Neurologic function
Lithium (**Li**)	Antidepressant drug monitoring
Lumbar puncture (**LP**)	Cerebrospinal fluid analysis
Magnetic resonance imaging (MRI)	Soft tissue examination
Myelogram	Spinal cord examination
X-ray	Organ examination

TABLE 3–12   **Commonly Used Medications for the Nervous System**

Type	Generic and Trade Names	Purpose
Analgesics	Non-narcotic: Levoprome, Nubain, and Stadol	Relieve pain
	Narcotic: codeine, Darvon, Demerol, Dilaudid, and morphine sulfate	
Anesthetics	Local: Novocain, Nupercainal, Solarcaine, Tronolane, and Xylocaine	Produce loss of sensation
	General: Fluothane, nitrous oxide, Penthrane, and Pentothal	
Anticonvulsants	Depakene, Diamox, Dilantin, Mesantoin, and Tridione	Reduce the severity of convulsive seizures
Antipyretics	Aspirin, ibuprofen, Naprosyn, and Tylenol	Reduce fever and relieve pain
Sedatives and hypnotics	Nonbarbiturates: Ambien, Dalmane, Halcion, Noctec, Placidyl, and Restoril	Calm nerves and induce sleep
	Barbiturates: Amytal, Buticaps, Luminal, Nembutal, and Seconal	

- Shingles—an acute viral disease caused by varicella-zoster, the virus that causes chickenpox, which can remain dormant in the body and reappear in the form of shingles; painful herpes blister eruptions occur along the peripheral nerves at or above the waist.

Diagnostic Tests

The most frequently ordered diagnostic tests associated with the nervous system and their clinical correlations are presented in Table 3–11.

Medications

Table 3–12 lists the names and purpose of the most commonly used medications for the nervous system.

RESPIRATORY SYSTEM

KEY TERMS

- *Deoxyhemoglobin* Oxygen-poor hemoglobin
- *External respiration* Exchange of O_2 and CO_2 at the lungs
- *Hemoglobin* Red blood cell protein that transports O_2 and CO_2 in the bloodstream
- *Internal respiration* Exchange of O_2 and CO_2 between the blood and the cells of the body
- *Oxyhemoglobin* Hemoglobin with O_2 attached
- *Pleura* Double-folded membrane surrounding each lung

The respiratory system in conjunction with the circulatory system furnishes the oxygen (O_2) for individual tissue cells and removes carbon dioxide (CO_2). Crucial to the survival of cells, this process is accomplished by breathing air in and out of the lungs, where respiration, the exchange of oxygen and carbon dioxide, occurs.

Function

The function of the respiratory system is to exchange the gases, oxygen and carbon dioxide, between the circulating blood and the air and tissues. Oxygen is a colorless, odorless, combustible gas found in the air, and carbon dioxide is a colorless, odorless, incombustible gas that is a waste product of cell metabolism.

The exchange of gases involves two types of respiration processes: *external respiration* and *internal respiration*. External respiration is the exchange of gases in the blood by the lungs, and internal respiration is the exchange of gases in the body between the blood and the tissue cells. In external respiration, ventilated lungs receive oxygen from the air that enters the bloodstream through capillaries in the lungs; at the same time, carbon dioxide leaves the bloodstream and is expelled into the air by the lungs. In internal respiration the oxygen leaves the blood and enters the tissue cells, and carbon dioxide from the tissue cells enters the bloodstream (Fig. 3–10).

Components

The respiratory system consists of the upper respiratory tract, which includes the organs outside the chest cavity, and the lower respiratory tract, which includes the organs within the chest cavity. The nose, **pharynx**, **larynx**, and upper **trachea** make up the upper respiratory tract. The lower trachea, **bronchi**, and lungs constitute the lower respiratory tract (Fig. 3–11).

Air enters and leaves the respiratory system through the nose, which acts as the primary filter. The nose moistens and warms the inhaled air, helps to produce sound, and contains the **olfactory receptors** (sensory organs for smell).

Air from the nose passes into the pharynx (throat), which is a tubelike structure that acts as a passageway for food and air. The pharynx is divided into three portions: the nasopharynx, the oropharynx, and the laryngopharynx. The laryngopharynx opens anteriorly to the larynx (voice box) and posteriorly into the esophagus. Food passes to the esophagus, which leads to the stomach, and air passes to the larynx, which leads to the lungs.

Located in the larynx are vocal cords, which determine the quality of voice sounds. A leaf-shaped piece of cartilage on top of the larynx, the **epiglottis**, blocks the opening to the larynx during swallowing to prevent food or liquid from entering the trachea.

From the larynx, the air passes to the trachea (windpipe), which provides the opening through which outside air can reach the lungs. The trachea divides into two main branches called primary bronchi that lead to the right and left lungs. These bronchi continue to subdivide into smaller and smaller treelike secondary branches until they reach the smallest branches, called **bronchioles**, which extend to all parts of the lung. Attached to the bronchioles are alveolar ducts that terminate in clusters of air sacs called **alveoli**.

The lungs lie on either side of the heart, enclosed in a serous membrane called the *pleura*. The right lung is divided into three lobes and the left lung, into two lobes. The main function of the lung is to bring air into contact with the blood to exchange oxygen and carbon dioxide. To facilitate this exchange, each lung contains approximately 300 million alveoli. Effective gas exchange occurs between the alveoli and the surrounding capillaries because the walls of the alveoli and capillaries are composed of a one-cell layer of epithelium. Surfactant, a fluid to coat the thin walls, reduces surface tension to stabilize the walls and allow inflation of the alveoli. Blood in the lung capillaries is low in oxygen and high in carbon dioxide. Oxygen from the alveoli diffuses into the blood in the capillaries while carbon dioxide diffuses from the capillaries into alveoli to be exhaled.

Blood transports oxygen and carbon dioxide via the *hemoglobin* in red blood cells. Hemoglobin with oxygen attached is called *oxyhemoglobin* and is carried to the tissues for use by the body cells. When oxygen is released, carbon dioxide attaches

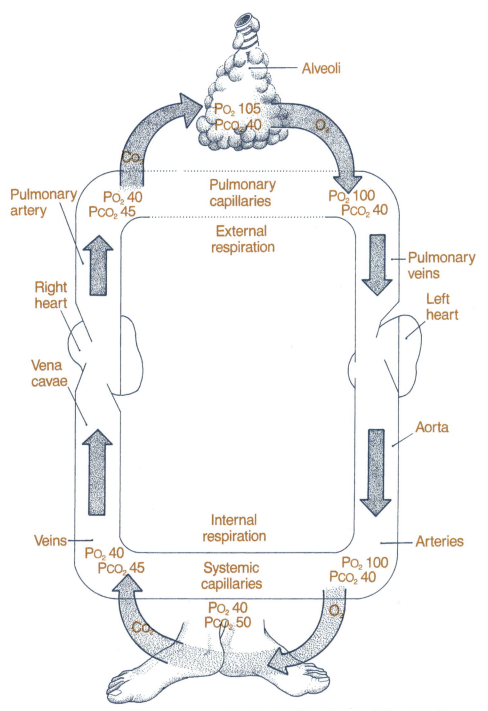

FIGURE 3–10 External and internal respiration. (From Scanlon, VC, and Sanders, T: Essentials of Anatomy and Physiology, ed. 2. FA Davis, Philadelphia, 1995, p. 346, with permission.)

to hemoglobin to form **deoxyhemoglobin**, which is carried to the lungs, where the carbon dioxide is expelled.

Gaseous pressure determines how oxygen or carbon dioxide associates with (attaches to) or dissociates (releases) from hemoglobin. The concentration of each gas in a particular site is expressed as a value called partial pressure. In the lungs, the partial pressure of oxygen is high and the partial pressure of carbon dioxide is low. Therefore, in the lungs, oxygen attaches to hemoglobin and carbon dioxide dissociates from hemoglobin. In the tissues, the partial pressure of oxygen is low and the partial pressure

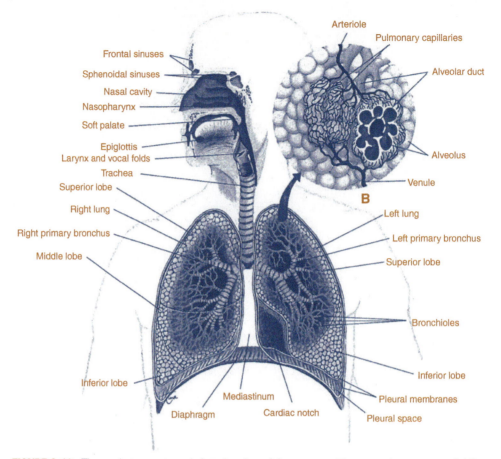

FIGURE 3–11   The respiratory system. *A*, Anterior view of the upper and lower respiratory tracts. *B*, Microscopic view of alveoli and pulmonary capillaries. (From Scanlon, VC, and Sanders, T: Essentials of Anatomy and Physiology, ed. 2. FA Davis, Philadelphia, 1995, p. 338, with permission.)

of carbon dioxide is high, so that oxygen dissociates from hemoglobin and carbon dioxide attaches to hemoglobin. Arterial blood gases measure the partial pressure of oxygen and carbon dioxide in the blood.

Disorders

The following are disorders of the respiratory system:

- Asthma—wheezing, a feeling of chest constriction, and difficulty in breathing caused by swelling or constriction of the bronchial tubes; most common in children and adolescents and triggered by infection, emotional upset, cold air, air pollution, or allergens.
- Bronchitis—chronic inflammation of the bronchial tubes, causing a deep cough that can produce sputum.
- Chronic obstructive pulmonary disease (**COPD**)—inflammation or obstruction of the bronchi and/or alveoli over a long period of time; wheezing and progressive, irreversible damage occur with chronic bronchitis and emphysema.
- Cystic fibrosis—a hereditary disorder causing production of viscous mucus that blocks the bronchioles; can result in chronic respiratory infections and pulmonary failure.
- Emphysema—chronic inflammation resulting in destruction of the bronchioles, caused by cigarette smoke or air pollutants; symptoms are shortness of breath (**SOB**) and enlargement of the chest cavity.

- Infant respiratory distress syndrome (**IRDS**)—a condition affecting prematurely born infants, caused by a lack of surfactant in the alveolar air sacs in the lungs. Surfactant coats the alveolar walls to lower the surface tension so that air moves easily in and out of the lungs. Without surfactant, alveoli collapse and breathing is difficult.
- Lung cancer—masses form and block air passages; most frequent site is the bronchi, and the cancer can spread rapidly to other parts of the body. Symptoms are coughing and sputum production.
- Pleurisy—inflammation of the pleural membrane covering the chest cavity and the outer surface of the lungs; symptoms are chest pain and worsening pain with a deep breath or cough.
- Pneumonia—acute infection of the alveoli of the lungs, in which the alveoli fill with fluid so that the air spaces are blocked and it is difficult to exchange oxygen and carbon dioxide; characterized by fever, chills, cough, and headache.
- Pulmonary edema—accumulation of fluid in the lungs; frequently a complication of congestive heart failure.
- Rhinitis—inflammation of the nasal mucous membranes; a runny nose caused by viruses, allergies, or prolonged used of nose drops.
- Strep throat—inflammation of the pharynx caused by streptococcal group A bacteria; symptoms are a sore throat, fever, swollen lymph glands, scarlet fever rash, or abdominal pain.
- Tuberculosis (**TB**)—infectious disease decreasing respiratory function caused by the bacterial organism *Mycobacterium tuberculosis*.
- Upper respiratory infection (**URI**)—infection of the nose, pharynx, or larynx, including the common cold; symptoms include sore throat, runny nose, congested ears, hoarseness, swollen glands, or fever.

Diagnostic Tests

The most frequently ordered diagnostic tests associated with the respiratory system and their clinical correlations are presented in Table 3–13.

Medications

Table 3–14 lists the names and purpose of the most commonly used medications for the respiratory system.

TABLE 3–13 **Diagnostic Tests Associated with the Respiratory System**

Test	Clinical Correlation
Arterial blood gases (**ABGs**)	Acid-base balance
Bronchoalveolar lavage	Microbial infection
Bronchoscopy	Lung examination or biopsy
Cold agglutinins	Atypical pneumonia
Complete blood count (**CBC**)	Pneumonia
Computerized axial tomography (CAT scan)	Soft tissue examination
Electrolytes (**Lytes**)	Acid-base balance
Gram stain	Microbial infection
Lung biopsy (Bx)	Malignancy
Magnetic resonance imaging (MRI)	Soft tissue examination
Pleural fluid analysis	Infection or malignancy
Pulmonary function tests (**PFTs**)	Respiratory disorders
Purified protein derivative (**PPD**)	Tuberculosis (TB) screening
Thoracentesis	Pleural effusions
Throat and sputum cultures	Bacterial infection
X-ray	Organ examination

TABLE 3–14 **Commonly Used Medications for the Respiratory System**

Type	Generic and Trade Names	Purpose
Antihistamines	Allegra, Benadryl, Claritin, Hismanal, Periactin, Seldane, and Zyrtec	Relieve nasal passage swelling and inflammation
Antituberculosis agents	Myambutol, Nydrazid, and Rifamate	Treat tuberculosis
Antitussives	Non-narcotic: Benylin, Delsym, Robitussin, and Tessalon Narcotic: codeine, endal-HD, and Tussar	Suppress coughing
Bronchodilators	Aminophylline, ephedrine sulfate, and Proventil	Improve bronchial airflow
Decongestants	Afrin, Coricidin, Sinutab, and Sudafed	Reduce nasal congestion
Expectorants	Deconsal, Entex, Isoclor, and Robitussin	Remove lower respiratory tract secretions
Inhalation corticosteroids	Azmacort, Beclovent, and Decadron	Treat allergies and bronchial asthma
Mucolytics	Duratuss, Humibid, and Mucomyst	Liquefy mucus

DIGESTIVE SYSTEM

KEY TERMS

- ***Alimentary tract***   Digestive tract
- ***Amino acids***   "Building blocks" for protein
- ***Bile***   Digestive juice to break up fat
- ***Bilirubin***   Yellow pigmented hemoglobin degradation product
- ***Diarrhea***   Watery stools
- ***Digestion***   Breakdown of complex foods to simpler forms so they can be used by cells
- ***Feces***   Waste product of digestion
- ***Insulin***   Hormone produced by the pancreas to promote the use of glucose by the body
- ***Nausea***   Unpleasant sensation producing the urge to vomit
- ***Peristalsis***   Wavelike muscular contractions to propel material through the digestive tract

Food provides the energy required for the growth, repair, and maintenance of body cells. A meal of meat and mashed potatoes with butter provides complex proteins, carbohydrates, and fat. The body cells cannot absorb food in this complex form. The digestive system converts the protein from meat to ***amino acids***, the carbohydrate from the potatoes to a simple sugar (glucose), and the fat from the butter to fatty acids and triglycerides, simple molecules that are absorbed and used by the body. The digestive system eliminates waste products formed during this process as ***feces***.

Function

The digestive system performs three major functions: ***digestion***, absorption of nutrients, and elimination of waste products. Digestion occurs by both mechanical and chemical processes. The mechanical breakdown begins in the mouth, where the teeth and tongue physically alter the food into smaller pieces. Saliva moistens and lubricates the food to facilitate swallowing. The food continues to mechanically break down by churning in the stomach, where it mixes with digestive fluids. Digestive enzymes and acids further break down the larger molecules into smaller molecules in chemical digestion. Enzymes in the saliva, gastric fluid, pancreatic fluid, and intestinal fluid speed up these chemical reactions, while specific enzymes exist to break down carbohydrates, proteins, and fats. Carbohydrates such as starch are broken down to simple sugars by the enzyme **amylase**, proteins are digested to amino acids by the peptidase enzymes, and fats are converted to fatty acids and glycerol by the enzyme **lipase**. Other chemicals facilitate the process and help food pass through the digestive tract.

Absorption of the digested products of food occurs through the walls of the small intestine into the blood and lymph, which transport the nutrients to the other parts of the body to produce energy and nourish body cells. Sugars and amino acids are absorbed into the bloodstream; fatty acids and triglycerides enter the lymphatic vessels.

Elimination of waste products is the third function of the digestive system. Unusable products of digestion are concentrated as feces in the large intestine, from which they pass out of the body through the anus.

Components

The components of the digestive system (Fig. 3–12) form a 30-ft (in adults) continuous tube that begins with the mouth and ends at the anus. This is commonly known as the gastrointestinal tract or *alimentary tract*. The organs of the gastrointestinal tract include the mouth, pharynx, esophagus, stomach, small intestine, large intestine, **rectum**, and anus. The pharynx and esophagus act as a passageway through which food is propelled to the stomach by wavelike muscular contractions called *peristalsis*. The stomach is a large saclike organ that stores food and continues to digest it with hydrochloric acid and other gastric juices. The small intestine has three parts: the **duodenum**, the **jejunum**, and the **ileum**. Digestion takes place in the mouth, stomach, and small intestine; nutrient absorption occurs mainly in the small intestine. The large intestine is divided into the **cecum**, colon, rectum, and anal canal. The **appendix** is attached to the cecum and does not have a known function in the digestive process. The

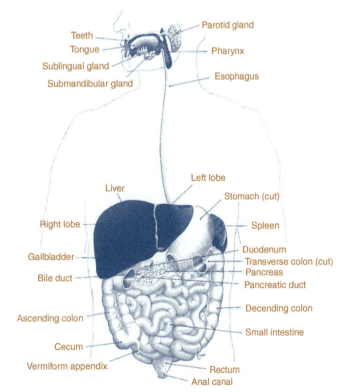

FIGURE 3–12   The digestive system. (From Scanlon, VC, and Sanders, T: Essentials of Anatomy and Physiology, ed. 2. FA Davis, Philadelphia, 1995, p. 361, with permission.)

colon consists of four parts: the ascending, transverse, descending, and sigmoid colons. Elimination of waste products begins in the colon and ends at the rectum and anus.

Accessory organs that assist in the breakdown of food include the teeth, salivary glands, tongue, liver, gallbladder, and pancreas. The teeth and tongue break food into small pieces. The salivary glands (the parotid, submandibular, and sublingual) provide saliva to dissolve and moisten food and produce salivary amylase. The liver secretes ***bile*** to aid in fat digestion and absorption. The gallbladder concentrates and stores excess bile. The pancreas secretes the digestive enzymes lipase, amylase, and trypsin and produces ***insulin***. The liver, the largest internal organ in the body, has several important functions. It converts glucose to glycogen and back to glucose as needed; assists in protein breakdown; manufactures fibrinogen, prothrombin, heparin, and the blood-clotting proteins; stores vitamins; forms ***bilirubin***; and detoxifies harmful substances such as alcohol.

Disorders

The following are disorders of the digestive system:

- Appendicitis—inflammation of the appendix requiring surgical removal; symptoms are acute pain in the RLQ of the abdomen, ***nausea*** or vomiting, and fever.
- Cholecystitis—inflammation of the gallbladder caused by gallstones blocking the bile duct; if gallstones cannot pass out of the gallbladder, severe pain radiating to the right shoulder and obstructive jaundice may occur.
- Cirrhosis—chronic inflammation of the liver caused by alcoholism, hepatitis, or malnutrition, resulting in degeneration of liver cells; jaundice and liver failure may occur.
- Colitis—acute or chronic inflammation of the colon; causes abdominal cramping, ***diarrhea***, or possible ulceration, producing blood- and mucus-streaked stools.
- Crohn's disease—autoimmune disorder producing chronic inflammation of the intestinal tract accompanied by diarrhea and malabsorption.
- Diverticulosis—inflammation of the pouches in the walls of the colon with pain presenting in the LLQ of the abdomen, tenderness, and fever.
- Gastritis—inflammation of the stomach lining.
- Gastroenteritis—inflammation of the stomach and intestinal tract, producing nausea, vomiting, diarrhea, and abdominal cramps and pain.
- Hemorrhoids—enlargement of the veins in the anus and rectum; may be internal or external and produce bleeding, inflammation, and pain.
- Hepatitis—acute inflammation of the liver caused by exposure to toxins or to hepatitis viruses A, B, or C; symptoms include loss of appetite, nausea, fatigue, and jaundice.
- Hernia—protrusion of an organ or structure through the wall of the body cavity in which it is contained.
- Pancreatitis—inflammation of the pancreas, resulting from abdominal injury, toxins, gallstones, drugs, or alcoholism; results in pancreatic tissue destruction due to an accumulation of pancreatic digestive fluids.
- Peritonitis—inflammation of the lining of the abdominal cavity, the peritoneum; frequently caused by a ruptured appendix or a perforated ulcer.
- Ulcer—open lesion in the gastric mucosa caused by increased acid secretion or bacterial infection that may cause pain, hemorrhage, or perforation of the walls of the stomach or duodenum; contributing factors are anxiety, alcohol, caffeine, or smoking.

Diagnostic Tests

The most frequently ordered diagnostic tests associated with the digestive system and their clinical correlations are presented in Table 3–15.

TABLE 3–15   **Diagnostic Tests Associated with the Digestive System**

Test	Clinical Correlation
Alanine aminotransferase (**ALT[SGPT]**)	Liver disorders
Albumin	Malnutrition or liver disorders
Alcohol	Intoxication
Alkaline phosphatase (ALP)	Liver disorders
Ammonia	Severe liver disorders
Amylase	Pancreatitis
Aspartate aminotransferase (**AST[SGOT]**)	Liver disorders
Barium enema (**BaE**)	Colon abnormalities
Bilirubin	Liver disorders
Carcinoembryonic antigen (**CEA**)	Carcinoma detection and monitoring
Cholecystogram	Gallbladder function
Colonoscopy	Colon examination or biopsy
Complete blood count (CBC)	Appendicitis or other infection
Computerized axial tomography (CAT scan)	Soft tissue examination
Gamma glutamyltransferase (**GGT**)	Early liver disorders
Gastrin	Gastric malignancy
Gastrointestinal (**GI**) series	Gastrointestinal tract obstruction or abnormalities
Hepatitis B surface antigen (**HBsAg**)	Hepatitis B screening
Lactic dehydrogenase (**LD[LDH]**)	Liver disorders
Lipase	Pancreatitis
Liver biopsy (Bx)	Malignancy
Magnetic resonance imaging (MRI)	Soft tissue examination
Occult blood	Gastrointestinal bleeding or intestinal malignancy
Ova and parasites (**O & P**)	Parasitic infection
Peritoneal fluid analysis	Bacterial infection
Peritoneal lavage	Hemorrhage
Stool culture	Pathogenic bacteria
Sweat chloride test	Cystic fibrosis
Total protein (**TP**)	Liver disorders
Ultrasonogram	Organ examination

Medications

Table 3–16 lists the names and purpose of the most commonly used medications for the digestive system.

URINARY SYSTEM

KEY TERMS

- *Nephron*   Functional unit of the kidney that forms urine
- *Renal*   Pertaining to the kidney
- *Renal dialysis*   Procedure to remove waste products from the blood when the kidneys are not functioning
- *Uremia*   Increased urea in the blood

The urinary system removes waste products of metabolism, excess dietary chemicals, and excess water from the body in the form of urine. Urine is continually produced by the kidney, flows through the **ureters** to the bladder, and leaves the body through the **urethra**. This process maintains normal homeostasis of body fluids.

TABLE 3–16 **Commonly Used Medications for the Digestive System**

Type	Generic and Trade Names	Purpose
Antacids	Amphojel, Mylanta, sodium bicarbonate, and Tums	Neutralize excess stomach acid and relieve indigestion
Antidiarrheal agents	Imodium, Kaopectate, Lomotil, and Pepto-Bismol	Relieve diarrhea
Antiemetics	Antivert, Compazine, Dramamine, Phenergan, and Tigan	Suppress vomiting
Laxatives	Dulcolax, Ex-Lax, Metamucil, Milk of Magnesia, and Senokot	Relieve constipation

Function

Urine is formed in the **nephrons** of the kidney by a process of filtration and reabsorption. Blood enters the kidney through the **renal** artery, which branches into arterioles leading to the nephrons, and then into a collection of capillaries called the **glomerulus**. The filtration process takes place in the glomerulus, where small substances such as water, sodium and chloride ions, urea, creatinine, and uric acid are filtered out of the blood and collect in the **Bowman's capsule**. Large proteins and cells remain in the blood.

Reabsorption of water, glucose, sodium, and other essential nutrients required by the body begins as the glomerular filtrate passes through the **proximal convoluted tubule** and continues in the descending and ascending **loop of Henle**. The final adjustment of urinary composition occurs in the **distal convoluted tubule** and **collecting duct** (Fig. 3–13). Substances not filtered by the glomerulus are secreted by the tubules into the urinary filtrate. Urine consists of 95% water and 5% solid substances. Normal urine is clear yellow to amber, with a specific gravity of 1.010 to 1.025 and a slightly acid pH.

The actual amount of urine produced depends upon the body's state of hydration and normally averages about 1000 mL per 24 hours. An average adult bladder can retain about 800 mL of urine. Normally, an adult feels the urge to void when the bladder contains around 300 mL of urine.

The ability of the kidneys to reabsorb previously filtered substances from the blood into the bloodstream regulates the acid-base and fluid balances of the body.

The kidneys also produce hormones, such as renin to control blood pressure and erythropoietin to regulate the production of red blood cells.

Components

The urinary system consists of two kidneys, two ureters, urinary bladder, and urethra.

The kidneys are bean-shaped organs containing an outer cortex region and an inner medulla region. The functioning unit of the kidney is the nephron, which consists of the Bowman's capsule, glomerulus, proximal convoluted tubule, loop of Henle, distal convoluted tubule, and collecting duct. Each kidney contains approximately 1 million nephrons.

The ureters are muscular tubes that conduct urine from the kidney to the bladder. The urinary bladder is an expandable sac located in the anterior portion of the pelvic cavity. The bladder stores the urine formed by the nephron. When the bladder becomes full, muscles in the bladder walls squeeze urine into the urethra for elimination. The urethra is a tube extending from the bladder to an external opening called the *urinary meatus*. The male urethra transports urine and semen. The female urethra carries only urine.

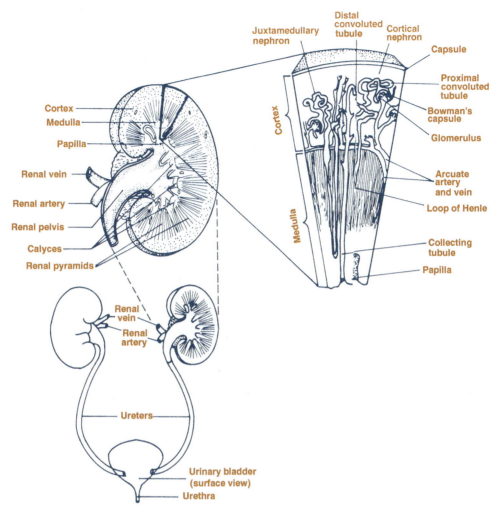

FIGURE 3–13   The relationship of the nephron to the urinary system. (From Strasinger, SK: Urinalysis and Body Fluids, ed. 3. FA Davis, Philadelphia, 1994, p. 14, with permission.)

Disorders

The following are disorders of the urinary system:

- Cystitis—inflammation of the urinary bladder, usually caused by a bacterial infection; the most common symptoms are pain or burning on urination, frequent urgent urination, or blood in the urine.
- Glomerulonephritis—inflammation of the glomerulus of the kidney, caused by an immune disorder or infection; dark brown (cola)-colored urine with hematuria and albuminuria, headache, elevated blood pressure, renal failure, and ***uremia*** are characteristics of this disorder; acute glomerulonephritis can be caused by a delayed immune response to a streptococcal infection.
- Pyelonephritis—inflammation of the renal pelvis and connective tissue of the kidney usually caused by a bacterial infection; symptoms at onset are chills, fever, nausea, and vomiting. Urine examination reveals bacteria, white blood cells, and red blood cells.
- Renal calculi—stones composed of calcium phosphate, uric acid, oxalate, or other chemicals that crystallize within the kidney.
- Renal failure—complete cessation of renal function, resulting in the need for ***renal dialysis*** and kidney transplantation.

- Uremia—excess urea, creatinine, and uric acid in the blood.
- Urinary tract infection (**UTI**)—bacterial infection involving any of the organs of the urinary system, including urethritis, cystitis, and pyelonephritis.

Diagnostic Tests

The most frequently ordered diagnostic tests associated with the urinary system and their clinical correlations are presented in Table 3–17.

Medications

Table 3–18 lists the names and purpose of the most commonly used medications for the urinary system.

ENDOCRINE SYSTEM

KEY TERMS

■	*Endocrine*	Pertaining to ductless glands that secrete hormones directly into the bloodstream to affect other organs
■	*Gland*	Organ that secretes a substance
■	*Homeostasis*	State of equilibrium in the body
■	*Hormone*	Substance that is produced by a ductless gland and transported to parts of the body via the blood to control and regulate body functions
■	*Hyperglycemia*	Elevated glucose levels in the blood
■	*Polydipsia*	Excessive thirst
■	*Polyphagia*	Excessive desire to eat

TABLE 3–17 **Diagnostic Tests Associated with the Urinary System**

Test	Clinical Correlation
Albumin	Kidney disorders
Antistreptolysin O (**ASO**) titer	Acute glomerulonephritis
Blood urea nitrogen (**BUN**)	Kidney disorders
Computerized axial tomography (CAT scan)	Soft tissue examination
Creatinine	Kidney disorders
Creatinine clearance	Glomerular filtration
Cystoscopy	Bladder examination or biopsy
Electrolytes (Lytes)	Fluid balance
Intravenous pyelogram	Kidney structure
Kidney biopsy (Bx)	Malignancy
Magnetic resonance imaging (MRI)	Soft tissue examination
Osmolality	Fluid and electrolyte balance
Routine urinalysis (**UA**)	Renal or metabolic disorders
Total protein (TP)	Kidney disorders
Ultrasonogram	Organ examination
Uric acid	Kidney disorders
Urine culture	Bacterial infection

TABLE 3–18   **Commonly Used Medications for the Urinary System**

Type	Generic and Trade Names	Purpose
Antibacterial agents	Bactrim, Cipro, Floxin, Gantanol, Gantrisin, Septra, and Thiosulfil	Treat UTI
Diuretics	Aldactone, Bumex, Demadex, Diuril, Dyrenium, HydroDIURIL, and Lasix	Promote urination

The ***endocrine*** system produces and regulates ***hormones***. Hormones regulate activities such as metabolism, growth and development, reproduction, and responses to stress. Hormones maintain ***homeostasis*** through the regulation of body fluids, acid-base balance, and energy production.

Function

The endocrine system interacts with the nervous system to communicate, regulate, and control body functions. Unlike the nervous system, which commands and controls with nerve impulses, the ***glands*** of the endocrine system direct long-term changes in body activities by secreting chemical substances called hormones. Endocrine glands are ductless glands that secrete hormones directly into the bloodstream to circulate throughout the body until they reach a target organ. Hormones bind to a specific receptor site located on the cell membrane of a target organ and cause specific chemical reactions to occur. A feedback system regulated by supply and demand stimulates or decreases the release of hormones.

Components

The endocrine glands include the thyroid gland, four parathyroid glands, two adrenal glands, pancreas, pituitary gland, two female ovaries, two male testes, thymus, and pineal gland (Fig. 3–14). Each gland produces hormones that perform a specific function, as listed in Table 3–19.

The secretions of the gastrointestinal mucosa, the placenta, and the kidney also provide endocrine function. The stomach lining secretes **gastrin** to stimulate gastric acid secretion; the placenta secretes **chorionic gonadotropin** hormone, estrogen, and progesterone during pregnancy; and the kidney secretes **erythropoietin** to stimulate red blood cell production and **renin,** which increases blood pressure.

Disorders

The following are disorders of the endocrine system:

Pituitary

- Acromegaly—marked enlargement of the bones in the hands, feet, and face caused by hypersecretion of growth hormone in adulthood.
- Diabetes insipidus (**DI**)—hyposecretion of antidiuretic hormone, causing a failure of the kidneys to reabsorb water, which results in excessive urination and thirst.
- Dwarfism—abnormally small body size caused by hyposecretion of growth hormone in childhood; bones are underdeveloped but well-proportioned to the body; sexual immaturity.
- Gigantism—marked increase in body size caused by hypersecretion of growth hormone in childhood.

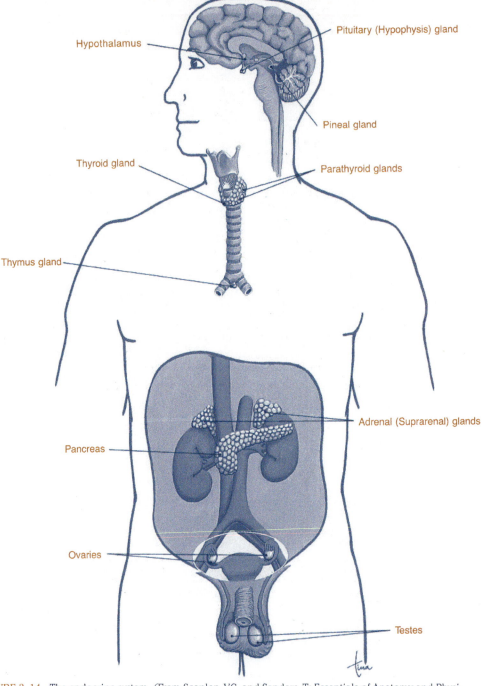

FIGURE 3–14   The endocrine system. (From Scanlon, VC, and Sanders, T: Essentials of Anatomy and Physiology, ed. 2. FA Davis, Philadelphia, 1995, p. 219, with permission.)

Thyroid

- Cretinism—congenital deficiency in the secretion of the thyroid hormones triiodothyronine and thyroxine (hypothyroidism), resulting in mental retardation, impaired growth, and abnormal bone formation.
- Goiter—an enlargement of the thyroid gland caused by hyperthyroidism; sometimes caused by dietary deficiency of iodine.
- Grave's disease—increased cellular metabolism caused by excessive production of the thyroid hormones T_3 and T_4 (hyperthyroidism); characteristics in-

TABLE 3–19   **Summary of Endocrine Hormones**

Gland	Hormone	Function
Anterior pituitary	**Growth hormone (GH)** (Somatropin)	Stimulates bone and body growth
	Thyroid-stimulating hormone (TSH)	Stimulates the thyroid gland hormones thyroxine (T_4) and triiodothyronine (T_3)
	Adrenocorticotropic hormone (ACTH)	Stimulates adrenal cortex to secrete cortisol
	Follicle-stimulating hormone (FSH)	Stimulates growth of ovarian follicles in females and sperm production in males
	Luteinizing hormone (LH)	Stimulates ovulation in females and produces testosterone in males
	Prolactin (PRL)	Stimulates milk production by mammary glands and promotes growth of breast tissue
	Melanocyte-stimulating hormone (MSH)	Regulates melanin deposits that influence skin pigmentation
Posterior pituitary	**Antidiuretic hormone (ADH)**	Stimulates water reabsorption in the kidney to maintain body hydration
	Oxytocin	Stimulates uterine contraction and milk secretion by the mammary gland
Thyroid	**Triiodothyronine (T_3)** and **thyroxine (T_4)**	Regulate cell metabolism and increase energy production
	Calcitonin	Decreases the reabsorption of calcium and phosphate from bones into the blood
Parathyroid	**Parathyroid hormone (PTH)**	Increases the reabsorption of calcium and phosphate from the bones into the blood
Adrenal cortex	**Aldosterone**	Regulates sodium and potassium levels in the blood
	Cortisol	Regulates metabolism of proteins, carbohydrates, and fats and suppresses inflammation
	Androgens and **estrogens**	Maintain secondary sex characteristics
Adrenal medulla	**Epinephrine (adrenaline)**	Increases cardiac activity
	Norepinephrine (noradrenalin)	Constricts blood vessels and increases blood pressure
Pancreas	**Insulin**	Lowers blood sugar by transporting glucose from blood to the cells
	Glucagon	Increases blood sugar levels by converting glycogen to glucose
Ovaries	**Estrogen** and **progesterone**	Maintain female reproductive system and develop secondary female sex characteristics
Testes	**Testosterone**	Promotes maturation of spermatozoa and development of male secondary sex characteristics
Thymus	**Thymosin**	Promotes maturation of T lymphocytes and development of the immune system
Pineal	**Melatonin**	Regulates the body's internal clock

clude **exophthalmos** (a protrusion of the eyeballs due to swelling behind the eyes), weight loss, increased appetite, nervousness, excessive perspiration, rapid heart rate, and fatigue.

- Myxedema—a condition of subcutaneous tissue swelling caused by hypothyroidism that develops in adulthood; symptoms of the lowered metabolic rate lead to lethargy, weight gain, loss of hair, mental apathy, muscle weakness, slow heart rate, and puffiness of the face.

Parathyroid

- Hyperparathyroidism—excessive parathyroid hormone secretion often caused by a benign tumor, leading to kidney stones, bone weakness, osteoporosis, and hypercalcemia (increased blood calcium levels).

- Hypoparathyroidism—deficient parathyroid hormone secretion caused by injury or surgical removal of the gland; decreases blood calcium levels (hypocalcemia), resulting in muscle spasms called tetany.

Adrenal

- Addison's disease—caused by hyposecretion of the adrenal cortex hormone cortisol, resulting in decreased blood sugar levels, muscle weakness, weight loss, nausea, low blood pressure, and dehydration.
- Cushing's disease—hypersecretion of the adrenal cortex hormone cortisol because of an increased adrenal cortex stimulation by adrenocorticotropic hormone (ACTH) from the pituitary gland, caused by a tumor of the pituitary gland or adrenal cortex gland or by excessive administration of corticosteroids for medical reasons. Patients develop a round "moonface" and a buffalo hump on the thoracic region of the back due to the redistribution of fat. Skin and bones become thin and fragile.

Pancreas

- Diabetes mellitus (**DM**)—insulin deficiency that prevents sugar from leaving the blood and entering the body cells, resulting in *hyperglycemia* and **glucosuria**; symptoms include frequent urination (**polyuria**), excessive thirst (*polydipsia*), extreme hunger (*polyphagia*), weight loss, fatigue, and blurred vision.
- Hyperinsulinism—increased secretion of insulin by the pancreas, decreasing the blood sugar level.
- Hypoglycemia—abnormally decreased blood sugar level that is associated with nervousness, headaches, and confusion.

Diagnostic Tests

The most frequently ordered diagnostic tests associated with the endocrine system and their clinical correlations are presented in Table 3–20.

Medications

Table 3–21 lists the names of the most commonly used medications for the endocrine system and their purpose.

REPRODUCTIVE SYSTEM

KEY TERMS

■	*Gamete*	Male or female sex cell
■	*Gonads*	Ovaries and testes
■	*Menopause*	Permanent end of the monthly menstrual cycle
■	*Menstruation*	Monthly shedding of the uterine lining
■	*Ova*	Female sex cells
■	*Ovulation*	Release of the egg cell from the ovary
■	*Semen*	Fluid containing spermatozoa
■	*Spermatozoa*	Male sex cells

TABLE 3–20   **Diagnostic Tests Associated with the Endocrine System**

Test	Clinical Correlation
Adrenocorticotropic hormone (ACTH)	Adrenal and pituitary gland function
Calcium (Ca)	Parathyroid function
Catecholamines	Adrenal function
Computerized axial tomography (CAT scan)	Soft tissue examination
Cortisol	Adrenal cortex function
Glucose	Hypoglycemia or diabetes mellitus
Glucose tolerance test (**GTT**)	Hypoglycemia or diabetes mellitus
Growth hormone (GH)	Pituitary gland function
Insulin	Glucose metabolism and pancreatic function
Magnetic resonance imaging (MRI)	Soft tissue examination
Parathyroid hormone (PTH)	Parathyroid function
Phosphorus (P)	Endocrine disorders
Testosterone	Testicular function
Thyroid function (T_3, T_4, TSH) studies	Thyroid function
Thyroid scan	Thyroid tumors

The purpose of the reproductive system is the perpetuation of future generations of the human species. The organs and hormones specific to the male and female reproductive systems ensure sexual reproduction and development of male and female secondary sex characteristics.

Function

The vital functions of the male and female reproduction systems are to produce ***gametes***, to enable fertilization, and to provide a nourishing environment for the developing embryo/fetus. The male and female reproductive glands, called the ***gonads***, produce and store the gametes or sex cells. In men the testes produce the gametes called ***spermatozoa***, and in women the ovaries produce the gametes called ***ova*** or eggs. Reproduction occurs through the **fertilization** between the ovum and the spermatozoon, usually in the fallopian tubes, producing an embryo that develops for 9 months in the uterus during pregnancy. If fertilization does not occur, the uterine lining sheds, indicated by bleeding called ***menstruation***.

Release of ova from the ovaries (***ovulation***) begins at puberty and continues until ***menopause***. Hormones from the pituitary gland stimulate the ovaries to secrete **estrogen** and **progesterone**. These hormones facilitate menstruation, pregnancy, and development of the secondary sex characteristics. During pregnancy the placenta produces the hormone **human chorionic gonadotropin (HCG)**. Detection of HCG in serum or urine provides the diagnostic test to confirm pregnancy.

Beginning at puberty and continuing throughout life, the male testes produce billions of spermatozoa and secrete the hormone testosterone for the development of secondary male sex characteristics.

TABLE 3–21   **Commonly Used Medications for the Endocrine System**

Type	Generic and Trade Names	Purpose
Antithyroid hormone	Tapazole	Increases metabolic rate
Insulin	Humulin, Nonolin, and Velosulin	Lowers blood sugar level
Oral hypoglycemics	DiaBeta, Glucophage, Glucotrol, Micronase, and Tolinase	Stimulate insulin secretion
Thyroid hormones	Cytomel, Euthroid, Levothroid, Synthroid, and Thyrolar	Increase metabolic rate

Components

The female reproductive system consists of two **ovaries** that produce ova (eggs); two **fallopian tubes** that transport an egg, or fertilized embryo, to the **uterus**; a uterus that allows embryo development; a vagina that receives sperm during intercourse, discharges menstrual blood, and acts as a birth canal during delivery of a fetus; external genitalia (vulva) that allow sexual stimulation and lubrication; and mammary glands (breasts) that produce milk for a newborn (Fig. 3–15).

The male reproductive organs are shown in Figure 3–16 and include: two **testes** (enclosed in the **scrotum**) that manufacture sperm and produce **testosterone**, two **epididymides** that allow sperm maturation and storage, two **vas deferens** that convey sperm to the ejaculatory duct, two **seminal vesicles** that produce fluid to nourish the sperm, the **prostate gland** that secretes fluid to maintain sperm motility, two **bulbourethral glands** that secrete fluid prior to ejaculation, and the urethra within the penis that carries the sperm out of the body. *Semen* is the transporting medium for the sperm discharged during ejaculation. Sperm and the secretions of the seminal vesicles, prostate gland, and the bulbourethral glands constitute semen.

Disorders

The following are disorders of the reproductive system:

- Carcinoma—malignant tumors of the cervix(**Cx**), ovary, prostate, or testes.
- Endometriosis—increased endometrial (uterine lining) tissue that migrates outside the uterus; associated with dysmenorrhea, pelvic pain, and the inability to become pregnant.
- Fibroids—**benign** uterine tumors that may cause excessive uterine bleeding.
- Pelvic inflammatory disease (**PID**)—inflammation of the ovaries, cervix, uterus, or fallopian tubes caused by infection; may result in infertility or septicemia.
- Premenstrual syndrome (**PMS**)—symptoms are depression, irritability, mood swings, weight gain, breast tenderness, water retention, and nervousness, occurring 7 to 14 days before menstruation.
- Sexually transmitted diseases (**STDs**)—diseases transmitted by sexual contact such as chlamydia, gonorrhea, herpes genitalis, syphilis, trichomoniasis, and AIDS.

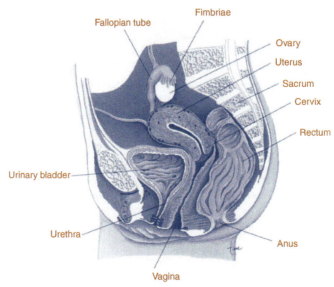

FIGURE 3–15   The female reproductive system. (Adapted from Scanlon, VC, and Sanders, T: Essentials of Anatomy and Physiology, ed. 2. FA Davis, Philadelphia, 1995, p. 463, with permission.)

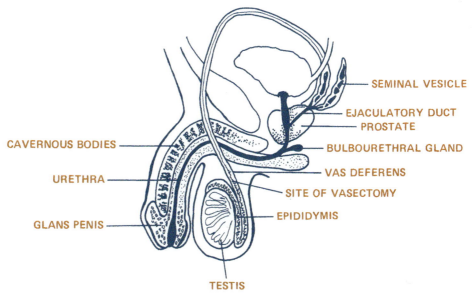

FIGURE 3–16   The male reproduction system. (Adapted from Strasinger, SK: Urinalysis and Body Fluids, ed. 3. FA Davis, Philadelphia, 1994, p. 160, with permission.)

- Toxic shock syndrome (**TSS**)—systemic shock symptoms usually caused by a *Staphylococcus aureus* infection in menstruating women using superabsorbent tampons; characterized by high fever, confusion, syncope, headache, skin rash, and decreased blood pressure.

Diagnostic Tests

The most frequently ordered diagnostic tests associated with the reproductive system and their clinical correlations are presented in Table 3–22.

TABLE 3–22   **Diagnostic Tests Associated with the Reproductive System**

Test	Clinical Correlation
Amniocentesis	Fetal maturity or genetic defects
Chorionic villus sampling (**CVS**)	Genetic defects
Computerized axial tomography (CAT scan)	Soft tissue examination
Estradiol, estriol, and estrogen	Ovarian or placental function
Fluorescent treponemal antibody—absorbed (**FTA-ABS**)	Syphilis
Genital culture	Bacterial infection
Gram stain	Microbial infection
Human chorionic gonadotropin (HCG)	Pregnancy
Laparoscopy	Abdominal exploration or ovarian or fallopian tube disorders
Magnetic resonance imaging (MRI)	Soft tissue examination
Mammogram	Breast cancer detection
Pap smear (**Pap**)	Cervical or vaginal carcinoma
Prostate-specific antigen (**PSA**)	Prostatic cancer
Prostatic acid phosphatase (**PAP**)	Prostatic cancer
Rapid plasma reagin (**RPR**)	Syphilis
Rubella titer	Immunity to German measles
Semen analysis	Fertility or effectiveness of a vasectomy
Toxoplasma antibody screening	*Toxoplasma* infection
Ultrasonogram	Organ examination
Vaginal wet prep	Microbial infection
Venereal Disease Research Laboratory (**VDRL**)	Syphilis

TABLE 3–23 **Commonly Used Medications for the Reproductive System**

Type	Generic and Trade Names	Purpose
Contraceptives	Brevicon, Demulen, Lo/Ovral, Micronor, Norplant System, Ortho-Novum, Ovulen, and Triphasil	Prevent ovulation
Female hormones	Aygestin, Estrace, Estraderm, Gesterol, Norinyl, Norulate, Premarin, Provera, and TACE	Treat amenorrhea, dysfunctional bleeding, and menopausal replacement therapy
Uterine relaxants	Ethanol and Yutopar	Delay labor
Uterine stimulants	Oxytocin and Pitocin	Control postpartum bleeding and induce labor

Medications

Table 3–23 lists the names and purpose of the most commonly used medications for the reproductive system.

BIBLIOGRAPHY

Gylys, BA, and Wedding, ME: Medical Terminology: A Systems Approach, ed. 3. FA Davis, Philadelphia, 1995.

Rice, J: Medical Terminology with Human Anatomy, ed. 3. Appleton & Lange, Norwalk, CT, 1995.

Scanlon, VC, and Sanders, T: Essentials of Anatomy and Physiology, ed. 2. FA Davis, Philadelphia, 1995.

Strasinger, SK: Urinalysis and Body Fluids, ed. 3. FA Davis, Philadelphia, 1994.

Strasinger, SK, and DiLorenzo, MA: Phlebotomy Workbook for the Multiskilled Healthcare Professional. FA Davis, Philadelphia, 1996.

STUDY QUESTIONS

1. Name and define the four types of tissue in the body.

   a. _____

   b. _____

   c. _____

   d. _____

2. Name the body system associated with each of the following functions:

   a. Directs body activities through hormones _____

   b. Protects the body against the invasion of harmful pathogens and chemicals

   _____

   c. Provides skeletal movement _____

   d. Exchanges oxygen and carbon dioxide between the air and blood _____

   e. Removes urea from the blood _____

3. Name the plane that divides the body into equal right and left halves.

   _____

4. Define the following directional terms:

   a. Anterior _____

   b. Posterior _____

   c. Proximal _____

   d. Distal _____

   e. Dorsal _____

5. Name the cavity lined by each of the following membranes:

   a. Parietal pleura _____

   b. Peritoneum _____

   c. Meninges _____

6. Define homeostasis.

   _____

   _____

7. Describe the two layers of skin.

   a. _____

   _____

   b. _____

   _____

8. Name the pigment that determines skin color and the cell that produces it.

   a. Pigment _____

   b. Cell _____

9. Name the two types of skin glands and the function of each.

   Type   **Function**

   a. _____   _____

   b. _____   _____

10. The vitamin produced by the skin is _____.

11. List four classifications of bones and give an example of each.

   Classification   **Example**

   a. _____   _____

   b. _____   _____

   c. _____   _____

   d. _____   _____

12. The fluid within the joint cavity that prevents friction is _____.

13. The action of moving a body part toward the midline is _____.

14. Name the three types of muscle tissue.

   a. _____

   b. _____

   c. _____

15. The connective tissues that attach skeletal muscle to bones are _____.

16. Name the two divisions of the nervous system.

   a. _____

   b. _____

17. List and describe the three major parts of the neuron.

   Part   **Description**

   a. _____   _____

   b. _____   _____

   c. _____   _____

18. Name the two types of neurons and describe their function.

   Type   **Function**

   a. _____   _____

   b. _____   _____

19. The tissue fluid that circulates through the brain and spinal cord is _____.

20. Differentiate between external and internal respiration.

_____

_____

21. The air sacs of the lung are the _____.

22. The cartilage that blocks the larynx during swallowing is the

_____.

23. Name three digestive enzymes.

a. _____

b. _____

c. _____

24. State four functions of the liver.

a. _____

b. _____

c. _____

d. _____

25. Name the organ in the gastrointestinal tract where absorption mainly occurs.

_____

26. The functioning unit of the kidney is the _____.

27. The organs that transport urine from the kidneys to the bladder are the

_____.

28. Define and state the function of an endocrine gland.

_____

_____

29. The chemical substances secreted by endocrine glands are _____.

30. The hormone that maintains normal blood sugar is _____.

31. The endocrine gland that produces the most hormones is the _____.

32. The male sex hormone produced by the testes is _____.

33. The gonad for the female reproductive system is the _____.

34. List the three functions of the reproductive system.

a. _____

b. _____

c. _____

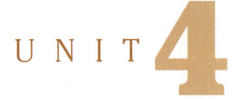

U N I T 4

BLOOD AND THE CIRCULATORY AND LYMPHATIC SYSTEMS

Circulatory System

KEY TERMS

■ **Antecubital**	Area of the arm opposite the elbow (location of the large veins used in phlebotomy)
■ **Antibody**	Protein produced by exposure to antigen
■ **Antigen**	Substance that stimulates the formation of antibodies
■ **Arteriole**	Small arterial branch leading into a capillary
■ **Artery**	Blood vessel carrying oxygenated blood from the heart to the tissues
■ **Atrium**	One of two upper chambers of the heart
■ **Capillary**	Small blood vessel connecting arteries and veins that allows the exchange of gases and nutrients between the cells and the blood
■ **Cardiovascular**	Pertaining to the heart and the blood vessels

▪ *Erythrocyte*	Red blood cell
▪ *Hemostasis*	Stoppage of blood flow from a damaged blood vessel
▪ *Leukocyte*	White blood cell
▪ *Pulmonary circulation*	Flow of blood from the heart to the lungs and back to the heart
▪ *Systemic circulation*	Flow of blood between the heart and the tissues
▪ *Thrombocyte*	Blood-clotting cell
▪ *Vascular*	Pertaining to blood vessels
▪ *Vein*	Blood vessel carrying deoxygenated blood from the tissues to the heart
▪ *Ventricle*	One of two lower chambers of the heart
▪ *Venule*	Small vein leading from a capillary

The circulatory (**cardiovascular**) system, in conjunction with blood and the lymphatic system, acts as the transportation system for the body. Blood circulates through the blood vessels by the action of the heart, whereas lymph is propelled by skeletal muscle contraction through the lymph vessels and drains into the circulatory system.

FUNCTION

Through the circulatory system, blood delivers oxygen, nutrients, enzymes, and hormones to the cells and transports carbon dioxide and waste products to the organs that expel them from the body. To facilitate the process, the heart acts as two pumps with two separate circulations that work in unison. The **pulmonary circulation** carries deoxygenated blood from the right ventricle of the heart to the lungs and returns oxygenated blood from the lungs to the left atrium of the heart. The **systemic circulation** conveys oxygenated blood from the left ventricle of the heart throughout the body to the tissue cells and transports carbon dioxide and waste products away from the tissue cells.

COMPONENTS

The organs of the circulatory system are the **arteries**, **veins**, **capillaries**, and heart.

Blood Vessels

The three types of blood vessels that transport blood throughout the body are the arteries, veins, and capillaries. Arteries and veins are composed of three layers. The outer layer is a connective tissue called **tunica adventitia**. The middle layer is a smooth muscle tissue called **tunica media**. The inner layer is called the **tunica intima** and is composed of endothelial cells. The space within a blood vessel through which the blood flows is called the **lumen**. Figure 4–1 shows the differences between arteries, veins, and capillaries.

Arteries are large, thick-walled, tubelike blood vessels that propel oxygen-rich blood away from the heart to the capillaries. Arteries branch into smaller, thinner vessels called **arterioles** that connect to capillaries. The walls of arteries consist of tough connective tissue, elastic fibers, and an inner layer of endothelial cells. The thicker

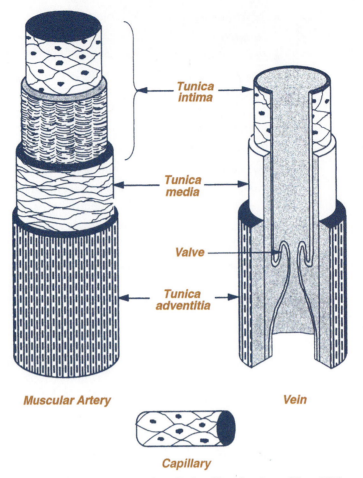

FIGURE 4–1   Comparison of arteries, veins, and capillaries. (From Strasinger, SK, and Di Lorenzo, MA: Phlebotomy Workbook for the Multiskilled Healthcare Professional. FA Davis, Philadelphia, 1996, p. 92, with permission.)

walls aid in the pumping of blood, maintaining normal blood pressure, and giving arteries the strength to resist the high pressure caused by the contraction of the heart ventricles. The elastic walls expand as the heart pushes blood through the arteries. A **pulse** is the wave of increased pressure felt along arteries each time the heart ventricle contracts. The pulse rate equals the heart rate and can be felt by placing two fingers against an artery.

The radial artery, located near the thumb side of the wrist, is the most common site for obtaining a pulse rate. The brachial artery, located in the *antecubital* space of the elbow, is the most common site to obtain a blood pressure. The carotid artery, located near the side of the neck, is the most accessible site in an emergency, such as cardiac arrest, to check for a pulse rate. The femoral artery, located near the groin, and the temporal artery, located at the temple, are other major arteries. The aorta is the largest artery and branches into the smaller arteries to distribute oxygen-rich blood throughout the body. The pulmonary artery is the only artery that does not carry oxygenated blood. Figure 4–2 shows the major arteries in the body.

Capillaries are the smallest vessels, one epithelial cell thick, that connect arterioles and *venules*. The blood in capillaries consists of a mixture of arterial and venous blood. The thin walls of capillaries allow the exchange of oxygen, carbon dioxide, and nutrients between the blood and the tissue cells.

Venules are small veins that join to become larger veins. Veins have thinner walls than arteries and carry oxygen-poor blood, carbon dioxide, and other waste products back to the heart. No gaseous exchange takes place in the veins, only in the capillaries.

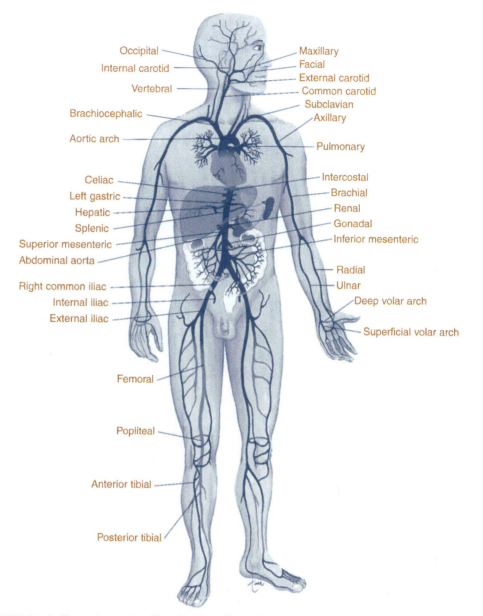

FIGURE 4–2   The major arteries. (From Scanlon, VC, and Sanders, T: Essentials of Anatomy and Physiology, ed. 2. FA Davis, Philadelphia, 1995, p. 288, with permission.)

The thinner walls of veins have less elastic tissue and less connective tissue than arteries because the blood pressure in the veins is very low. Veins have one-way **valves** to keep blood flowing in one direction because the blood flows through the veins by skeletal muscle contraction. Leg veins have numerous valves to return the blood to the heart against the force of gravity.

The main veins in the arm are the basilic, cephalic, and median cubital veins. The great saphenous vein is the principal vein in the leg and the longest vein in the body. The largest veins, the superior and inferior venae cavae, carry the oxygen-poor blood back to the heart. The pulmonary vein is the only vein that carries oxygenated blood. Figure 4–3 shows the principal veins of the body.

Most blood tests are performed on venous blood. Venipuncture is the procedure for removing blood from a vein for analysis. The veins of choice for venipuncture are the basilic, cephalic, and median cubital veins, located in the antecubital area of the elbow, as shown in Figure 4–4.

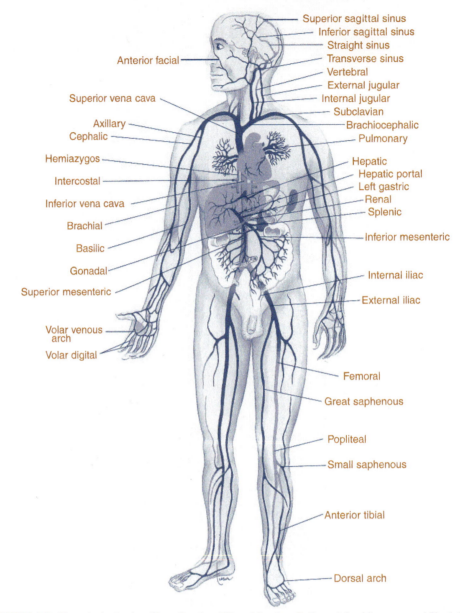

FIGURE 4–3 The principal veins. (From Scanlon, VC, and Sanders, T: Essentials of Anatomy and Physiology, ed. 2. FA Davis, Philadelphia, 1995, p. 289, with permission.)

Heart

The heart is a hollow muscular organ, located in the thoracic cavity between the lungs and slightly to the left of the body midline, that circulates blood throughout the circulatory system. The heart has three layers of tissue. The thin outer layer of the heart is the **epicardium**. Lining the walls of each heart chamber is a thick muscle tissue called the **myocardium**, and lining the cavities of the heart is a smooth tissue called the **endocardium**. The **pericardium** is a fibrous membrane sac surrounding the heart to hold it in position.

The heart has four chambers and is divided into right and left halves by a partition called the **septum**. Each side has an upper chamber called the *atrium* to collect blood and a lower chamber called the *ventricle* to pump blood from the heart. The right side is the "pump" for the pulmonary circulation, and the left side is the "pump" for the systemic circulation. The heart contracts and relaxes to pump deoxygenated blood through the heart to the lungs and to return oxygenated blood to the heart for

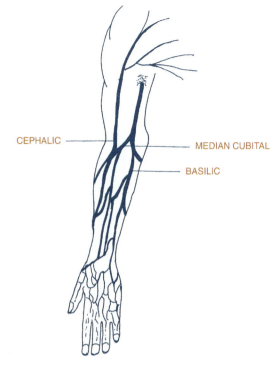

CEPHALIC

MEDIAN CUBITAL

BASILIC

FIGURE 4–4   Veins in the arm used for venipuncture. (From Strasinger, SK, and Di Lorenzo, MA: Phlebotomy Workbook for the Multiskilled Healthcare Professional. FA Davis, Philadelphia, 1996, p. 94, with permission.)

distribution throughout the body. Refer to Figure 4–5 to follow the circulation of blood through the heart.

Valves located at the entrance and exit of each ventricle prevent a backflow of blood and keep the blood flowing in one direction. The right **atrioventricular (AV) valve**, or **tricuspid valve**, located at the entrance to the right ventricle, lets blood flow into the right ventricle and prevents backflow into the right atrium. The **pulmonary semilunar valve**, located at the exit of the right ventricle, allows blood to flow from the right ventricle through the pulmonary artery to the lungs. The left AV valve or **bicuspid valve**, also called the **mitral valve**, located at the entrance of the left ventricle, prevents the backflow of blood to the left atrium, forcing blood into the left ventricle. The **aortic semilunar valve**, located at the exit of the left ventricle, permits blood to leave the left ventricle and flow into the aorta. Heart sounds created by the cardiac cycle are the "lubb-dupp" sounds heard with a **stethoscope**. The first sound, the "lubb," is the closure of the AV valves as the ventricles contract. The second sound, the "dupp," is the closure of the semilunar valves. A heart murmur is an abnormal heart sound that occurs when the valves close incorrectly.

The heart has its own vascular system to nourish the heart muscle. The right and left coronary arteries branch off the aorta to deliver blood carrying oxygen and nutrients to the heart. When coronary arteries become obstructed, heart muscle dies and a heart attack can occur because of a diminished oxygen supply to the heart.

Pathway of Blood through the Heart

Two large veins, the superior vena cava and the inferior vena cava, transport blood to the right atrium of the heart. The superior vena cava collects blood from the upper portion of the body, and the inferior vena cava collects blood from the lower portion of the body. The blood passes through the tricuspid valve to the right ventricle. The right ventricle contracts to pump the blood through the pulmonary semilunar valve into the right and left pulmonary arteries, which carry it to each lung. In the lung capillaries, blood releases carbon dioxide and acquires oxygen. The right and left pulmonary veins carry the oxygenated blood from the lungs to the left atrium of the heart. The

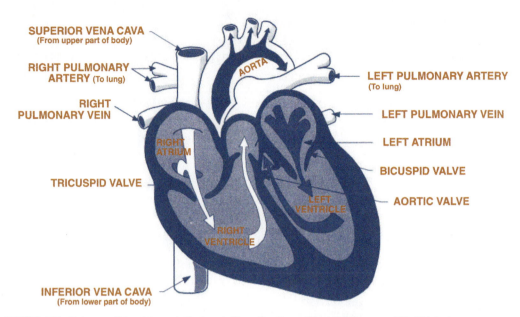

FIGURE 4–5   Pathway of blood through the heart. (From Strasinger, SK, and Di Lorenzo, MA: Phlebotomy Workbook for the Multiskilled Healthcare Professional. FA Davis, Philadelphia, 1996, p. 96, with permission.)

blood flows through the mitral valve into the left ventricle, which contracts to pump blood through the aortic semilunar valve into the aorta. Blood travels throughout the body to the capillaries by arteries that branch off the aorta.

The cardiac cycle comprises the contraction phase (**systole**) and the relaxation phase (**diastole**) that occur in one heartbeat. Specialized cardiac conductive tissue ini-

SUMMARY OF BLOOD CIRCULATION

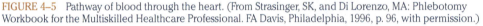

- Oxygen-poor blood from the venae cavae enters the right atrium of the heart.
- The right atrium contracts to force the blood through the tricuspid valve to the right ventricle.
- The right ventricle contracts to force the blood through the pulmonary semilunar valve into the pulmonary artery, which divides to each lung.
- The red blood cells release carbon dioxide and absorb oxygen in the lungs.
- The oxygen-rich blood returns to the heart through the pulmonary veins and enters the left atrium.
- The left atrium contracts to force the blood through the mitral valve into the left ventricle.
- The left ventricle contracts to force the blood through the semilunar valve into the aorta.
- The aorta divides into arteries that branch into arterioles to deliver blood throughout the body.
- The arterioles connect to capillaries, where oxygen and nutrients leave the blood and carbon dioxide and waste products enter the blood.
- The blood from the capillaries returns to the heart through venules that fuse into larger veins.
- The blood enters the heart through the largest veins, the superior and the inferior venae cavae.

tiates electrical impulses that cause the heart muscle to rhythmically contract. The **sinoatrial (SA) node**, located in the upper right atrium, is the pacemaker of the heart and initiates the heartbeat. An electrical impulse travels from the SA node to the AV node located in the lower right atrium. This causes the right and left atria to contract, forcing blood through the AV valves into the ventricles. The impulse travels to the AV bundle (**bundle of His**), located in the upper interventricular septum, where it divides into right and left branches. The impulse continues to travel to the **Purkinje fibers** in the ventricles, causing them to contract. This forces blood through the semilunar valves into the pulmonary artery and the aorta. After a brief relaxation, the cycle starts again.

The heart contracts approximately 72 to 80 times per minute, which represents the heart or pulse rate. The cardiac output is the quantity of blood pumped by the heart ventricle in 1 minute and averages about 5 liters of blood per minute. Cardiac output increases to meet the body's need for more oxygen.

An electrocardiogram (**ECG**) detects and records the electrical activity of the atria and ventricles by placing leads on the patient's skin. An ECG detects cardiac abnormalities and heart muscle damage. ECGs and the electrical system of the heart are discussed in detail in Unit 13.

Blood pressure (**BP**) is the pressure exerted by the blood on the walls of blood vessels during contraction and relaxation of the ventricles. Systolic and diastolic readings are taken and reported in millimeters of mercury (mm Hg). The systolic pressure is the higher of the two numbers and indicates the blood pressure during contraction of the ventricles. The diastolic pressure is the lower number and is the blood pressure when the ventricles are relaxed.

To measure blood pressure, a blood pressure cuff called a **sphygmomanometer** is placed around the upper arm, and a stethoscope is placed over the brachial artery to listen for heart sounds. The blood pressure cuff is inflated to restrict the blood flow in the brachial artery and then slowly deflated until loud heart sounds are heard with the stethoscope. The first heart sounds represent the systolic pressure during contraction of the ventricles. This is the top number of a blood pressure reading. The cuff continues to be deflated until the sound is no longer heard; this represents the diastolic pressure during the relaxation of the ventricles and is the bottom number of a blood pressure reading. The average blood pressure for an adult is 120/80, representing a systolic pressure of 120 mm Hg and a diastolic pressure of 80 mm Hg. The blood pressure procedure will be discussed further in Unit 14.

BLOOD

Blood is the body's main fluid for transporting nutrients, waste products, gases, and hormones through the circulatory system. Blood assists in regulating body temperature; protecting against pathogens; maintaining acid-base, fluid, and electrolyte balance; and regulating blood clotting. An average adult has a blood volume of 5 to 6 liters. Blood consists of two parts: a liquid portion called plasma and a cellular portion called the formed elements.

Plasma makes up approximately 55% of the total blood volume. It is a clear, straw-colored fluid that is about 91% water and 9% dissolved substances. It is the transporting medium for plasma proteins (albumin, globulin, fibrinogen, and prothrombin), nutrients (glucose and lipids), minerals (sodium, potassium, calcium, and magnesium), gases (oxygen, carbon dioxide, and nitrogen), and vitamins, hormones, and blood cells, as well as waste products of metabolism (blood urea nitrogen, creatinine, and uric acid).

The formed elements constitute 45% of the total blood volume and include the *erythrocytes* (red blood cells), *leukocytes* (white blood cells), and *thrombocytes* (**platelets**). Blood cells are produced in the bone marrow, which is the spongy material that fills the inside of the major bones of the body. Cells originate from stem cells in the bone marrow, differentiate, and mature through several stages in the bone marrow and lymphatic tissue until they are released to the circulating blood. Examination of the bone marrow is used to diagnose many blood disorders.

Erythrocytes

Erythrocytes, or red blood cells (**RBCs**), are anuclear biconcave disks that are approximately 7.2 microns in diameter. Erythrocytes contain the protein hemoglobin to transport oxygen and carbon dioxide. Hemoglobin consists of two parts: heme and globin. The heme portion requires iron for its synthesis.

Erythrocytes mature in the bone marrow through several stages and enter the circulating blood as reticulocytes that contain fragments of nuclear material. There are approximately 4.5 to 6.0 million erythrocytes per microliter of blood, with men having slightly higher values than women. The normal life span for an erythrocyte is 120 days. **Macrophages** in the liver and spleen remove the old erythrocytes from the bloodstream and destroy them. The iron is reused in new cells.

The surface of erythrocytes contains ***antigens*** that determine the blood group and blood type of an individual, frequently referred to as a person's **ABO** group and **Rh** type. As shown in Table 4–1, four blood types exist based on the antigens present on the erythrocyte membrane. Type A blood has the "A" antigen (**Ag**) and type B blood has the "B" antigen. Type AB blood has both the "A" and the "B" antigens, and type O blood has neither the "A" nor the "B" antigen. Types O and A are the most common blood types, and type AB is the least common.

The plasma of an individual contains naturally occurring ***antibodies*** for those antigens not present on the erythrocytes. Type A blood has anti-B antibodies in the plasma and type B blood has anti-A antibodies. Type O blood has both the anti-A and the anti-B antibodies, and type AB blood has neither anti-A nor anti-B antibody. The naturally occurring antibodies will react with erythrocytes carrying antigens that are not present on the individual's own erythrocytes.

A transfusion reaction may occur when a person receives a different type of blood because a person's natural antibodies will destroy the donor red blood cells that contain the antigen specific to the donor's antibody. For example, if a person with type A blood receives type B blood, the anti-B antibodies of the type A person would bind to the B antigens of the type B donor blood. This causes the blood cells to rupture. Patients receive type-specific blood to avoid this transfusion reaction. Misidentification of patients during phlebotomy is a major cause of transfusion reactions.

The presence or absence of the red blood cell antigen called the Rh factor determines whether a person is Rh positive or Rh negative. Approximately 85% of the population has the Rh factor. Rh negative people do not have natural antibodies to the Rh factor but will form antibodies if they receive Rh positive blood. A second transfusion of Rh positive blood will cause a transfusion reaction. **Hemolytic disease of the newborn (HDN)** occurs when an incompatibility exists between maternal and fetal blood.

Leukocytes

Leukocytes, or white blood cells (**WBCs**), provide immunity from certain diseases by producing antibodies, and they destroy harmful pathogens by **phagocytosis**. Leuko-

TABLE 4–1 **ABO Blood Group System**

Blood Type	RBC Antigen	Plasma Antibodies
A	A	Anti-B
B	B	Anti-A
AB	A and B	Neither Anti-A nor Anti-B
O	Neither	Anti-A and Anti-B

cytes are produced in the red bone marrow from a stem cell and develop in the thymus and bone marrow. They differentiate and mature through several stages before being released into the bloodstream. Leukocytes circulate in the peripheral blood for several hours and then migrate to the tissues through the capillary walls. The normal number of leukocytes for an adult is 4500 to 11,000/μL of blood.

Five types of leukocytes are present in the blood, each with a specific function. They are distinguished by their morphology, as shown in Figure 4–6. When stained with Wright's stain, the cells are examined microscopically for the presence of granules in the cytoplasm, the shape of the nucleus, and the size of the cell. A differential cell count determines the percentage of each type of leukocyte. The five normal types of leukocytes are neutrophils, eosinophils, basophils, lymphocytes, and monocytes.

Neutrophils (40% to 60%)

Neutrophils, the most numerous leukocytes, provide protection against infection through phagocytosis. Neutrophils are called segmented, or polymorphonuclear, cells because the nucleus has several lobes. The nucleus stains dark purple, and the cytoplasm stains pink with fine granules. The number of neutrophils increases in bacterial infections.

Eosinophils (1% to 3%)

The granules in the cytoplasm of eosinophils stain red-orange, and the nucleus has only two lobes. Eosinophils detoxify foreign proteins and increase in number in allergies, skin infections, and parasitic infections.

Basophils (0% to 1%)

Basophils are the least common of the leukocytes. The cytoplasm contains large granules that stain purple-black and release histamine in the inflammation process and heparin in the prevention of abnormal blood clotting.

Lymphocytes (20% to 40%)

Lymphocytes, the second most numerous leukocyte, provide the body with immune capability. The lymphocyte has a large, round, purple nucleus with a rim of sky-blue cytoplasm. There are two main types of lymphocytes: B cells and T cells. The B lymphocyte develops in the bone marrow, becomes a **plasma cell**, and produces antibodies

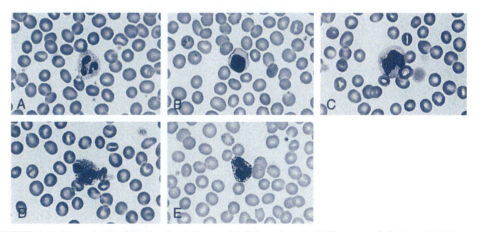

FIGURE 4–6   Normal white blood cells. *A*, Neutrophil. *B*, Lymphocyte. *C*, Monocyte. *D*, Eosinophil. *E*, Basophil. (Courtesy of Karen Lofsness, University of Minnesota, Minneapolis.)

for defense against bacterial infections. T lymphocytes mature in the thymus, act in delayed hypersensitivity reactions and graft rejections, and assist B lymphocytes in the production of antibodies. The number of lymphocytes increases in viral infections.

Monocytes (3% to 8%)

Monocytes are the largest circulating leukocytes and act as powerful phagocytes that differentiate into macrophages to digest foreign material. The cytoplasm has a fine, blue-gray appearance with vacuoles and a large, irregular nucleus. A tissue monocyte is known as a macrophage. The number of monocytes increases in intracellular infections and tuberculosis.

Thrombocytes

Thrombocytes or platelets are small, irregularly shaped disks formed from particles of a very large cell in the bone marrow called the megakaryocyte. Platelets have a life span of 9 to 12 days. The average number of platelets is 140,000 to 440,000/μL of blood. Platelets play a vital role in blood clotting in all stages of the coagulation mechanism.

Coagulation

A complex coagulation mechanism that involves blood vessels, platelets, and coagulation factors maintains ***hemostasis***. Hemostasis is the process of forming a blood clot to stop the leakage of blood when injury occurs and lysing the clot when the injury has been repaired. The process of coagulation occurs as primary hemostasis, secondary hemostasis, and **fibrinolysis**.

Primary Hemostasis

Primary hemostasis forms a temporary platelet plug. It is the ***vascular*** platelet phase because blood vessels and platelets are the first to respond to an injury. Blood vessels constrict to slow the flow of blood to the injured area. Platelets become sticky, clump together (platelet aggregation), and adhere to the injured blood vessel wall (platelet adhesion) to stop bleeding. The bleeding time test evaluates primary hemostasis.

Secondary Hemostasis

Secondary hemostasis involves interaction of the coagulation factors to convert the primary platelet plug to a stable **fibrin** clot to stop bleeding in larger vessel injuries. This interaction is called the coagulation cascade. In this cascade one factor becomes activated and activates the next factor in a specific sequence. Substances released during an injury activate the coagulation factors, which in combination with calcium and platelet factor 3 (**PF3**) produce a tough fibrin clot. This clot stabilizes the platelet plug and stops the bleeding. The coagulation cascade can be initiated by two pathways, the intrinsic and the extrinsic, which come together in a common pathway (Fig. 4–7).

   The intrinsic system is initiated when large molecules in the bloodstream called contact factors activate factor XII and platelets release the phospholipid PF3. The release of tissue thromboplastin from an injured area activates factor VII, which initiates the extrinsic pathway. Both systems react with factors X and V to convert **prothrombin** (factor II) to **thrombin**. Thrombin converts **fibrinogen** (factor I) to the fibrin that forms the basis of the fibrin clot. Factor XIII stabilizes the fibrin clot.

   The activated partial thromboplastin time and the activated clotting time tests evaluate the intrinsic pathway and monitor **heparin** therapy. The prothrombin time test evaluates the extrinsic pathway and monitors warfarin (**Coumadin**) therapy.

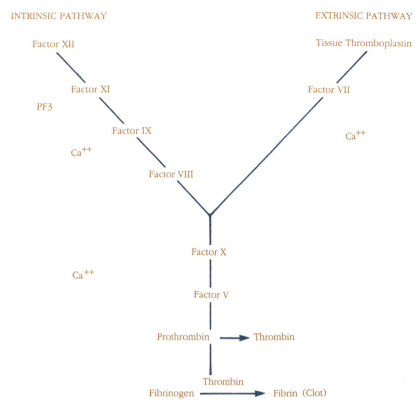

FIGURE 4–7   The coagulation cascade. (Ca^{++} = calcium; PF3 = platelet factor 3.) (Adapted from Strasinger, SK, and Di Lorenzo, MA: Phlebotomy Workbook for the Multiskilled Healthcare Professional. FA Davis, Philadelphia, 1996, p. 101, with permission.)

Fibrinolysis

The breakdown and removal of a clot after healing is the process of fibrinolysis. Fibrin in the clot is broken down into small fragments called fibrin degradation products (**FDPs**) that are cleared from the circulation by the liver. The measurement of FDPs or **D-dimers** monitors fibrinolysis.

DISORDERS

The following are disorders of the circulatory system:

Blood Vessels

- Aneurysm—bulge formed by a weakness in the wall of a blood vessel, usually an artery, that can burst and cause severe hemorrhaging.
- Arteriosclerosis—hardening of the arteries that contributes to aneurysm or stroke.
- Atherosclerosis—form of arteriosclerosis characterized by the accumulation of lipids and other materials in the walls of arteries, causing the lumen of the vessel to narrow and stimulate clot formation.
- Embolism—obstruction of a blood vessel by a moving blood clot or other foreign matter in the vascular system; tissue destruction and/or death occurs if the emboli lodge in an organ.
- Phlebitis—inflammation of the vein wall, causing pain and tenderness.
- Thrombosis—obstruction of a blood vessel by a stationary blood clot, causing an aching pain.
- Varicose veins—swollen peripheral veins caused by damaged valves, allowing backflow of blood that causes swelling (**edema**) in the tissues.

Heart

- Angina pectoris (angina)—sharp chest pain caused by decreased blood flow to the heart, usually because of an obstruction in the coronary arteries.
- Bacterial endocarditis—inflammation of the inner lining of the heart caused by a bacterial infection, usually streptococcal.
- Congestive heart failure (**CHF**)—a chronic disorder that impairs the ability of the heart to pump blood efficiently, causing fluid accumulation in the lungs and other tissues.
- Myocardial infarction (**MI**)—death (**necrosis**) of the heart muscle, caused by a lack of oxygen to the myocardium because of an occluded coronary artery; commonly known as a heart attack. Symptoms are a feeling of pressure on the chest just inside the breastbone, pain in the jaw or down part of either arm, nausea, sweating, dizziness, shortness of breath, and irregular pulse.
- Pericarditis—inflammation of the membrane surrounding the heart (the pericardium), induced by bacteria, virus, trauma, or malignancy; throbbing pain may occur with each heartbeat.
- Rheumatic heart disease—an autoimmune disorder affecting heart tissue following a streptococcal infection, generally seen in childhood; it can result in painful, swollen joints; unusual rashes; and heart damage.

Blood

- Anemia—decrease in the number of erythrocytes or the amount of hemoglobin in the circulating blood; a variety of anemias exist, such as aplastic anemia, iron deficiency anemia, hemolytic anemia, pernicious anemia, sickle cell anemia, and thalassemia; symptoms include difficulty in breathing, rapid heartbeat, paleness, and low blood pressure.
- Leukemia—marked increase in the number of abnormal white blood cells in the bone marrow and circulating blood. Leukemias are named for the particular type of leukocyte that is increased: An acute leukemia is characterized by the presence of immature cell forms and a rapidly progressing disease course, and chronic leukemia is characterized by the presence of mature cell forms and a slower disease progression.
- Leukocytosis—abnormal increase in the number of normal leukocytes in the circulating blood, as seen in infections.
- Leukopenia—decrease below normal in the number of leukocytes, caused by viral infections, exposure to radiation, or chemotherapy.
- Polycythemia—consistent increase above normal in the number of erythrocytes and other formed elements, causing the blood to have a viscous consistency; frequently treated by therapeutic phlebotomy.
- Thrombocytopenia—decrease below normal in the number of circulating platelets, frequently seen in patients receiving chemotherapy; spontaneous bleeding can result.
- Thrombocytosis—increase above normal in the number of circulating platelets.

Coagulation

- Disseminated intravascular coagulation (**DIC**)—spontaneous activation of the coagulation system by certain foreign substances entering the circulatory system, causing a depletion of platelets and coagulation factors and elevated fibrin degradation products, resulting in hemorrhage.
- Hemophilia—a hereditary disorder characterized by excessive bleeding because of the lack of a coagulation factor, usually factor VIII.

DIAGNOSTIC TESTS

The most frequently ordered diagnostic tests associated with the circulatory system and their clinical correlations are presented in Table 4–2.

MEDICATIONS

Table 4–3 lists the names and purpose of the most commonly used medications for the circulatory system.

TABLE 4–2 **Diagnostic Tests Associated with the Circulatory System**

Test	Clinical Correlation
Activated clotting time (**ACT**)	Heparin therapy
Activated partial thromboplastin time (**APTT[PTT]**)	Heparin therapy or coagulation disorders
Angiogram	Blood vessel integrity
Antibody (**Ab**) screen	Blood transfusion
Antistreptolysin O (ASO) titer	Rheumatic fever
Antithrombin III	Coagulation disorders
Aspartate aminotransferase (AST[SGOT])	Cardiac muscle damage
Bilirubin	Hemolytic disorders
Bleeding time (**BT**)	Platelet function
Blood culture	Microbial infection
Blood group and type	ABO group and Rh factor
Bone marrow	Blood cell disorders
C-reactive protein (**CRP**)	Inflammatory disorders
Cardiac catheterization	Coronary artery examination
Cholesterol	Coronary artery disease
Complete blood count (CBC)	Bleeding disorders, anemia, or leukemia
Computerized axial tomography (CAT scan)	Soft tissue examination
Creatine kinase (CK[CPK])	Myocardial infarction
Creatine kinase isoenzymes (CK-MB)	Myocardial infarction
Direct antihuman globulin test (**DAT**) or direct Coombs'	Anemia or hemolytic disease of the newborn
Echocardiogram	Cardiac abnormalities
Electrocardiogram (ECG)	Myocardial damage
Erythrocyte sedimentation rate (**ESR**)	Inflammatory disorders
Fibrin degradation products (FDP)	Disseminated intravascular coagulation
Fibrinogen	Coagulation disorders
Hematocrit (**Hct**)	Anemia
Hemoglobin (**Hgb**)	Anemia
Hemoglobin (Hgb) electrophoresis	Hemoglobin abnormalities
High-density lipoprotein (**HDL**)	Coronary risk
Iron	Anemia
Lactic dehydrogenase (LD[LDH])	Myocardial infarction
Low-density lipoprotein (**LDL**)	Coronary risk
Platelet (**Plt**) count	Bleeding tendencies
Prothrombin time (**PT**)	Coumadin therapy and coagulation disorders
Reticulocyte (**Retic**) count	Bone marrow function
Sickle cell screening	Sickle cell anemia
Stress test	Cardiac function
Total iron-binding capacity (**TIBC**)	Anemia
Triglycerides	Coronary artery disease
Type and crossmatch (**T & C**)	Blood transfusion
Type and screen	Blood transfusion
Ultrasonogram	Organ examination
White blood cell (WBC) count	Infections or leukemia

TABLE 4–3   **Commonly Used Medications for the Circulatory System**

Type	Generic and Trade Names	Effect
Antiarrhythmics	Inderal, Lanoxin, Quinidex, Tambocor, and Tonocard	Treat cardiac arrhythmias
Anticoagulants	Athrombin-K, Coumadin, and heparin sodium	Inhibit blood clotting
Antihypertensive agents	Aldomet, Capoten, Cardizem, Catapres, Lopressor, and Procardia	Lower blood pressure
Digitalis compounds	Cedilanid-D and Crystodigin	Strengthen heart muscle and alter heart contractions
Hematinic agents	Feosol, ferrous fumarate, ferrous gluconate, ferrous sulfate, Niferex, and Triniscon	Treat iron deficiency anemia
Hemostatic agents	Amicar, Humafac, Proplex, Protamine, Surgicel, and vitamin K	Stop bleeding
Hypolipidemics	Atromid-S, Lescol, Lipitor, Lopid, Mevacor, niacin, Pravachol, Questran, and Zocor	Lower lipid blood levels
Thrombolytic agents	Activase, Eminase, streptokinase, and urokinase	Dissolve clots
Vasodilators	Apresoline, Cardilate, nitroglycerin, and Sorbitrate	Lower blood pressure
Vasopressors	Aramine, dopastat, and levorphanol tartrate	Raise blood pressure

Lymphatic System

KEY TERMS

- ***B lymphocytes*** Lymphocytes that transform into plasma cells to produce antibodies
- ***Cell-mediated immunity*** Immune response by T lymphocytes to directly destroy foreign antigens
- ***Humoral immunity*** Immune response that produces antibodies
- ***Immunoglobin*** Antibody that circulates in the bloodstream to attack foreign cells
- ***Lymph*** Fluid in the lymphatic vessels
- ***Lymph nodes*** Lymph tissue that filters lymph as it passes to the circulatory system
- ***T lymphocytes*** Lymphocytes that act directly on an antigen to destroy it

The lymphatic system is the body's "other" vessel system that connects to the circulatory system. Lymphatic vessels, called capillaries and veins, extend throughout the body to propel **lymph** fluid back to the circulatory system. Lymph forms from **interstitial fluid**, the tissue fluid that leaks from blood capillaries and surrounds the body cells. It is a clear, colorless fluid consisting of 95% water, proteins, salts, sugar, lymphocytes, monocytes, and waste products of metabolism. It does not contain platelets or red blood cells. Lymph flows through the lymphatic vessels, entering the bloodstream through ducts that connect to veins in the upper chest.

FUNCTION

The lymphatic system has three major functions. (1) It drains excess fluid from the tissue spaces and transports nutrients and waste products back to the bloodstream. (2) It provides a defense mechanism against disease by storing lymphocytes and monocytes that protect the body from foreign substances through phagocytosis and the immune response. (3) It acts as the passageway for the absorption of fats from the small intestine into the bloodstream.

COMPONENTS

The parts of the lymphatic system are the lymph vessels, **right lymphatic duct**, **thoracic duct**, *lymph nodes*, tonsils, thymus, and spleen. Lymph capillaries collect the fluid from the interstitial spaces and join with larger lymph vessels, the venules and veins, where the lymph enters two terminal vessels, the right lymphatic duct and the thoracic duct. The right lymphatic duct receives lymph from the right upper quadrant (RUQ) of the body and empties into the right subclavian vein. The thoracic duct receives lymph from the left quadrant of the body and lower body and returns it to the blood in the left subclavian vein. Valves in the lymph vessels allow the lymph to flow in only one direction toward the chest cavity by skeletal muscle contraction. Figure 4–8 displays the relationship between the lymphatic and the circulatory systems.

Lymph nodes located along the lymphatic pathway filter the lymph as it flows through the lymphatic vessels. Lymph nodes store lymphocytes and monocytes to phagocytize bacteria and foreign substances, stimulate the immune response, and recognize and destroy cancer cells. The major lymph nodes are the cervical (neck), axillary (armpit), inguinal (groin), and mediastinal (chest).

The tonsils, thymus gland, and spleen also contain lymphoid tissue to store lymphocytes and monocytes. The tonsils, located in the pharynx, filter bacteria at the entrance of the respiratory and digestive tracts. The thymus gland, located between the lungs, controls the immune system and produces T cells to provide cellular immunity. The spleen, located in the left upper quadrant (LUQ) of the abdomen, filters cell debris, bacteria, parasites, and old red blood cells.

IMMUNE SYSTEM

The lymphatic system controls the body's **immune** system by the recognition of foreign antigens filtered through the lymph nodes and spleen and by the maintenance of a high concentration of *B* and *T lymphocytes*. An antigen is a large molecule located on cells that stimulates the formation of antibodies. Cells are recognized as "self" or foreign by the antigens present on the cell membrane. Foreign antigens include bacteria, toxins, viruses, and fungi that cause the B or T lymphocytes to activate either a humoral or a cellular immune response.

An antibody (*immunoglobulin*) is a protein that is produced by exposure to antigens. *Humoral immunity* or antibody-mediated immunity involves the production of antibodies to specific antigens by B lymphocytes in the spleen and lymph nodes. Helper T cells recognize foreign antigens and then activate B cells to transform into plasma cells, producing specific antibodies to the antigens and destroying them. Humoral immunity is the major immune response against bacterial infections.

T lymphocytes produce chemical substances (**lymphokines**) rather than antibodies for the destruction of foreign antigens in cellular or *cell-mediated immunity*. T cells differentiate into helper T cells to recognize a foreign antigen and suppressor T cells to control the immune response by stopping the immune response once the foreign antigen has been destroyed. Natural killer (NK) cells chemically destroy foreign cells, cells infected with viruses, and cancer cells by disrupting the cell membrane.

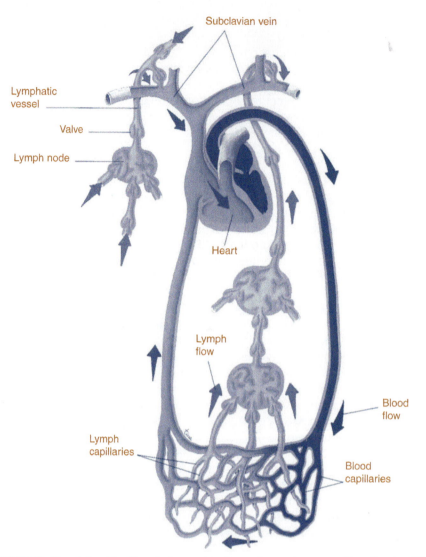

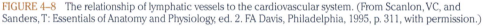

FIGURE 4–8   The relationship of lymphatic vessels to the cardiovascular system. (From Scanlon, VC, and Sanders, T: Essentials of Anatomy and Physiology, ed. 2. FA Davis, Philadelphia, 1995, p. 311, with permission.)

Cell-mediated immunity is the major protection against intracellular microorganisms, such as viruses, and tumor cells. It also can cause rejection of transplanted tissue.

In acquired immunodeficiency syndrome (AIDS), the helper T cells are infected by human immunodeficiency virus (HIV). Without the helper T cells, the immune system is severely compromised. Foreign antigens are not recognized, B cells are not activated, and natural killer, or NK, cells are not stimulated to proliferate.

DISORDERS

The following are disorders of the lymphatic system:

- AIDS—a suppressed immune system caused by the pathogen HIV, transmitted through sexual contact or infected blood products or from mother to infant **prenatally**; conditions frequently associated with AIDS are *Pneumocystis carinii* pneumonia, Kaposi's sarcoma, and a variety of fungal and viral diseases.
- Hodgkin's disease—a malignant tumor of the lymphatic tissue, producing painless, enlarged lymph nodes, splenomegaly, fever, weakness, anemia, weight loss, and night sweats.

TABLE 4–4 **Diagnostic Tests Associated with the Lymphatic System**

Test	Clinical Correlation
Anti-HIV	Human immunodeficiency virus
Antinuclear antibody (ANA)	Systemic lupus erythematosus
Complete blood count (CBC)	Infectious mononucleosis
Computerized axial tomography (CAT scan)	Soft tissue examination
Fluorescent antinuclear antibody (FANA)	Systemic lupus erythematosus
Immunoglobulin (**Ig**) levels	Immune system function
Lymph node biopsy (Bx)	Malignancy
Magnetic resonance imaging (MRI)	Soft tissue examination
Monospot	Infectious mononucleosis
Protein electrophoresis	Multiple myeloma
T-cell count	Immune function/AIDS monitoring
Western blot	Human immunodeficiency virus

- Infectious mononucleosis (**IM**)—infectious disease caused by the Epstein-Barr virus, characterized by enlarged lymph nodes, increased lymphocytes, weakness, fatigue, fever, and sore throat; occurs mostly in young adults.
- Lymphoma—a solid tumor, frequently malignant, of the lymphatic tissue, such as Burkitt's lymphoma or non-Hodgkin's lymphoma.
- Lymphosarcoma—a diffuse malignant tumor of the lymphatic tissue.
- Multiple myeloma—a malignant proliferation of plasma cells in the bone marrow, producing painful nodules, impaired hematologic and immune system functions, and destruction of bone.

DIAGNOSTIC TESTS

The most frequently ordered diagnostic tests associated with the lymphatic system and their clinical correlations are presented in Table 4–4.

MEDICATIONS

Table 4–5 lists the names and purpose of the most commonly used medications for the lymphatic system.

TABLE 4–5 **Commonly Used Medications for the Lymphatic System**

Type	Generic and Trade Names	Effect
Acquired immunodeficiency syndrome agents	ddC, ddI, indinavir, lamivudine, nevirapine, and zidovudine (AZT)	Inhibit viral replication
Antihistamines	Atarax, Benadryl, Periactin, and Zyrtec	Relieve allergic symptoms
Anti-inflammatories	Decadron, Feldene, Indocin, and Lodine	Relieve swelling
Antineoplastics	Cytoxan, methotrexate, Nolvadex (tamoxifen), and Taxol	Destroy malignant cells, prevent metastasis
Biologicals	Gamulin, Hep-B-Gammagee, and vaccines	Provide immunity
Immunosuppressives	Imuran, Prograf, and Sandimmune (cyclosporine)	Prevent transplant rejection
Multiple sclerosis agents	Betaseron	Inhibit autoimmune myelin destruction

BIBLIOGRAPHY

Gylys, BA, and Wedding, ME: Medical Terminology: A Systems Approach, ed. 3. FA Davis, Philadelphia, 1995.

McKenzie, SB: Textbook of Hematology. Lea & Febiger, Philadelphia, 1996.

Rice, J: Medical Terminology with Human Anatomy, ed. 3. Appleton & Lange, Norwalk, CT, 1995.

Scanlon, VC, and Sanders, T: Essentials of Anatomy and Physiology, ed. 2. FA Davis, Philadelphia, 1995.

Strasinger, SK, and Di Lorenzo, MA: Phlebotomy Workbook for the Multiskilled Healthcare Professional. FA Davis, Philadelphia, 1996.

STUDY QUESTIONS

1. Give the function for each of the three major types of blood vessels.

   a. _____

   b. _____

   c. _____

2. The most common site to check a blood pressure is the _____.

3. The procedure for removing blood from a vein is called a _____.

4. The _____ divides the heart into right and left halves.

5. Name the three layers of the heart.

   a. _____

   b. _____

   c. _____

6. Name the vein that carries oxygenated blood. _____

7. The contraction phase of the heart is called the _____.

8. The left atrioventricular valve in the heart is also called the

   _____ or _____ valve.

9. The chamber of the heart that receives blood from the venae cavae is the

   _____.

10. The pacemaker of the heart is the _____.

11. Trace the flow of blood through the heart starting with the vena cava. The pathway should include four chambers, two veins, two arteries, four valves, and one accessory organ.

    a. _____   h. _____

    b. _____   i. _____

    c. _____   j. _____

    d. _____   k. _____

    e. _____   l. _____

    f. _____   m. _____

    g. _____

12. Name the three formed elements of the blood and state their function.

    Element   *Function*

    a. _____   _____

    b. _____   _____

    c. _____   _____

13. Name the leukocyte for each of the following functions:

    a. Recognizes foreign antigens _____

    b. Increases in allergies _____

    c. Phagocytizes bacteria _____

    d. Becomes a macrophage _____

    e. Produces antibodies _____

    f. Releases histamine _____

14. List two types of T lymphocytes.

    a. _____

    b. _____

15. Define the following:

    a. Leukocytosis _____

    b. Leukemia _____

    c. Anemia _____

16. Describe what will occur when a person with type B positive blood receives a unit of type A negative blood.

    _____

    _____

    _____

17. The process of forming a blood clot to stop bleeding is _____ .

18. The breakdown and removal of a clot is called _____ .

19. The predominant lymphocyte produced in humoral immunity is the

    _____ .

20. The immune response that is stimulated in an organ transplant is

    _____ .

21. Label the indicated parts of the heart.

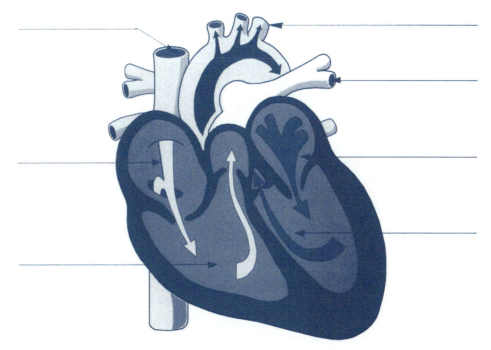

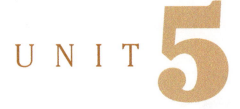

UNIT 5

VENIPUNCTURE EQUIPMENT

LEARNING OBJECTIVES

Upon completion of this unit, the reader will be able to:

1 Define the key terms associated with venipuncture equipment.
2 List 10 items that may be carried on a phlebotomy tray.
3 Differentiate among the various needle sizes as to gauge and purpose.
4 Discuss methods to safely dispose of contaminated needles.
5 Differentiate between a vacuum collection tube, syringe, and winged infusion apparatus, and know the advantages and disadvantages of each.
6 Identify the types of vacuum tubes by color code, and state the anticoagulants and additives present, any special characteristics, and the purpose of each.
7 State the mechanism of action, advantages, and disadvantages of the anticoagulants EDTA, sodium citrate, potassium oxalate, and heparin.
8 List the correct order of draw for vacuum tubes and the correct order of fill for tubes collected by syringe.
9 Describe three types of tourniquets.
10 Name two substances used to cleanse the skin prior to venipuncture.
11 Discuss the use of sterile gauze, bandages, gloves, and slides when performing venipuncture.
12 Describe the quality control of venipuncture equipment.

KEY TERMS

- *Anticoagulant*   Substance that prevents blood from clotting
- *Antiseptic*   Substance that destroys or inhibits the growth of microorganisms
- *Bacteriostatic*   Capable of inhibiting the growth of bacteria
- *Butterfly*   Winged infusion set used for small veins
- *Plasma*   Liquid portion of blood
- *Serum*   Clear yellow fluid that remains after blood has been centrifuged and separated
- *Sterile*   Free of microorganisms

In facilities that have decentralized their phlebotomy department, a primary responsibility of PCTs is the collection of blood samples (performing phlebotomy).

Becoming proficient at performing a phlebotomy requires considerable time and effort because of the noticeable differences among people's veins, the numerous laboratory tests with their specific specimen requirements, and the variety of collection equipment. Properly collected specimens are essential for accurate test results, and when they are collected incorrectly, they must be redrawn. The re-collection of blood specimens negatively affects both efficiency of patient care and patient satisfaction. Therefore, several units of this text are devoted to detailed explanations of the techniques used to collect appropriate specimens by both venipuncture and dermal puncture and the correct handling of specimens after they are collected.

The first step in learning to perform a venipuncture is knowledge of the needed equipment. An adequate amount of the necessary equipment is essential whenever performing venipuncture. Therefore, this unit covers the types of equipment used when performing venipunctures with evacuated systems, syringes, and winged infusion sets. Discussion includes the advantages and disadvantages of the various pieces of equipment, the situations in which they are used, and, when appropriate, the mechanisms by which the equipment works.

The equipment necessary to perform venipunctures includes needles, needle disposal containers, needle holders, collection tubes, syringes, winged infusion sets, tourniquets, **antiseptic** cleansing solutions, gauze pads, bandages, and gloves.

Organization of Equipment

Equipment for phlebotomy is usually organized in a collection tray similar to the one shown in Figure 5–1. In outpatient settings, the phlebotomy tray or a more permanent arrangement is located at the drawing station (Fig. 5–2). The phlebotomy tray provides a convenient way for the PCT to carry equipment to the patients' rooms. Except in isolation situations, the tray is carried into the patient's room. It should be placed on a solid surface, such as a nightstand, and not on the patient's bed, where it could be knocked off. Only the needed equipment should be brought directly to the patient's bed.

Maintaining an adequate supply of phlebotomy equipment, checking the expiration dates on applicable equipment, and disinfecting and restocking phlebotomy trays may be a duty of the PCT. Trays should be emptied totally and disinfected on a weekly basis.

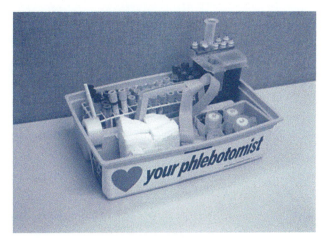

FIGURE 5–1 Phlebotomy collection tray. (From Strasinger, SK, and Di Lorenzo, MA: Phlebotomy Workbook for the Multiskilled Healthcare Professional. FA Davis, Philadelphia, 1996, p. 174, with permission.)

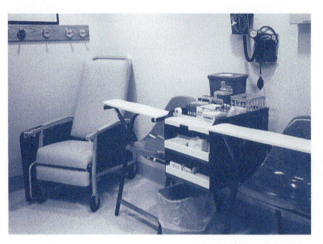

FIGURE 5–2 Phlebotomy drawing station, including a reclining chair. (From Strasinger, SK, and Di Lorenzo, MA: Phlebotomy Workbook for the Multiskilled Healthcare Professional. FA Davis, Philadelphia, 1996, p. 175, with permission.)

Needles

All needles used in venipuncture are disposable and are used only once. Needle size varies by both length and gauge (diameter). For routine venipuncture, 1- and 1.5-inch lengths are used.

Manufacturers package needles individually in *sterile* containers that are color coded by gauge for easy identification.

Needle **gauge** refers to the diameter of the needle bore and varies from large (16-gauge) needles used to collect units of blood for transfusion to much smaller (23-gauge) needles used for very small veins. Notice that the smaller the gauge number, the bigger the diameter of the needle. Needles with gauges smaller than 23 are available, but they can cause **hemolysis** when used for drawing blood specimens. They are most frequently used for injections and intravenous (**IV**) solutions.

As shown in Figure 5–3, needle structure varies to adapt to the type of collection equipment being used. All needles consist of a **beveled** point, shaft, **lumen**, and hub. Needles should be visually examined prior to use to determine if they have any structural defects, such as nonbeveled points or bent shafts.

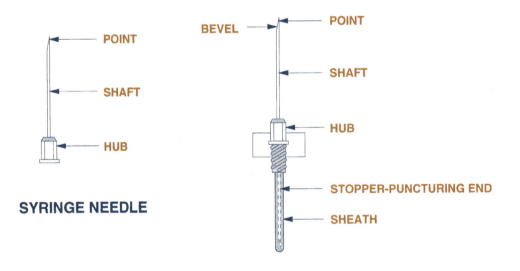

SYRINGE NEEDLE

EVACUATED TUBE NEEDLE

FIGURE 5–3 Needle structure. (From Strasinger, SK, and Di Lorenzo, MA: Phlebotomy Workbook for the Multiskilled Healthcare Professional. FA Davis, Philadelphia, 1996, p. 175, with permission.)

The most frequently used needles in venipuncture collections are those for evacuated collection systems. These are often referred to as Vacutainer needles (Becton Dickinson, Franklin Lakes, NJ). They are double-ended needles designed so that one end is used for phlebotomy and the other end punctures the rubber stopper of the collection tube. Vacutainer needles are designated as single-draw and multi-draw needles. Single-draw needles have a visible stopper-puncturing needle and are used when only one tube of blood is required. The puncturing needle of multi-draw needles is covered by a rubber sheath that is pushed back when a tube is attached and returns to full needle coverage when the tube is removed. This feature prevents leakage of blood when tubes are being changed. The increased possibility of blood contamination when using single-draw needles, even when only one tube of blood is being drawn, has caused most institutions to use multi-draw needles for all venipunctures. PCTs should check the type of needle when working in an unfamiliar setting.

Needles used with syringes are attached to a plastic hub designed to fit onto the barrel of the syringe. They are also individually packaged, sterile, and color coded as to gauge. Syringe needles routinely used for venipuncture range from 20 to 23 gauge with 1- and 1.5-inch lengths. An advantage when using syringe needles is that blood will appear in the hub of the needle when the vein has been entered successfully. Blood is not visible when using vacuum system needles.

Needle Adapters

Needles used in the evacuated tube collection systems are designed to be screwed into an adapter that holds the collection tube. Adapters are made of clear, rigid plastic and may be reused, or they may be designed to act as a safety shield for the used needle, in which case they are discarded. Nondisposable adapters must be disinfected whenever they become visually contaminated.

Adapters are available to accommodate collection tubes of different sizes. To provide proper puncturing of the rubber stopper and maximum control, tubes should fit securely in the adapter. Needles and adapters should be from the same manufacturer. The Hemogard Vacutainer System (Becton Dickinson, Franklin Lakes, NJ) has standardized the diameter of all its collection tubes to 13 mm to allow the use of a single adapter.

The flared ends of the needle adapters aid during the transfer of tubes in multi-draw situations. A marking near the top of the adapter indicates the distance an evacuated tube may be advanced into the stopper-puncturing needle without entering the tube and losing the vacuum (Fig. 5–4).

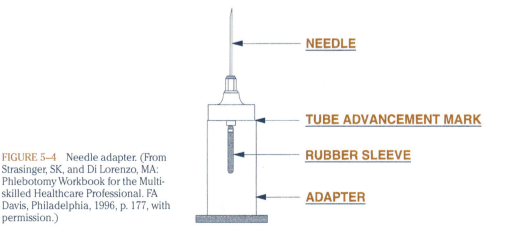

FIGURE 5–4 Needle adapter. (From Strasinger, SK, and Di Lorenzo, MA: Phlebotomy Workbook for the Multi-skilled Healthcare Professional. FA Davis, Philadelphia, 1996, p. 177, with permission.)

NEEDLE

TUBE ADVANCEMENT MARK

RUBBER SLEEVE

ADAPTER

Needle Disposal Systems

To protect healthcare personnel from accidental needle sticks by contaminated needles, a means of safe disposal must be available whenever phlebotomy is performed. Because of the increased concern over exposure to blood-borne pathogens, many disposal systems have been developed in recent years.

Needle disposal systems include basic needle recapping devices, puncture-resistant containers for manual unscrewing of the needle or disposal of the entire assembly, needle holders that become disposable puncture-resistant shields, and automatic needle removal devices (Fig. 5–5).

Blunting needles in which the safety device is engaged before the needle is removed from the arm are also available. PCTs should become familiar with the types of disposal systems used in their institutions. They should also remember that the rubber-sheathed puncturing end of a vacuum tube needle causes many accidental punctures.

Under no circumstances should a needle be recapped without using a safety device.

Collection Tubes

The primary tubes used for blood collection are evacuated (vacuum) tubes, often referred to as Vacutainers (Becton Dickinson, Franklin Lakes, NJ), although they are also available from other manufacturers. Use of vacuum tubes with their corresponding needles and adapters provides a means of collecting blood directly into the tube,

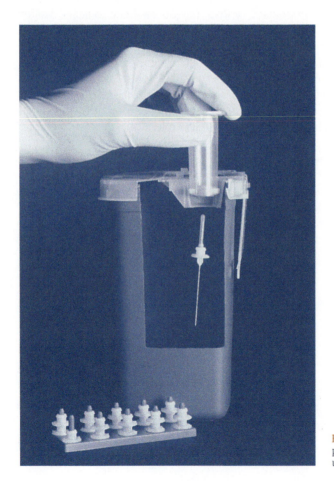

FIGURE 5–5 AutoDrop needle disposal system. (Courtesy of Sage Products, Inc., Crystal Lake, IL.)

thereby minimizing accidental contact with blood. Laboratory instrumentation is also available for direct sampling from the vacuum tubes, providing additional protection for laboratory workers.

The amount of blood collected in a vacuum tube ranges from 2 to 15 mL and is determined by the size of the tube and the amount of vacuum present. As shown in Figure 5–6, a wide variety of sizes is available to accommodate both adult and pediatric patients. When selecting the appropriate size of tube, the PCT must consider the amount of blood needed and the size and condition of the patient's veins. Using a 23-gauge needle with a large vacuum tube can produce hemolysis, because red blood cells are damaged when the large amount of vacuum causes the cells to be pulled rapidly through the small lumen of the needle. Therefore, if it is necessary to use a small-gauge needle, the PCT should collect two small tubes instead of one large tube.

Most vacuum tubes are sterile, and many are silicon coated to prevent cells from adhering to the tube or to prevent the activation of clotting factors in coagulation studies. Information about the characteristics of a tube is contained on the write-on label attached to the tube and should be verified by the PCT when special collection procedures are needed. Tubes may also contain **_anticoagulants_** and additives.

As shown in Figure 5–7, vacuum tubes have thick rubber stoppers with a thinner central area to allow puncture by the Vacutainer needle. To aid the PCT in identifying the many types of vacuum tubes, the tops are color coded. Color coding for routinely used tubes is uniform among manufacturers, and instructions for sample collection usually refer to the tube color.

> **EXAMPLE:** Draw one red top tube, one light-blue top tube, and one lavender top tube.

Two types of color-coded tops are available. Rubber stoppers may be colored, or a color-coded plastic shield may cover the stopper, as with the Hemogard Vacutainer System. Removing the rubber stoppers from vacuum tubes can be hazardous because an aerosol of blood can be produced if the stopper is quickly "popped off." Stoppers should be covered with a gauze pad and slowly loosened, with the opening facing

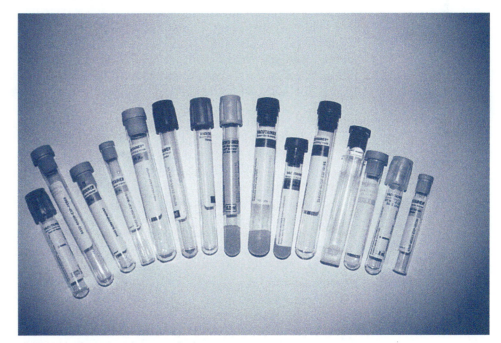

FIGURE 5–6 Examples of evacuated tubes.

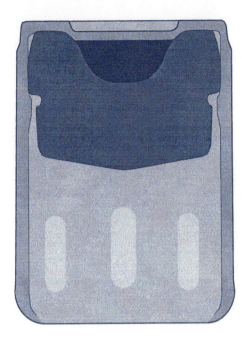

FIGURE 5–7 Cut-away view of a vacuum tube stopper (Hemogard closure). (Adapted from Product Literature, Becton Dickinson, Franklin Lakes, NJ.)

away from the body. Hemogard closures provide additional protection by allowing the stoppers to be easily twisted and pulled off and having a shield over the stopper.

PRINCIPLES OF COLOR-CODED TUBES

Color coding indicates the type of specimen that will be obtained when a particular tube is used. Laboratory tests may be run on ***plasma***, ***serum***, or whole blood. For tests on whole blood and plasma, an anticoagulant must be in the collection tube. Plasma is the liquid portion of blood that has not been allowed to clot. If the blood is allowed to clot, the liquid portion is called serum. The major difference between plasma and serum is that plasma contains fibrinogen and serum does not. Figure 5–8 illustrates the role of fibrinogen in the coagulation process. Figure 5–9 illustrates the differences between plasma and serum. It is important to differentiate between plasma and serum because many laboratory tests are designed to be performed specifically on either plasma or serum. Tests may also require the presence of preservatives, inhibitors, clot activators, or barrier gels. To produce the necessary conditions, some tubes will contain anticoagulants or additives and others will not. PCTs must be able to relate the color of the collection tubes to the types of specimens needed and to any special techniques, such as tube inversion, that may be required. This section discusses the routinely used tubes with regard to anticoagulants, additives, types of tests for which they are used, and special handling required.

Lavender top tubes contain the anticoagulant sodium or potassium ethylenediaminetetraacetic acid (**EDTA**) in either liquid or powdered form. Coagulation is prevented by the binding of calcium in the specimen to sites on the large EDTA molecule, thereby preventing the participation of the calcium in the coagulation cascade (see Fig. 5–8). All tubes containing anticoagulants or additives should be inverted immediately after drawing to ensure uniform mixing with the specimen. Lavender top tubes should be gently inverted eight times. When using powdered anticoagulants, the bottom of the tube should be gently tapped to loosen the powder from the tube prior to drawing the specimen.

For hematology procedures that require whole blood, such as the complete blood count (CBC), EDTA is the anticoagulant of choice because it maintains cellular integrity better than other anticoagulants, inhibits platelet clumping, and does not interfere with routine staining procedures. Lavender top tubes cannot be used for coagula-

INTRINSIC PATHWAY

EXTRINSIC PATHWAY

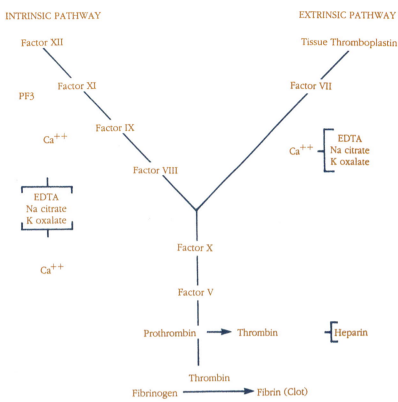

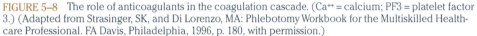

FIGURE 5–8   The role of anticoagulants in the coagulation cascade. (Ca^{++} = calcium; PF3 = platelet factor 3.) (Adapted from Strasinger, SK, and Di Lorenzo, MA: Phlebotomy Workbook for the Multiskilled Health-care Professional. FA Davis, Philadelphia, 1996, p. 180, with permission.)

tion studies because EDTA interferes with factor V and the thrombin-fibrinogen reaction.

Light-blue top tubes contain the anticoagulant sodium citrate, which also prevents coagulation by binding calcium. Centrifugation of the anticoagulated light-blue top tubes provides plasma used for coagulation tests. Sodium citrate is the required anticoagulant for coagulation studies because it preserves coagulation factors. Tubes should be inverted eight times.

The ratio of blood to liquid sodium citrate is critical and should be 9:1 (for example, 4.5 mL blood:0.5 mL sodium citrate). Therefore, to ensure accurate results light-blue top tubes must be completely filled. When drawing coagulation tests on patients with **polycythemia** or hematocrit readings, higher than 55% the amount of anticoagulant must be decreased, because the lower volume of plasma in these patients will be diluted by the standard volume of sodium citrate. Likewise, the amount of anticoagulant may be increased for severely anemic patients because of the larger amount of plasma. The clinical laboratory should be contacted to provide appropriate tubes and instructions in these situations.

A special light-blue top tube containing thrombin and a soybean trypsin inhibitor must be used when drawing blood for determinations of certain fibrin degradation products.

Black top tubes containing sodium citrate may be used for Westergren sedimentation rates. They differ from light-blue top tubes in that they provide a ratio of blood to liquid anticoagulant of 4:1.

Red/gray rubber stoppers and *gold* Hemogard closures are found on tubes containing a clot activator and a separation gel. They are frequently referred to as serum separator tubes (**SST**). Clot activators such as glass particles, silica, and celite increase platelet activation, thereby shortening the time required for clot formation. Tubes should be inverted five times to expose the blood to the clot activator. A nonreactive

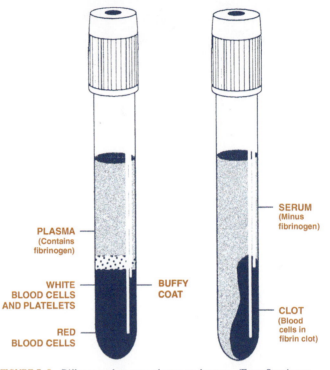

PLASMA
(Contains
fibrinogen)

SERUM
(Minus
fibrinogen)

WHITE
BLOOD CELLS
AND PLATELETS

BUFFY
COAT

CLOT
(Blood
cells in
fibrin clot)

RED
BLOOD CELLS

FIGURE 5–9   Differences between plasma and serum. (From Strasinger, SK, and Di Lorenzo, MA: Phlebotomy Workbook for the Multiskilled Healthcare Professional. FA Davis, Philadelphia, 1996, p. 40, with permission.)

thixotropic gel that undergoes a temporary change in viscosity during centrifugation is in the bottom of the tube. As shown in Figure 5–10, when the tube is centrifuged, the gel forms a barrier between the cells and the serum to prevent contamination of the serum with cellular materials. To produce a solid separation barrier, specimens must be allowed to clot completely before they are centrifuged. Specimens should be centrifuged as soon as clot formation is complete.

SSTs are used for most chemistry tests and prevent contamination of the serum by cellular chemicals. They are not suitable for use in the blood bank.

Green top tubes contain the anticoagulant **heparin** combined with either sodium, lithium, or ammonium ion. Heparin prevents clotting by inhibiting thrombin in the coagulation cascade (see Fig. 5–8). Green top tubes are used for chemistry tests performed on plasma, including ammonia, carboxyhemoglobin, and **stat** electrolytes. Interference by sodium and lithium heparin with their corresponding chemical tests and by ammonium heparin in blood urea nitrogen (BUN) determinations must be avoided. In general, lithium heparin has been shown to produce the least interference. Tubes should be inverted eight times. Green top tubes are not used for hematology because heparin interferes with the Wright's-stained blood smear.

Green/black top tubes containing lithium heparin and a separation gel are called **plasma separator tubes (PST)** and are available with Hemogard closures that are *light-green*. They are well-suited for potassium determinations because heparin prevents the release of potassium by platelets during clotting, and the gel prevents contamination by red blood cell potassium.

Red top tubes are often referred to as "plain" vacuum tubes because they contain no anticoagulants or additives. Blood drawn in red top tubes clots by the normal coagulation process in about 30 minutes. Centrifuging then yields serum as the liquid portion. Red top tubes are used for serum chemistry and serology tests and in the blood bank, where both serum and red blood cells are used. There is no need to invert red top tubes. Plastic red top tubes contain a clot activator and should be inverted.

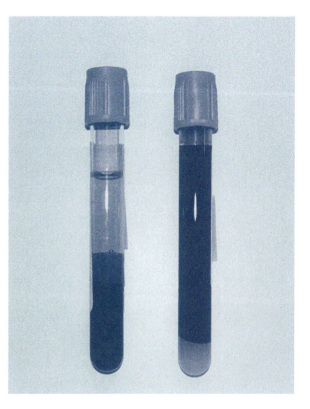

FIGURE 5–10   Centrifuged and uncentrifuged SSTs.

Plain pink top tubes are also available and are used specifically for the blood bank in some facilities. Using a designated tube for the blood bank is believed to help prevent the testing of specimens from the wrong patient.

Yellow/gray rubber stoppers and *orange* Hemogard closures are found on tubes containing the clot activator thrombin. Notice in Figure 5–8 that thrombin is generated near the end of the coagulation cascade; the addition of thrombin to the tube results in faster clot formation, usually within 5 minutes. Tubes should be inverted eight times. Tubes containing thrombin are used for stat serum chemistry determinations and for patients receiving anticoagulant therapy.

Gray top tubes are available with a variety of additives and anticoagulants for the primary purpose of preserving glucose. All gray top tubes contain a glucose preservative (**antiglycolytic agent**), either sodium fluoride or lithium iodoacetate. Sodium fluoride maintains glucose stability for 3 days, and iodoacetate maintains it for 24 hours. Sodium fluoride and iodoacetate are not anticoagulants; therefore, if plasma is needed for analysis, an anticoagulant must also be present, and the tubes must be inverted eight times. In gray top tubes the anticoagulant is potassium oxalate, which, like EDTA and sodium citrate, prevents clotting by binding calcium. When patient glucose levels are being monitored, tubes for the collection of plasma and serum should not be interchanged. Sodium fluoride will interfere with some enzyme analyses; therefore, gray top tubes should not be used for other chemical analyses.

Blood alcohol levels are drawn in gray top tubes containing sodium fluoride because sodium fluoride inhibits microbial growth, which could produce alcohol as a metabolic end product. Tubes with or without potassium oxalate can be used, depending on the need for plasma or serum in the test procedure.

Dark-blue top tubes are used for toxicology and trace metal and nutritional analyses. Because many of the elements analyzed in these studies are significant at very low levels, the tubes must be chemically clean, and the rubber stoppers are specially formulated to contain the lowest possible levels of metal. Dark-blue top tubes are available plain or with sodium heparin or disodium EDTA to conform to a variety of testing requirements.

Brown top tubes are used for lead determinations. They are certified to contain less than 0.1 µg/mL lead and contain sodium heparin.

Yellow top tubes are available for two different purposes and contain different additives. Yellow stoppers are found on tubes containing the red blood cell preservative acid citrate dextrose (**ACD**). Specimens drawn in these tubes are used for cellular studies in the blood bank.

Sterile yellow top tubes containing the anticoagulant sodium polyanetholesulfonate (**SPS**) are used to collect specimens to be cultured for the presence of microorganisms. SPS aids in the recovery of microorganisms because it inhibits the actions of complement, phagocytes, and certain antibiotics. Yellow top tubes should be inverted eight times.

Evacuated tubes are summarized in Table 5–1.

ORDER OF DRAW

When collecting multiple specimens and specimens for coagulation tests, the order in which tubes are drawn can affect some test results. As shown in Figure 5–8, the extrinsic pathway of the coagulation cascade is initiated by the presence of tissue thromboplastin. Release of tissue thromboplastin from the skin as it is punctured can result in its presence in the first tube collected, and this could interfere with coagulation tests.

TABLE 5–1 **Summary of Evacuated Tubes***

Stopper Color	Anticoagulant Additive	Laboratory Use
(1) Lavender (2) Lavender	Ethylenediaminetetraacetic acid (EDTA)	Whole blood for hematology tests
(1) Light-blue (2) Light-blue	Sodium citrate 0.105 M or 0.129 M	Plasma for coagulation tests
(1) Red/gray (2) Gold	Clot activator and thrixotropic gel	Serum separator tube for chemistry tests
(1) Green (2) Green	Sodium heparin, lithium heparin, or ammonium heparin	Plasma chemistry tests
(1) Green/black (2) Light-green	Lithium heparin and thrixotropic gel	Plasma chemistry tests
(1) Red (2) Red	None	Serum tests in chemistry, blood bank, and serology
(1) Yellow/gray (2) Orange	Thrombin	Stat serum chemistry tests
(1) Gray (2) Gray	Potassium oxalate/sodium fluoride, sodium fluoride, iodoacetate/lithium heparin, or iodoacetate	Glucose tests (glycolytic inhibitors stabilize values for up to 24 hours with iodoacetate and for 3 days with fluoride; oxalate and heparin produce plasma)
(1) Dark-blue (2) Dark-blue	Sodium heparin, EDTA, or none	Trace elements, toxicology, and nutrient analyses (special stopper provides a minimum of external contamination)
(1) Brown (2) Brown	Sodium heparin	Lead determinations (tube is certified to contain less than 0.01 µg/mL [ppm] lead)
(1) Yellow (2) Yellow	Sodium polyanetholesulfonate (SPS)	Blood cultures

*Note: (1) Conventional stopper and (2) Hemogard closure.

Therefore, a light-blue top tube should not be drawn first. If only a coagulation test is ordered, it is recommended that a small red top tube be drawn first; it can be discarded if it is not needed.

Transfer of anticoagulants among tubes resulting from possible contamination of the stopper-puncturing needle must be avoided. This is why the red top tube is drawn before the coagulation tube is drawn and why tubes containing other anticoagulants are drawn after the light-blue top tube is drawn. Also, tubes containing EDTA, which can bind calcium and iron, should not be drawn before a tube for chemistry tests is drawn.

When sterile specimens, such as blood cultures, are to be collected, they must be considered in the order of draw. Such specimens are always drawn first to prevent contamination.

Summarizing the previous discussion, the order of draw for multiple tubes using the vacuum tube system is as follows:

1 Sterile specimens
2 Nonadditive tubes (red) or SST (red/gray or gold), depending on institutional policy
3 Coagulation tubes (light-blue)

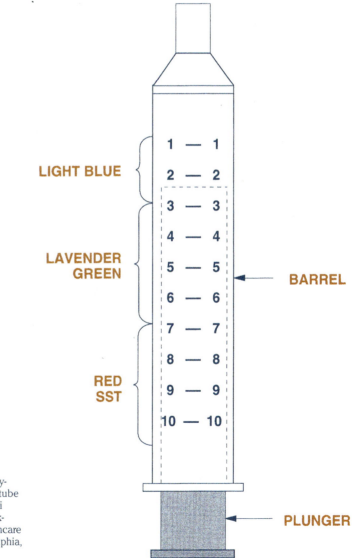

FIGURE 5–11 Diagram of a syringe, illustrating the order of tube fill. (From Strasinger, SK, and Di Lorenzo, MA: Phlebotomy Workbook for the Multiskilled Healthcare Professional. FA Davis, Philadelphia, 1996, p. 184, with permission.)

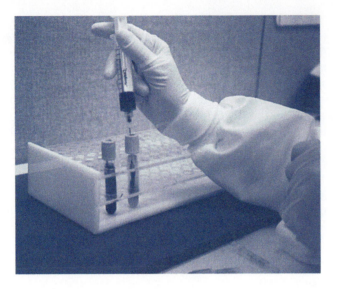

FIGURE 5–12   Transfer of blood from a syringe to an evacuated tube. (Note that the blood is being directed against the side of the tube.) (From Strasinger, SK, and Di Lorenzo, MA: Phlebotomy Workbook for the Multiskilled Healthcare Professional. FA Davis, Philadelphia, 1996, p. 185, with permission.)

4 Other anticoagulants and additives in this order: green (heparin), lavender (EDTA), gray (oxalate/fluoride), (SST and plastic [clot activator] red top tubes)

The order changes when tubes are being filled from a syringe because the portion of blood possibly contaminated by tissue thromboplastin is the first portion to enter the syringe and therefore, as shown in Figure 5–11, is the last to be expelled. The order of tube fill from a syringe is as follows:

1 Sterile specimens
2 Coagulation tubes
3 Other anticoagulants and additives (lavender, green, and gray)
4 Plain and SSTs

Syringes

Syringes are often preferred over vacuum tubes when drawing blood from patients with small or fragile veins. The suction pressure on the vein can be controlled by slowly withdrawing the syringe plunger.

Syringes routinely used for venipuncture range from 2 to 10 mL, and a size corresponding to the amount of blood needed should be used. Syringes consist of a plunger and a barrel graduated in **milliliters (mL)** or **cubic centimeters (cc)** (see Fig. 5–11). The technique for use of syringes is discussed in Unit 7.

Blood drawn in a syringe is transferred to appropriate evacuated tubes. It is acceptable to puncture the rubber stopper with the syringe needle and allow the blood to be drawn, but not forced, into the tube. Care must be taken to avoid hemolysis and needle punctures. As shown in Figure 5–12, the tube should be placed in a rack, not held in the free hand, and the needle should be angled toward the side of the tube for gentler transfer of the blood.

Winged Infusion Sets

Winged infusion sets, or "***butterflies***," as they are routinely called, are used for the infusion of IV fluids and for performing venipuncture from very small veins. Butterfly needles used for phlebotomy are usually 23 gauge with lengths of 1/2 or 3/4 inch. Plastic attachments to the needle that resemble butterfly wings are used for holding the

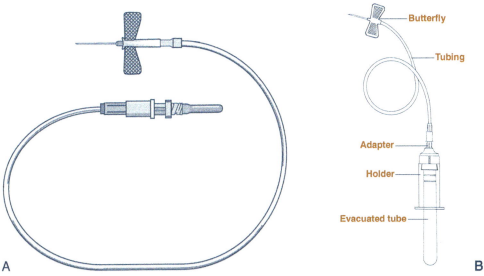

FIGURE 5–13 Winged infusion sets. *A*, Adaptable butterfly apparatus. *B*, Butterfly with evacuated tube. (*A* from Strasinger, SK, and Di Lorenzo, MA: Phlebotomy Workbook for the Multiskilled Healthcare Professional. FA Davis, Philadelphia, 1996, p. 186, with permission. *B* from Wedding, ME, and Toenjes, SA: Medical Laboratory Procedures, ed. 2. FA Davis, Philadelphia, 1998, p. 98, with permission.)

needle during insertion and to secure the apparatus during IV therapy (Fig. 5–13*A*). They also provide the ability to lower the needle insertion angle when working with very small veins. To accommodate the dual purpose of venipuncture and infusion, the needle is attached to a flexible plastic tubing that can then be attached to an IV setup, syringe, or specially designed Vacutainer adapter (Fig. 5–13*B*). Extreme care must be taken when working with winged infusion sets to avoid accidental needle punctures (see Unit 7).

Tourniquets

Tourniquets are used during venipuncture to make it easier to locate patients' veins. They do this by impeding venous, but not arterial, blood flow in the area just below the tourniquet application site.

The most frequently used tourniquets are flat latex strips (Fig. 5–14). They are inexpensive and may be disposed of between patients or reused if disinfected. Tourniquets

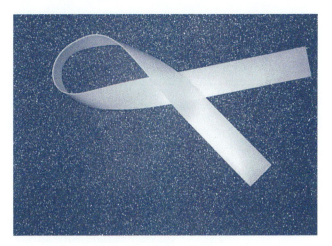

FIGURE 5–14 Latex strip tourniquet. (From Strasinger, SK, and Di Lorenzo, MA: Phlebotomy Workbook for the Multiskilled Healthcare Professional. FA Davis, Philadelphia, 1996, p. 186, with permission.)

with Velcro and buckle closures are easier to apply but are more difficult to decontaminate. Rubber tubing may be used for pediatric patients and persons allergic to latex.

Blood pressure cuffs can be used as tourniquets. They are used primarily for veins that are difficult to locate. The cuff should be inflated to a pressure below the patient's systolic blood pressure reading and above the diastolic reading to allow blood to flow into but not out of the affected veins.

The application of tourniquets and the effects on blood tests are discussed in Units 6 and 7.

Puncture Site Protection Supplies

The primary antiseptic used for cleansing the skin in routine phlebotomy is 70% isopropyl alcohol. This is a **bacteriostatic** antiseptic used to prevent contamination by normal skin bacteria during the short period required to perform collection of the specimen.

For collections that require additional sterility, such as blood cultures and arterial punctures, stronger antiseptics, including iodine or chlorhexidine gluconate (for patients allergic to iodine), are used to cleanse the area. To prevent skin discomfort, iodine should always be removed from the patient's skin with alcohol after a phlebotomy procedure.

Sterile 2- by 2-inch gauze pads are used for applying pressure to the puncture site after the needle has been removed. Gauze pads can also provide additional pressure when folded in quarters and placed under a bandage. Bandages or adhesive tape are placed over the puncture site when the bleeding has stopped. Patients should be instructed to remove the bandage in about 1 hour.

Additional Supplies

All healthcare workers must have an adequate supply of gloves at all times. Gloves are required for phlebotomy and must be changed after each patient. To provide maximal manual dexterity, they should fit securely. Gloves are available in several varieties, including powdered and unpowdered and latex and nonlatex. Allergy to latex is increasing among healthcare workers. Persons developing symptoms of allergy to latex should avoid these gloves and other latex products, such as tourniquets, at all times.

Clean glass slides may be needed to prepare blood films for certain hematology tests. This procedure is discussed in Unit 10.

The final piece of equipment needed is a pen for labeling tubes, initialing computer-generated labels, or noting unusual circumstances on the requisition form.

Quality Control

Ensuring the sterility of needles and puncture equipment devices and the stability of evacuated tubes, anticoagulants, and additives is essential to patient safety and specimen quality.

Disposable needles and puncture devices are individually packaged in tightly sealed sterile containers. PCTs should not use puncture equipment if the seal has been broken. Visual inspection for nonpointed or barbed needles may detect manufacturing defects.

Manufacturers of evacuated tubes must ensure that tubes, anticoagulants, and additives meet the standards established by the National Committee for Clinical Laboratory Standards. These standards specify the acceptable concentrations to provide quality specimens. Evacuated tubes produced at the same time are referred to as a "**lot**" and have a distinguishing lot number printed on the packages. There is also an expiration date printed on each package. The expiration date represents the last day the manufacturer guarantees the stability of the specified amount of vacuum in the tube and the reactivity of the anticoagulants and additives. The expiration date should be checked each time a new package of tubes is opened, and outdated tubes should not be used.

Use of expired tubes may cause incompletely filled tubes (short draws), clotted anticoagulated specimens, improperly preserved specimens, and insecure gel barriers. Short draws in tubes containing anticoagulants and additives affect specimen quality because the amount of anticoagulant or additive present in the tube is based on the assumption that the tube will be completely filled. Possible errors include excessive dilution of the specimen by liquid anticoagulants and distortion of cellular structures by increased chemical concentrations.

Defects in the manufacturing of evacuated tubes are possible and, when present, frequently affect an entire lot of tubes. When a new lot of tubes is opened, the tubes should be checked for vacuum by measuring the amount of water drawn into the tube. They should also be checked for the presence of small clots in anticoagulated tubes, the visual appearance of additives, stability during centrifugation, and stopper integrity and ease of stopper removal. The results of these checks should be documented, and testing may need to be repeated if problems with tube integrity develop at a later date. Manufacturers must be notified when defects are discovered.

BIBLIOGRAPHY

Becton Dickinson: Order of Draw. Lab Notes 7(2):7, Franklin Lakes, NJ, 1997.

Calam, RR, and Cooper, MH: Recommended "Order of Draw" for collecting blood specimens into additive-containing tubes. Clin Chem 28:1399, 1982.

National Committee for Clinical Laboratory Standards Approved Standard H1-A4: Evacuated Tubes and Additives for Blood Specimen Collection. NCCLS, Villanova, PA, 1996.

National Committee for Clinical Laboratory Standards Approved Guideline H21-A2: Collection, Transport and Processing of Blood Specimens for Coagulation Testing and Performance of Coagulation Assays. NCCLS, Villanova, PA, 1991.

STUDY QUESTIONS

1. State a purpose for which a PCT would use each of the following:

   a. 21-gauge needle _____

   b. 23-gauge needle _____

2. Using a 25-gauge needle to perform phlebotomy may cause _____ .

3. List three parts common to all needles.

   a. _____

   b. _____

   c. _____

4. How do evacuated tube systems accommodate both adult and pediatric patients?

   _____

   _____

   _____

5. How does the anticoagulant in a green top tube work?

   _____

6. Name three anticoagulants that prevent clotting by binding calcium and state their color-coded top.

Anticoagulant	*Color-Coded Top*
a. _____	_____
b. _____	_____
c. _____	_____

7. What is the purpose of sodium fluoride in a gray top tube?

   _____

8. Why is EDTA the anticoagulant of choice for a CBC?

   _____

   _____

9. The stopper color of the tube that must always be completely filled is

   _____ .

10. Which of the following tubes will clot first: red, red/gray, or yellow/gray?

   _____ .

11. List the order of draw using a vacuum tube system for the following tests using the numbers 1 through 5:

   a. _____ CBC

   b. _____ Blood culture

   c. _____ Plasma glucose

   d. _____ Serum iron

   e. _____ Coagulation studies

12. List the order of tube fill from a syringe for the tests in study question 11.

   a. _____

   b. _____

   c. _____

   d. _____

   e. _____

13. Under what circumstance should the amount of anticoagulant in a light-blue top tube be decreased?

   _____

14. Why are dark-blue top tubes used for collecting trace metal analyses?

   _____

15. List an advantage and a disadvantage of syringe use.

   _____

   _____

16. When are winged infusion sets used in phlebotomy?

   _____

   _____

17. Syringes are graduated in _____.

18. When a blood pressure cuff is used as a tourniquet, how should the pressure be adjusted?

   _____

   _____

19. List two antiseptics used in venipuncture and state a situation in which each is used.

Antiseptic	Used For
a. _____	_____
b. _____	_____

20. Fill in the blanks in the following chart:

Tube Color	Anticoagulant/Additive	Test
Red	None	RPR
	EDTA	
		Prothrombin
Orange		
		Ammonia
	Sodium fluoride	
Brown		

21. Define a "lot" of evacuated tubes.

_____

22. Define expiration date. How will the performance of an expired evacuated tube be affected?

_____

_____

_____

23. List four parameters that are checked when performing quality control on a new lot of evacuated tubes.

a. _____

b. _____

c. _____

d. _____

VENIPUNCTURE EQUIPMENT SELECTION EXERCISE

Instructions: State or assemble (if requested) the appropriate equipment for the situations described below. Include the number and color of evacuated tubes, needle size, syringe size, or butterfly, if appropriate. Instructors may specify the inclusion of supplies.

1. Collection of a CBC from a 35-year-old woman.

   _____

   _____

   _____

2. Collection of a CBC from a 3-year-old boy.

   _____

   _____

   _____

3. Collection of a stat CBC and electrolytes from a 40-year-old man.

   _____

   _____

   _____

4. Collection of a cholesterol from the hand of an obese patient.

   _____

   _____

   _____

5. Collection of a coagulation test from an elderly patient.

   _____

   _____

   _____

6. Assemble the equipment to collect a type and crossmatch on a 50-year-old man.

   _____

   _____

   _____

7. Assemble the equipment to collect a cardiac risk profile and erythrocyte sedimentation rate (ESR) from a patient with fragile veins.

   _____

   _____

   _____

8. Assemble the equipment to collect a lead level from a 2-year-old patient.

_____

_____

_____

EVALUATION OF EQUIPMENT SELECTION AND ASSEMBLY

RATING SYSTEM   2 = Satisfactory   1 = Needs improvement   0 = Incorrect/did not perform

_____ **1.** Collects all necessary equipment and supplies

_____ **2.** Selects appropriate tubes for requested tests

_____ **3.** Selects correct number of tubes and/or syringe size

_____ **4.** Correctly attaches needle to adapter or syringe

_____ **5.** Does not uncap needle prematurely

_____ **6.** Advances tube correctly into adapter or checks plunger movement

_____ **7.** Arranges supplies and extra tubes conveniently

Total points _____

Maximum points = 14

COMMENTS

U N I T 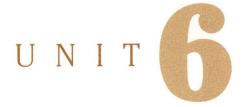6

ROUTINE VENIPUNCTURE

LEARNING OBJECTIVES

Upon completion of this unit, the reader will be able to:

1 Define the key terms associated with routine venipuncture.
2 List the required information on a requisition form.
3 Discuss the appropriate procedure to follow when greeting and reassuring a patient.
4 Describe correct patient identification procedures.
5 Describe patient preparation and positioning.
6 Correctly assemble venipuncture equipment and supplies.
7 Name and locate the three most frequently used veins for venipuncture.
8 Correctly apply a tourniquet.
9 Describe vein palpation.
10 Discuss the venipuncture site cleansing procedure.
11 Correctly perform a routine venipuncture using an evacuated tube system.
12 Safely dispose of contaminated needles and supplies.
13 List the information required on a specimen tube label.

KEY TERMS

- ***Hematoma*** Discoloration produced by leakage of blood into the tissues
- ***Hemoconcentra-tion*** Increase in the ratio of formed elements to plasma
- ***ID band*** Bracelet worn by patients that contains specific identification information
- ***Palpation*** Examination by touch
- ***Petechiae*** Small red spots appearing on the skin
- ***Venipuncture*** Procedure to collect blood by puncturing a vein with a needle

The most frequently performed procedure in phlebotomy is the ***venipuncture***, and the ability to perform this technique in an organized, patient-considerate manner is the key to success. Each healthcare worker develops his or her own style for dealing with patients and performing the actual venipuncture. Administrative protocols vary among institutions, and, of course, every patient is different; however, many basic rules are the same in all situations. These basic rules must be followed to ensure the safety of the patient and the person performing the procedure, to produce specimens that are representative of the patient's condition, and to create efficient phlebotomy for the institution.

In this unit the routine venipuncture technique is presented for the beginning PCT in the recommended step-by-step procedure. The procedure is outlined again in Unit 7, with a presentation of the complications that may occur at each step.

Requisitions

All phlebotomy procedures begin with the receipt of a test requisition form generated by or at the request of a physician. The requisition is essential to provide the PCT with the information needed to correctly identify the patient, organize the necessary equipment, collect the appropriate specimens, and provide legal protection. PCTs should not collect a specimen without a requisition form.

The method by which a PCT receives a requisition form varies with the setting. Requisitions from outpatients may be hand carried by the patient, or requests may be telephoned to the collection area by someone on the physician's staff, requiring the generation of a requisition at the collection area. Inpatient requisitions are generated at the nursing station.

PCTs should carefully examine all requisitions for which they are responsible. They should check to be sure that all requisitions for a particular patient are together so that all tests are collected with one venipuncture. They must be certain that they have all the necessary equipment when entering a patient's room.

The actual format of a requisition form may vary. Patient information may be handwritten or imprinted on color-coded forms with test check-off lists for different departments. There may be multiple copies for purposes of record keeping and billing. Computer-generated forms can include not only the patient information and tests requested but also the tube labels and bar codes for specimen processing, the number and type of collection tubes needed, and special collection instructions. Figure 6–1 shows a sample computer-generated requisition form with accompanying labels.

Requisitions must contain certain basic information to ensure that the specimen drawn and the test results are correlated to the appropriate patient and that these can be correctly interpreted with regard to any special conditions, such as the time of collection. This information includes the following:

1 Patient's name and identification (ID) number. The ID number may be a hospital-generated number that is also present on the patient's wrist **ID band** and all hospital documents or, in an outpatient setting, may be a department-assigned number or the patient's social security number.
2 Patient's location.
3 Ordering physician's name.
4 Tests requested.
5 Date and time of specimen collection. When the specimen is collected, the PCT must write the actual date and time on the requisition and the specimen label and initial both. Most hospitals have adopted the military time system (0000 to 2400 hours) because they operate continuously for 24 hours.

Other information that may be present includes:

- Patient's date of birth
- Special collection information (such as fasting specimen)
- Special patient information (such as areas that should not be used for venipuncture)
- Number and type of collection tubes
- Status of specimen (such as stat or preop)

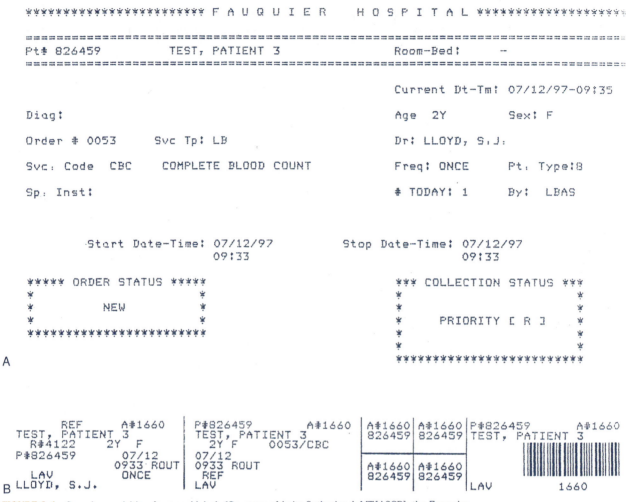

```
****************************** F A U Q U I E R    H O S P I T A L ****************************
===============================================================================================
Pt# 826459          TEST, PATIENT 3                    Room-Bed:        --
===============================================================================================
                                                       Current Dt-Tm: 07/12/97-09:35

Diag:                                                  Age   2Y        Sex: F

Order # 0053        Svc Tp: LB                         Dr: LLOYD, S.J.:

Svc: Code  CBC      COMPLETE BLOOD COUNT               Freq: ONCE      Pt. Type:8

Sp: Inst:                                              # TODAY: 1      By:  LBAS


            Start Date-Time: 07/12/97              Stop Date-Time: 07/12/97
                             09:33                                 09:33

    ***** ORDER STATUS *****                          *** COLLECTION STATUS ***
    *                      *                          *                        *
    *        NEW           *                          *      PRIORITY [ R ]     *
    *                      *                          *                        *
    ************************                          *                        *
                                                      *                        *
A                                                     **************************
```

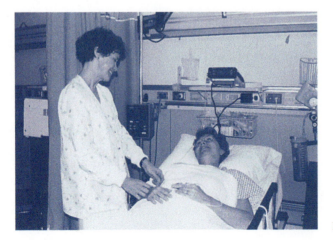

```
       REF       A#1660   │ P#826459          A#1660 │ A#1660│A#1660│ P#826459          A#1660
TEST, PATIENT 3           │ TEST, PATIENT 3          │ 826459│826459│ TEST, PATIENT 3
    R#4122     2Y  F      │    2Y  F       0053/CBC  │       │      │
P#826459         07/12    │ 07/12                    │       │      │
                 0933 ROUT│ 0933 ROUT                │ A#1660│A#1660│
    LAV          ONCE     │ REF                      │ 826459│826459│ LAV        ‖‖‖‖‖  1660
B LLOYD, S.J.            │ LAV                      │       │      │
```

FIGURE 6–1   Sample requisition form and label. (Courtesy of Anita Sutherland, MT[ASCP], the Fauquier Hospital, Warrenton, VA.)

Greeting the Patient

When approaching patients for whom they have not previously cared, PCTs should introduce themselves (Fig. 6–2) and explain that they will be collecting a blood specimen. In the outpatient setting, the patient usually knows what is about to take place.

FIGURE 6–2   PCT greeting patient.

When entering a patient's room, it is polite to knock lightly on the open or closed door. If the curtain is closed around the bed, speak to the patient first through the curtain. This will avoid any embarrassment if the patient happens to be bathing or using the bedpan. In the hospital setting a variety of other circumstances may be present that require additional consideration when greeting the patient. These will be discussed in Unit 7.

Patient Identification

The most important procedure in phlebotomy is correct identification of the patient. Serious diagnostic or treatment errors and even death can occur when blood is drawn from the wrong patient. The chance of misidentification is greatly reduced when PCTs are collecting specimens from patients for whom they have consistently been providing primary care; however, familiarity should not be used as the sole means of identification. Information from the patient's wrist ID band should still be compared with the requisition (Fig. 6–3).

PCTs will also collect blood specimens from patients who are unfamiliar to them. In this situation identification is made by comparing information obtained verbally from the patient and visually from the ID band with the information on the requisition form.

Verbal identification is made after the patient greeting by asking the patient to state his or her full name. Always have patients state their names. Do not ask "Are you John Jones?" because many patients have a tendency to say "yes" to anything. In an outpatient setting, comparison of verbal information with the requisition form may be the only means of verifying identification. Asking the patients for their date of birth or asking them to spell their name may be helpful in this situation.

Verbal identification is followed by examining the information on the patient's wrist ID band, which should be present on all hospitalized patients. Information on the wrist ID band should include patient's name, hospital ID number, date of birth, and physician. All information on the wrist ID band should match the information on the requisition form. Particular attention must be paid to the hospital ID number, because it is possible for two patients to have the same name, date of birth, and physician. They could not have the same ID number.

It is absolutely essential that identification of hospitalized patients be made from the ID band worn by the patient. Wrist bands are sometimes removed when IV fluids are being administered by way of the wrist or when fluids have infiltrated the area. They should be reattached around the patient's ankle. Ankle bands are frequently

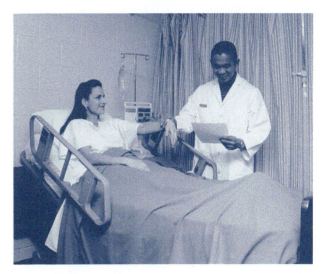

FIGURE 6–3 PCT checking a wrist ID band.

used for pediatric patients and newborns. A wrist band lying on the bedside table cannot be used for identification—it could belong to anyone. Likewise, a sign over the patient's bed or on the door cannot be relied on for identification because the patient could be in the wrong bed or room.

Patient Preparation and Positioning

When patient identification is completed, the patient must be positioned conveniently and safely for the procedure and given an explanation of the procedure.

Blood should never be drawn from a patient who is in a standing position. Outpatients are seated at a drawing station, as shown in Figure 5–2. In some drawing stations, the movable arm serves the dual purposes of providing a solid surface for the patient's arm and preventing a patient who faints from falling out of the chair. PCTs should always be alert for any changes in the patient's condition while the procedure is being performed. Some patients know that they experience difficulties during venipuncture, and provisions should be made for them to lie down for the procedure.

It may be necessary to move hospitalized patients slightly to make their arms more accessible or to place a pillow or towel under the patient's arm for better support. If bed rails are lowered, they must always be returned to the raised position prior to leaving the room.

Patients should remove any objects, such as gum or a thermometer, from their mouths prior to performance of the venipuncture.

Reassurance of the patient actually begins with the greeting and continues throughout the procedure. PCTs should demonstrate both concern for the patient's comfort and confidence in their own ability to perform the procedure. Patients should be given a brief explanation of the procedure, including any nonroutine techniques that will be used such as the additional site preparation performed when collecting blood cultures. Patients should not be told that the procedure will be painless.

Patients often question the PCT about what tests are being performed or why their blood is being drawn so frequently. The best policy is to politely suggest that patients ask their physicians these questions. Even listing the names of tests can cause problems because many medical books are available to the general public. Erroneous conclusions may be reached by the patient because many tests have several diagnostic purposes, or the patient may misunderstand the test name and look up an inappropriate test associated with a very severe condition.

If the PCT is not providing pretest preparation for the patient, the conversation should include verifying that the appropriate pretest preparation, such as fasting or abstaining from medications, has occurred. When these procedures have not been followed, it should be reported to a supervisor prior to drawing the blood. If the specimen is still required, the irregular condition, such as "nonfasting," should be noted on the requisition form and on the specimen.

Equipment Assembly

Before approaching the patient for the actual venipuncture, the PCT should put on gloves, collect all necessary supplies (including antiseptic pads, sterile gauze, bandages, and needle disposal system), and assemble the collection equipment (Fig. 6–4). The stopper-puncturing end of the double-ended vacuum tube needle is screwed into the needle adapter. The sterile cap is not removed from the other end of the needle. The requisition form is reexamined, and the appropriate number and type of col-

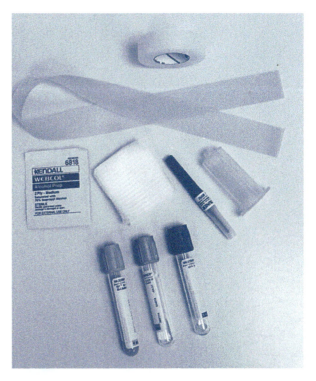

FIGURE 6–4   Venipuncture collection equipment.

lection tubes are selected. As described in Unit 5, the first tube to be collected can be inserted into the needle adapter up to the designated mark. Additional tubes should be readily available for possible use during the procedure. The assembled equipment and supplies are then carried to the patient.

Tourniquet Application

The tourniquet serves two functions in the venipuncture procedure. By causing blood to accumulate in the veins, the tourniquet causes the veins to be more easily located and provides a larger amount of blood for collection. Use of a tourniquet can alter some test results by increasing the ratio of cellular elements to plasma (***hemoconcentration***) and by causing hemolysis. Therefore, the maximum time the tourniquet should remain in place is 1 minute. This requires that the tourniquet be applied twice during the venipuncture procedure: first when vein selection is being made and then immediately before the puncture is performed.

The tourniquet should be applied 3 to 4 inches above the venipuncture site. Application of the commonly used latex strip requires practice to develop a smooth technique and can be difficult if properly fitting gloves are not worn. Figure 6–5 shows the technique used with latex strip tourniquets. To achieve adequate pressure, both sides of the tourniquet must be grasped near the patient's arm while the left side is being tucked under the right side. The loop formed should face downward, and the free end should be away from the venipuncture area but in a position that allows it to be easily pulled to release the pressure. This procedure would be reversed by left-handed persons.

Tourniquets that are folded or applied too tightly are uncomfortable for the patient and may obstruct blood flow to the area. The appearance of small, reddish discolorations (***petechiae***) on the patient's arm and the PCT's inability to feel a radial pulse are indications of a tourniquet tied too tightly.

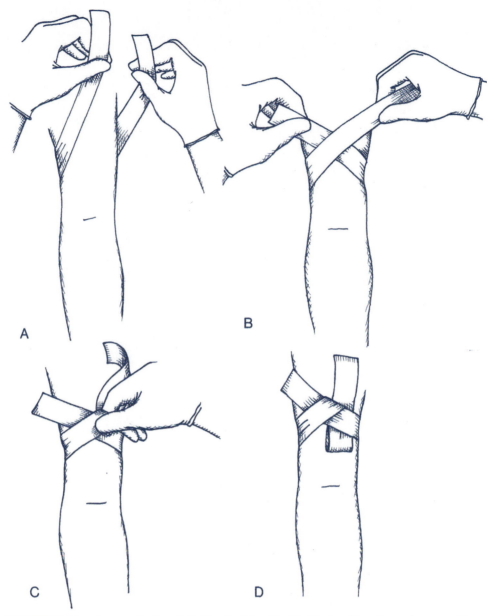

FIGURE 6–5   Tourniquet application. *A*, Position the latex strip 3 to 4 inches above the venipuncture site. *B*, Cross the tourniquet over the patient's arm. *C*, Tuck a portion of one end under the opposite end to form a loop. *D*, Properly applied tourniquet. (From Strasinger, SK, and Di Lorenzo, MA: Phlebotomy Workbook for the Multiskilled Healthcare Professional. FA Davis, Philadelphia, 1996, p. 203, with permission.)

Site Selection

The preferred site for venipuncture is the antecubital fossa located anterior to the elbow. As shown in Figure 6–6, three major veins—the **median cubital**, the **cephalic**, and the **basilic**—are located in this area, and in most patients at least one of these veins can be easily located. Notice that the veins continue down the forearm to the wrist area; however, in these areas the veins become smaller and less well anchored, and punctures are more painful to the patient. Small, prominent veins are also located in the back of the hand. When necessary, any of these veins can be used for venipuncture but may require a smaller needle or butterfly apparatus. The veins of the lower arm and hand are also the preferred sites for administering IV fluids because they allow the

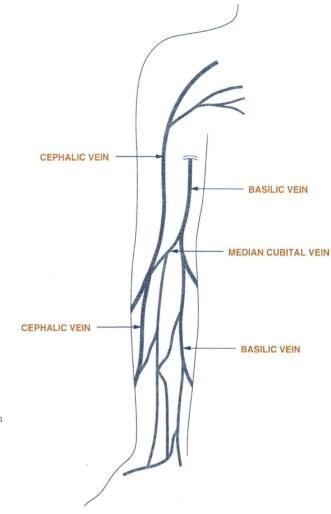

CEPHALIC VEIN

BASILIC VEIN

MEDIAN CUBITAL VEIN

CEPHALIC VEIN

BASILIC VEIN

FIGURE 6–6   The veins in the arm most often chosen for venipuncture. (From Strasinger, SK, and Di Lorenzo, MA: Phlebotomy Workbook for the Multiskilled Healthcare Professional. FA Davis, Philadelphia, 1996, p. 204, with permission.)

patient more arm flexibility. Frequent venipuncture in these veins could make them unsuitable for IV use.

Of the three veins located in the antecubital area, the median cubital is the vein of choice because it is large and does not tend to move when the needle is inserted. The cephalic vein is usually more difficult to locate, except in obese patients, and has more tendency to move. The basilic vein is the least firmly anchored and is located near the brachial artery. Care must be taken not to accidentally puncture the artery.

Two routine steps in the venipuncture procedure aid in locating a suitable vein: applying a tourniquet and asking a patient to clench his or her fist (Fig. 6–7A). Continuous clenching or pumping of the fist should not be encouraged because it will result in hemoconcentration and alter some test results. The difference in vein prominence before and after these procedures is usually remarkable, and PCTs examining an arm before these procedures have been performed should not become overly concerned if they cannot locate a vein at that time. Most practitioners prefer to apply the tourniquet before examining the arm. As discussed before, the tourniquet can be applied for only 1 minute; therefore, after the vein is located, the tourniquet should be removed while the site is being cleansed and then reapplied immediately before the venipuncture.

Veins are located by sight and touch (referred to as ***palpation***). The ability to feel a vein is much more important than the ability to see a vein—a concept that is often difficult to accept when first learning to perform venipuncture. Palpation is usually performed by using the index and second fingers of the nondominant hand to probe the

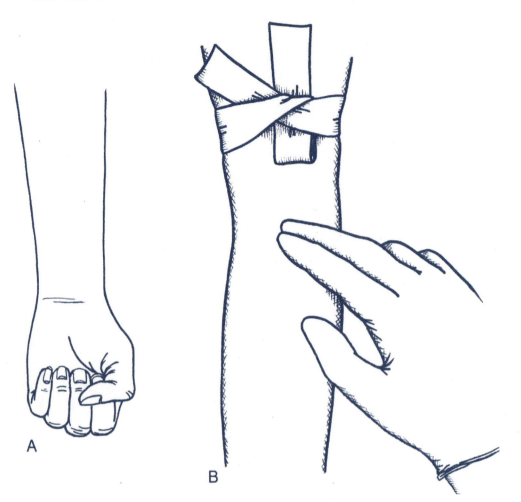

FIGURE 6–7   Locating a vein for venipuncture. *A*, Have the patient make a fist. *B*, Palpate the area, using the fingers, not the thumb. (From Strasinger, SK, and Di Lorenzo, MA: Phlebotomy Workbook for the Multi-skilled Healthcare Professional. FA Davis, Philadelphia, 1996, p. 205, with permission.)

antecubital area with a pushing rather than a stroking motion. The pressure applied by palpating locates deep veins; distinguishes veins, which feel like spongy cords, from rigid tendon cords; and differentiates veins from arteries, which produce a pulse (Fig. 6–7*B*). The thumb should not be used to palpate because it has a pulse beat. Once an acceptable vein is located, palpation is used to determine the direction and depth of the vein to aid in directing the needle during insertion.

Cleansing the Site

When an appropriate vein has been located, the tourniquet is released and the area cleansed using 70% isopropyl alcohol. Cleansing is performed with a circular motion starting at the inside of the venipuncture site and working outward (Fig. 6–8). For maximum bacteriostatic action to occur, the alcohol should be allowed to dry on the patient's arm rather than be wiped off with a gauze pad. Performing a venipuncture before the alcohol has dried causes a stinging sensation for the patient and may produce hemolysis in the specimen.

If additional palpation of the vein is needed after the cleansing process, the PCT should use alcohol to clean the gloved ends of the fingers to be used.

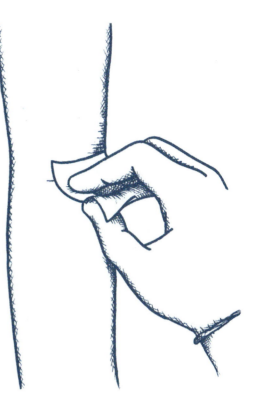

FIGURE 6–8   Cleansing the puncture site. (From Strasinger, SK, and Di Lorenzo, MA: Phlebotomy Workbook for the Multiskilled Healthcare Professional. FA Davis, Philadelphia, 1996, p. 206, with permission.)

While the alcohol is drying, make a final survey of the supplies at hand to be sure everything required for the procedure is present. The tourniquet is then reapplied and the suitability of the vein confirmed.

Examination of Puncture Equipment

Immediately prior to the needle's entering the vein, the plastic cap is removed and the point of the needle visually examined for any defects, such as a nonpointed or rough (barbed) end (Fig. 6–9). The needle is then positioned for entry into the vein with the bevel facing up.

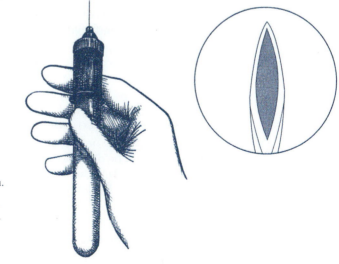

FIGURE 6–9   Needle inspection. (From Strasinger, SK, and Di Lorenzo, MA: Phlebotomy Workbook for the Multiskilled Healthcare Professional. FA Davis, Philadelphia, 1996, p. 207, with permission.)

Visual examination cannot detect all defective vacuum tubes; therefore, extra tubes should be at hand. It is not uncommon for the vacuum in a tube to be lost.

Performing the Venipuncture

The needle holder or syringe is held securely in the dominant hand with the thumb on top and the remaining fingers below. After insertion is made, the fingers can be braced against the patient's arm to provide stability while tubes are being moved in the holder or the plunger of the syringe is being pulled back. Figure 6–10 demonstrates the correct positioning of the hands during the venipuncture. Refer to these diagrams during the following discussion. Figure 6–11 provides additional illustration.

Use the thumb of the nondominant hand to anchor the selected vein while inserting the needle (Fig. 6–10A). Notice that the thumb is placed 1 or 2 inches below the insertion site. Anchoring the vein above and below the site using the thumb and index finger is not an acceptable technique because sudden patient movement could cause the index finger to be punctured. A vein that moves to the side is said to have "rolled." Patients often state that they have "rolling veins"; however, all veins will roll if they are not properly anchored. These patients are really saying that their blood has been drawn by practitioners who were not anchoring the veins well enough. As mentioned previously, the median cubital vein is the easiest to anchor and the basilic vein is the most difficult. In general, the closer a vein is to the surface, the more likely it is to "roll."

When the vein is securely anchored, the needle is inserted, bevel up, at an angle of 15 to 30 degrees depending on the depth of the vein (Figs. 6–10B and 6–11A). It should be done in a smooth movement so the patient feels the stick only briefly. A feeling of lessening of resistance to the needle movement is noticed when the vein has been entered.

Once the vein has been entered, the hand anchoring the vein can be moved and used to push the vacuum tube completely into the holder or to pull back on the syringe plunger (Figs. 6–10C and 6–11B). Some practitioners prefer to change hands at this point so that the dominant hand is free for performing the remaining tasks. This method of operating is usually better suited for use by experienced persons because holding the needle steady in the patient's vein is often difficult for beginners.

The hand used to hold the needle assembly should remain braced on the patient's arm. This is of particular importance when vacuum tubes are being inserted or removed from the holder because a certain amount of resistance is encountered and can cause the needle to be pushed through or pulled out of the vein. Tubes should be gently eased on and off the puncturing needle, using the flared ends of the adapter as an additional brace (Fig. 6–11C).

To prevent any chance of blood refluxing back into the needle, tubes should be held at a downward angle while they are being filled and have slight pressure applied. Be sure to follow the prescribed order of draw when multiple tubes are being collected and allow the tubes to fill completely before removing them. Mixing of evacuated tubes should be done as soon as the tube is removed, before another tube is placed in the assembly. The few required seconds does not cause additional discomfort to the patient and ensures that the specimen will be acceptable.

When the last tube has been filled, it is removed from the assembly and mixed prior to completing the procedure (Fig. 6–10D). Failure to remove the vacuum tube prior to removing the needle causes blood to drip from the end of the needle, resulting in unnecessary contamination and possible damage to the patient's clothes.

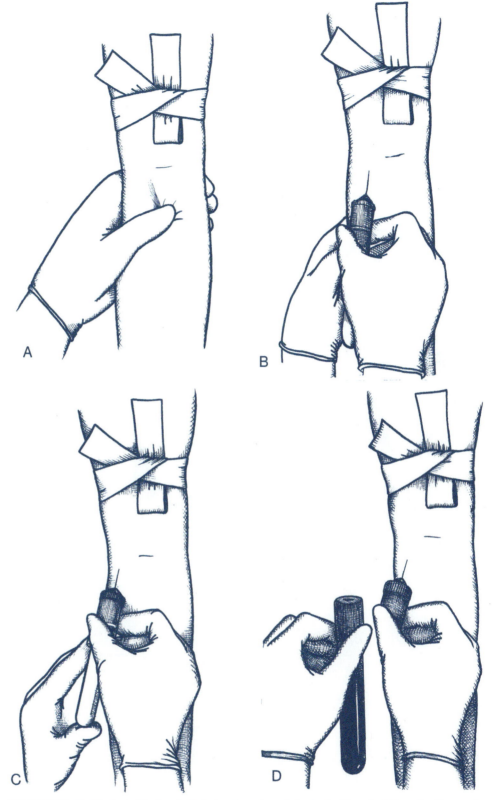

FIGURE 6–10   Positioning of the hands during venipuncture. *A*, Anchoring the vein. *B*, Inserting the needle (15- to 30-degree angle). *C*, Advancing the tube onto the needle. *D*, Removing the tube from the adapter. (From Strasinger, SK, and Di Lorenzo, MA: Phlebotomy Workbook for the Multiskilled Healthcare Professional. FA Davis, Philadelphia, 1996, p. 208, with permission.)

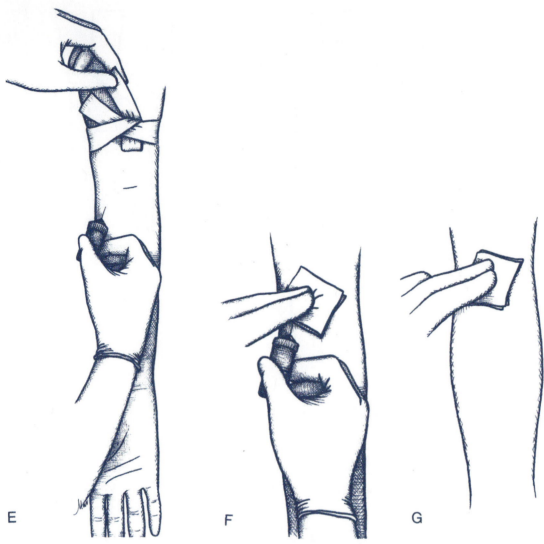

E   F   G

FIGURE 6–10   Continued. *E*, Removing the tourniquet before removing the needle. *F*, Removing the needle. *G*, Applying pressure to the puncture site. (From Strasinger, SK, and Di Lorenzo, MA: Phlebotomy Workbook for the Multiskilled Healthcare Professional. FA Davis, Philadelphia, 1996, p. 209, with permission.)

Removal of the Needle

Before removing the needle, remove the tourniquet by pulling on the free end and tell the patient to relax his or her hand (Fig. 6–10*E*). Failure to remove the tourniquet prior to removing the needle may produce a bruise (**hematoma**).

Place folded sterile gauze over the venipuncture site, withdraw the needle, and apply pressure to the site as soon as the needle is withdrawn (Figs. 6–10*F* and *G* and 6–11*D*). Do not apply pressure while the needle is still in the vein. To prevent blood from leaking into the surrounding tissue and producing a hematoma, pressure must be applied until the bleeding has stopped. The arm should be held in a raised, outstretched position. Bending the elbow to apply pressure allows blood to leak into the tissue more easily. A capable patient can be asked to apply the pressure, thereby freeing the PCT to dispose of the used needle and label the specimen tubes. If this is not possible the PCT must apply the pressure and perform the other tasks after the bleeding has stopped.

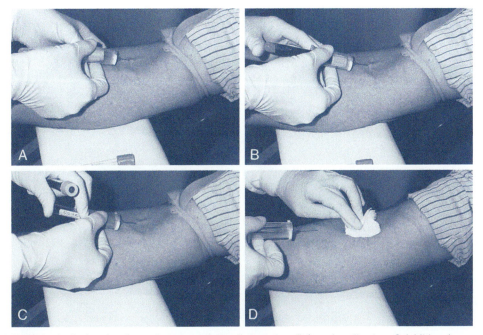

FIGURE 6–11   Performing the venipuncture. *A*, Needle insertion. *B*, Sample collection. *C*, Additional sample collection. *D*, Removal of needle, followed immediately by pressure to the puncture site. (From Strasinger, SK, and Di Lorenzo, MA: Phlebotomy Workbook for the Multiskilled Healthcare Professional. FA Davis, Philadelphia, 1996, p. 210, with permission.)

Disposal of the Needle

Upon completion of the venipuncture, the first thing the PCT must do is dispose of the contaminated needle in an appropriate sharps container located near the patient (Fig. 6–12). As discussed in Unit 5, the method by which this is done will depend on the type of disposal equipment selected by the institution. Remember, manual two-handed recapping of the needle is not acceptable. One-handed scooping of the cap onto the needle should be used only in extenuating circumstances.

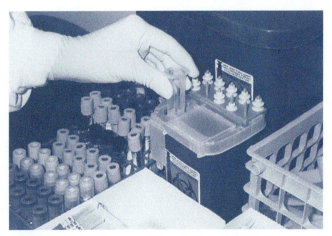

FIGURE 6–12   Needle disposal. (From Strasinger, SK, and Di Lorenzo, MA: Phlebotomy Workbook for the Multiskilled Healthcare Professional. FA Davis, Philadelphia, 1996, p. 211, with permission.)

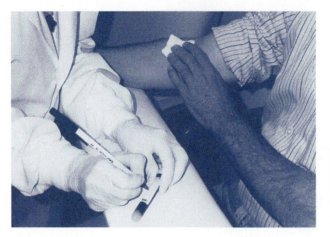

FIGURE 6–13 Labeling the tube. (From Strasinger, SK, and Di Lorenzo, MA: Phlebotomy Workbook for the Multiskilled Healthcare Professional. FA Davis, Philadelphia, 1996, p. 211, with permission.)

Labeling the Tubes

Tubes must be labeled at the time of specimen collection, prior to leaving the patient's room or accepting another requisition. Tubes are labeled by writing with a pen on the attached label or by applying a computer-generated label (Fig. 6–13). Tubes should not be labeled before the specimen is collected; it could result in confusion of specimens when more than one patient is having blood drawn or when a specimen cannot be collected. Preprinted labels should be verified prior to being attached to the specimen.

Information on the specimen label should include the patient's name and ID number, the date and time of collection, and the collector's initials. Additional information may be present on computer-generated labels. Specimens for the blood bank may require an additional label obtained from the patient's blood bank ID band.

Specimens requiring special handling, such as cooling or warming, are placed in the appropriate container when labeling is complete.

Bandaging the Patient's Arm

Bleeding at the venipuncture site should stop within 5 minutes. Before applying the bandage, the PCT should examine the patient's arm to be sure the bleeding has stopped. For additional pressure, the adhesive bandage or tape is applied over a folded gauze square (Fig. 6–14). The patient should be instructed to remove the

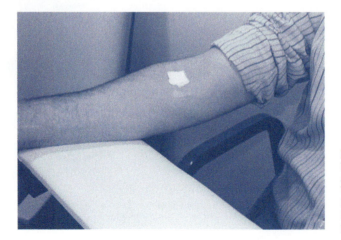

FIGURE 6–14 Patient's arm with bandage. (From Strasinger, SK, and Di Lorenzo, MA: Phlebotomy Workbook for the Multiskilled Healthcare Professional. FA Davis, Philadelphia, 1996, p. 212, with permission.)

bandage within 1 hour and to avoid using the arm to carry heavy objects during that period.

Leaving the Patient

Before leaving the patient's room, dispose of all contaminated supplies such as alcohol pads and gauze in a biohazard container, remove gloves and dispose of them in the biohazard container, and wash your hands.

In the outpatient setting, patients can be excused once the arm is bandaged. If patients have been fasting and no more procedures are scheduled, they should be instructed to eat. Before calling the next patient, clean up the area as described previously.

In both inpatient and outpatient settings, patients should be thanked for their cooperation.

Completing the Venipuncture

The venipuncture procedure is complete when the specimen is delivered to the laboratory in satisfactory condition and all appropriate paperwork has been completed. These procedures will vary, depending on institutional protocol and the types of specimens collected. The PCT must be familiar with these procedures.

Summary of Venipuncture Technique with a Vacuum Tube

1 Obtain and examine the requisition form.
2 Greet the patient.
3 Identify the patient.
4 Reassure the patient.
5 Position the patient.
6 Put on gloves.
7 Assemble equipment and supplies.
8 Apply the tourniquet.
9 Select the venipuncture site.
10 Release the tourniquet.
11 Cleanse the site.
12 Survey the supplies and equipment.
13 Reapply the tourniquet.
14 Confirm the venipuncture site.
15 Anchor the vein.
16 Insert the needle.
17 Push vacuum tube completely into adapter.
18 Mix the specimens as they are collected.
19 Remove last tube from the holder.
20 Release the tourniquet.
21 Place sterile gauze over the needle.
22 Remove the needle and apply pressure.
23 Dispose of the needle.
24 Label the tubes.

25 Perform appropriate specimen handling.
26 Examine the patient's arm.
27 Bandage the patient's arm.
28 Thank the patient.
29 Dispose of used supplies.
30 Remove and dispose of gloves.
31 Wash hands.
32 Complete any required paperwork.
33 Deliver specimens to appropriate locations.

BIBLIOGRAPHY   National Committee for Clinical Laboratory Standards Approved Standard H3-A3: Procedures for the Collection of Diagnostic Blood Specimens by Venipuncture. NCCLS, Villanova, PA, 1991.

STUDY QUESTIONS

1. List three reasons for requiring a requisition form before performing a venipuncture.

   a. _____

   b. _____

   c. _____

2. List five pieces of information that must be present on a requisition form.

   a. _____

   b. _____

   c. _____

   d. _____

   e. _____

3. List four pieces of information that must appear on a patient's ID band.

   a. _____

   b. _____

   c. _____

   d. _____

4. An outpatient enters the drawing area. The PCT asks, "Are you Sandra Brown?" The patient answers, "Yes." The PCT labels the tubes and performs the venipuncture. What is wrong with this situation?

   _____

   _____

5. The maximum length of time a tourniquet should be applied is

   _____.

6. List the three major veins located in the antecubital fossa.

   a. _____

   b. _____

   c. _____

7. The preferred vein for venipuncture is the _____.

8. The vein located on the thumb side of the arm is the _____.

9. List three reasons for vein palpation.

   a. _____

   b. _____

   c. _____

10. List three reasons for allowing the alcohol to dry on a patient's arm before performing the venipuncture.

a. _____

b. _____

c. _____

11. How does a PCT prepare for the possibility of encountering a defective vacuum tube?

_____

12. The cause of "rolling veins" is

_____

_____.

13. The angle of the needle during insertion is _____.

14. When should a specimen collected in a lavender top tube be mixed?

_____

15. Place the following steps in the venipuncture technique in the correct order by numbering them 1 through 10.

a. _____ Release the tourniquet.

b. _____ Identify the patient.

c. _____ Anchor the vein.

d. _____ Cleanse the site.

e. _____ Obtain and examine the requisition form.

f. _____ Label the tubes.

g. _____ Bandage the patient's arm.

h. _____ Insert the needle.

i. _____ Remove needle and apply pressure.

j. _____ Select and assemble equipment.

16. List five pieces of information that should be present on the specimen label.

a. _____

b. _____

c. _____

d. _____

e. _____

17. What should PCTs do immediately after removing their gloves?

_____

18. Determine whether the following are acceptable or not acceptable when performing a venipuncture and explain your reason in one sentence.

a. An outpatient with a sore back wishes to stand during the procedure.

_____

_____

b. The equipment is assembled before applying the tourniquet.

_____

_____

c. The procedure is explained to the patient.

_____

_____

d. Patients are requested to pump their fists during sample collection.

_____

_____

e. Palpation is performed with the thumb.

_____

_____

f. The site is cleansed in a circular motion from inside to outside.

_____

_____

g. The patient's elbow is bent while pressure is applied to the puncture site.

_____

_____

h. The hand holding the needle is braced against the patient's arm during specimen collection.

_____

_____

19. State an error in routine venipuncture technique that may cause

a. a hematoma _____

b. petechiae _____

EVALUATION OF TOURNIQUET APPLICATION AND VEIN SELECTION

RATING SYSTEM   2 = Satisfactory   1 = Needs improvement   0 = Incorrect/did not perform

_____ **1.** Positions correctly for vein selection

_____ **2.** Selects appropriate tourniquet application site

_____ **3.** Places tourniquet in flat position behind arm

_____ **4.** Smoothly positions hands when crossing and tucking tourniquet

_____ **5.** Fastens tourniquet at appropriate tightness

_____ **6.** Does not fold tourniquet into arm

_____ **7.** Ties tourniquet so loop and loose end do not interfere with puncture site

_____ **8.** Asks patient to clench fist

_____ **9.** Selects antecubital area to palpate

_____ **10.** Performs palpation using correct fingers

_____ **11.** Palpates entire area or both arms if necessary

_____ **12.** Checks depth and direction of veins

_____ **13.** Removes tourniquet smoothly

_____ **14.** Removes tourniquet in a timely manner

Total points _____

Maximum points = 28

COMMENTS

EVALUATION OF VENI-PUNCTURE TECHNIQUE USING AN EVACUATED TUBE

RATING SYSTEM   2 = Satisfactory   1 = Needs improvement   0 = Incorrect/did not perform

_____ **1.** Examines requisition form

_____ **2.** Greets patient and states procedure to be done

_____ **3.** Identifies patient verbally

_____ **4.** Examines patient's ID band

_____ **5.** Compares requisition information with ID band

_____ **6.** Puts on gloves

_____ **7.** Selects correct tubes and equipment for procedure

_____ **8.** Assembles and conveniently places equipment

_____ **9.** Positions patient's arm

_____ **10.** Applies tourniquet

_____ **11.** Identifies vein by palpation

_____ **12.** Releases tourniquet

_____ **13.** Cleanses site and allows it to air dry

_____ **14.** Reapplies tourniquet

_____ **15.** Does not touch puncture site with unclean finger

_____ **16.** Anchors vein below puncture site

_____ **17.** Smoothly enters vein at appropriate angle with bevel up

_____ **18.** Does not move needle when changing tubes

_____ **19.** Collects tubes in correct order

_____ **20.** Mixes anticoagulated tubes promptly

_____ **21.** Fills tubes completely

_____ **22.** Removes last tube collected from holder

_____ **23.** Releases tourniquet

_____ **24.** Covers puncture site with gauze

_____ **25.** Removes the needle smoothly and applies pressure

_____ **26.** Disposes of the needle in sharps container

_____ **27.** Labels tubes

_____ **28.** Examines puncture site

_____ **29.** Applies bandage

_____ **30.** Disposes of used supplies

_____ **31.** Removes gloves and washes hands

_____ **32.** Thanks patient

_____ **33.** Converses appropriately with patient during procedure

Total points _____

Maximum points = 66

COMMENTS

U N I T **7**

VENIPUNCTURE COMPLICATIONS

LEARNING OBJECTIVES

Upon completion of this unit, the reader will be able to:

1 Define the key terms associated with venipuncture complications.
2 State the procedure for obtaining requisition forms, patient identification, and labeling of tubes for unidentified patients.
3 Discuss the procedures to follow when patients are asleep or are being visited by a physician, member of the clergy, or family.
4 Discuss the procedure to follow when a patient develops syncope during the venipuncture procedure.
5 Recognize common laboratory tests that can be affected by patient activities prior to specimen collection.
6 State the policy regarding patients who refuse to have their blood drawn.
7 State the reasons why the tourniquet can be applied for only 1 minute.
8 List four methods used to locate veins that are not prominent.
9 List three conditions that make it inadvisable to draw from veins in the legs or feet.
10 State reasons why blood should not be drawn from a hematoma, a burned or scarred area, or an arm adjacent to the site of a mastectomy.
11 State three methods for obtaining blood from a patient by using an intravenous (IV) drip.
12 State the procedure to follow when drawing blood from a patient with a fistula.
13 Discuss cleansing of the venipuncture site prior to collecting a blood alcohol level.
14 Describe the venipuncture procedure using a syringe, including equipment examination, technique for exchanging syringes, transfer of blood to evacuated tubes, and disposal of the equipment.
15 Describe the venipuncture procedure using a butterfly, including technique involved and disposal of the equipment.
16 List six reasons why blood may not be immediately obtained from a venipuncture and the procedures to follow to obtain blood.
17 List 10 tests affected by hemolysis.
18 List seven venipuncture errors that may produce hemolysis.
19 List five causes of hematomas.
20 List five reasons for rejecting a specimen.

KEY TERMS

■ *Cannula*	Tube that can be inserted into a cavity, for example, to form a temporary connection between an artery and a vein
■ *Catheter*	Tube inserted into the body for injecting or withdrawing fluids
■ *Fistula*	Permanent surgical connection between an artery and a vein (used for dialysis)
■ *Hemolysis*	Destruction of red blood cells
■ *Heparin lock*	Device inserted into a vein for administering medications and collecting blood
■ *Indwelling line*	Tube inserted into an artery or vein (primarily for administering fluids)
■ *Infiltrated IV*	Fluid running into the tissues instead of into the vein
■ *Lymphostasis*	Blockage of lymph flow
■ *Occluded*	Obstructed
■ *Sclerosed*	Hardened
■ *Syncope*	Fainting
■ *Thrombi*	Clots formed on the inner walls of a vein
■ *Variable*	Measurable condition used to evaluate quality of a patient's specimen

The venipuncture procedure discussed in Unit 6 describes routine collection of blood. Complications with the routine procedure can occur at any step. In this unit, the procedure is reviewed in the same order, with emphasis on the complications that may be encountered.

Requisitions

When working in emergency care, a preprinted requisition form may not be available, making it necessary for the information to be written on a blank form. Be sure to transfer the ID number from the patient's wrist band when a temporary identification system has been used. When verbal orders are given, the name of the person giving the order should be documented.

Greeting the Patient

Patients are frequently asleep and should be awakened gently and given time to become oriented prior to performing the venipuncture. Unconscious patients should be greeted in the same manner as conscious patients, because they may be capable of hearing and understanding even though they cannot respond. In this circumstance, it may be necessary to request assistance from other members of the unit staff, because the patient may move when the needle is inserted.

Physicians, members of the clergy, and visitors may be present when the PCT enters the room. When a physician or clergy member is with the patient, it is preferable to return at another time unless the request is for a stat or timed specimen. When this occurs, the PCT should explain the situation and request permission to perform the procedure at that time. Visitors should be greeted in the same manner as the patient and given the option to step outside. If they choose to stay, the PCT should assess their possible reactions and may elect to pull the curtain around the bed. Visitors can sometimes be helpful, as in the case of pediatric or very apprehensive patients.

An advantage of using PCTs rather than laboratory-based phlebotomists is that collection of specimens can be better coordinated with other diagnostic procedures for which the patient is scheduled. PCTs should organize their specimen collections to correspond with other patient activities, particularly with respect to timed collections.

Patient Identification

The PCT should be alert for patients who do not have ID bands on either their wrist or their ankle. Patients without ID bands attached to their bodies should be rebanded following unit procedures prior to specimen collection. The name of the person identifying the patient should be documented.

Unidentified patients are sometimes brought into the emergency room, and a system must be in place to ensure they are correctly matched with their laboratory work. The American Association of Blood Banks requires that the patient be positively identified with a temporary but clear designation attached to the body. Some hospitals generate ID bands with an ID number and a tentative name, such as John Doe or Patient X. Commercial identification systems are particularly useful when blood transfusions are required. In these systems, the ID band that is attached to the patient comes with matching identification stickers. The stickers are placed on the specimen tubes, the requisition form, and any units of blood designated for the patient. Blood bank identification systems are used in addition to routine ID bands, not instead of them.

Patient Preparation and Positioning

It is not uncommon for patients to be extremely apprehensive about having their blood drawn. If you are not the patient's primary caregiver, it may be necessary to enlist the help of that caregiver to calm the patient's fears. It also may be necessary to ask for assistance from other staff members to hold the patient's arm steady during the procedure. Assistance from another healthcare person or a parent is frequently required when working with children.

Apprehensive patients may be prone to fainting (**syncope**), and the PCT should be alert to this possibility. It is sometimes possible to detect such patients during vein palpation, because their skin may feel cold and damp. Keeping their minds off the procedure through conversation can be helpful. If a patient begins to faint during the procedure, remove the tourniquet and needle and apply pressure to the venipuncture site. In the inpatient setting, report the incident to the nursing station as soon as possible. The PCT should be aware of visitors in a patient's room because they also may develop syncope. In the outpatient area, make certain the patient is supported and that the patient lowers his or her head. Cold compresses applied to the forehead and back of the neck and ammonia inhalants will help to revive the patient. Outpatients who have been fasting for prolonged periods should be given something sweet to drink and be required to remain in the area for 15 to 30 minutes. All incidents of syncope should be documented according to institutional policy. It is rare for patients to develop seizures during the venipuncture; if this happens, however, the needle and tourniquet should be removed, pressure applied to the site, and help summoned.

At all times, PCTs must be alert for changes in a patient's condition and should notify supervisors of any changes. Such changes include the presence of vomitus, urine, or feces; removed or **infiltrated IVs** (intravenous fluid lines); extreme difficulty in breathing; and, possibly, death.

TABLE 7–1 **Major Tests Affected by Patient Variables**

Variable	Increased Results	Decreased Results
Nonfasting	Glucose and triglycerides	—
Prolonged fasting	Bilirubin, fatty acids, and triglycerides	Glucose
Posture	Albumin, bilirubin, calcium, enzymes, lipids, total protein, RBCs, and WBCs	—
Short-term exercise	Creatinine, fatty acids, lactate, AST, CK, LD, and WBCs	—
Long-term exercise	Aldolase, creatinine, sex hormones, AST, CK, and LD	—
Stress	Adrenal hormones, fatty acids, lactate, and WBCs	—
Alcohol	Lactate, triglycerides, uric acid, GGT, HDL, and MCV	—
Tobacco	Catecholamines, cortisol, hemoglobin, MCV, and WBCs	—
Diurnal variation (A.M.)	Cortisol and serum iron	WBCs

Numerous *variables* associated with a patient's activities prior to specimen collection can affect the quality of the specimen. These variables can include diet, posture, exercise, stress, alcohol, smoking, time of day, and medications. Major tests affected by these variables are listed in Table 7–1. The PCT should be aware of the effect these conditions can have on test results and notify a supervisor of any concerns.

PATIENT REFUSAL

Some patients may refuse to have their blood drawn, and they have the right to do so. The PCT can stress to the patient that the results are needed by the physician for treatment and discuss the problem with the unit or nursing supervisor, who may be able to convince the patient to agree to have the test performed. If the patient continues to refuse, the patient's physician must be contacted. Performing a venipuncture without the patient's consent could result in charges of assault and battery.

Equipment Assembly

When positioning the needed equipment and supplies within easy reach, the PCT should include extra vacuum tubes. It is not uncommon to find a vacuum tube that does not contain the necessary amount of vacuum to collect a full tube of blood. Accidentally pushing a tube past the indicator mark on the needle holder before the vein is entered will also result in loss of vacuum.

As discussed in Unit 2, remember that only the necessary amount of equipment is brought into isolation rooms.

Tourniquet Application

As discussed in Unit 6, a blood pressure cuff is sometimes used to locate veins that are difficult to find. The cuff should be inflated to a pressure below the systolic and above the diastolic blood pressure readings of the patient.

When dealing with patients with skin conditions, it may be necessary to place the tourniquet over the patient's gown or to cover the area with gauze prior to application. If possible, another area should be selected for the venipuncture. Consideration should also be given to using a disposable tourniquet.

Application of the tourniquet for more than 1 minute will interfere with some test results. Tests most likely to be affected are those measuring large molecules, such as plasma proteins and lipids, or analytes affected by ***hemolysis***, including potassium, lactic acid, and enzymes. Therefore, during multiple tube collections, it may be necessary to release the tourniquet before the last tube has been filled. Tourniquet application and fist clenching are not recommended when drawing specimens for lactic acid determinations.

Hemoconcentration and hemolysis can be prevented by releasing the tourniquet as soon as blood begins to flow into the first tube. Difficulty filling additional tubes may be encountered, however, and the tourniquet may have to be retightened or pressure applied to the area with the free hand to increase the amount of blood present in the vein.

Site Selection

Not all patients have a median cubital, cephalic, or basilic vein that becomes immediately prominent when the tourniquet is applied. In fact, a high percentage of patients have veins that are not easily located, and the PCT may have to use a variety of techniques to locate a suitable puncture site. Many patients have prominent veins in one arm and not in the other; therefore, checking the patient's other arm should be the first thing done when a site is not easily located. Patients with veins that are difficult to locate often point out areas of previously successful phlebotomies. Palpation of these areas may prove beneficial and is also good for patient relations.

Other techniques to enhance the prominence of veins include gently tapping the antecubital area with the index finger, massaging the arm upward from the wrist to the elbow, briefly hanging the arm down, and applying heat to the site. Remember that the tourniquet should not remain tied for more than 1 minute at a time when performing these techniques.

If no palpable veins are found in the antecubital area, the wrist and hand should be examined. The tourniquet should be retied on the forearm. Because the veins in these areas are smaller, it may be necessary to change equipment and use a smaller needle with a syringe, a winged infusion set, or a smaller vacuum tube.

Veins in the legs and feet are sometimes used as venipuncture sites. They should be used only with physician approval. Leg veins are more susceptible to infection and the formation of clots (***thrombi***), particularly in patients with diabetes, cardiac problems, and coagulation disorders.

AREAS TO BE AVOIDED

Veins that contain thrombi or that have been subjected to numerous venipunctures often feel hard (***sclerosed***) and should be avoided because they may be blocked (***occluded***) and the circulation may be impaired. Areas that appear blue or are cold may also have impaired circulation.

The presence of a hematoma indicates that blood has accumulated in the tissue surrounding a vein. Puncturing into a hematoma not only is painful for the patient but also will result in the collection of old, hemolyzed blood from the hematoma rather than from circulating venous blood that is representative of the patient's current condition. If a vein containing a hematoma must be used, blood should be collected below the hematoma to ensure sampling of free-flowing blood. Drawing from areas containing excess tissue fluid (**edema**) is also not recommended because the sample will be contaminated with tissue fluid.

Extensively burned and scarred areas, including areas with tattoos, are more susceptible to infection; they also have decreased circulation and veins that are difficult to palpate.

Applying a tourniquet or drawing blood from an arm located on the same side of the body as a recent mastectomy can be harmful to the patient and produce erroneous test results. Removal of lymph nodes as part of the mastectomy procedure interferes with the flow of lymph fluid (**lymphostasis**) and increases the blood level of lymphocytes and waste products normally contained in the lymph fluid. The protective functions of the lymphatic system are also lost, so that the area becomes more prone to infection. Normal flow of lymph fluid usually returns in about 6 months. However, most patients have been told to never have blood drawn from the affected area, and their wishes should be respected. In cases of a double mastectomy, the side associated with the older surgery should be used. The physician should be consulted if both procedures are recent.

Frequently, the PCT encounters patients receiving IV fluids in an arm vein. Whenever possible, blood should then be drawn from the other arm. If an arm containing an IV drip must be used for specimen collection, the site selected must be below the IV insertion point and preferably from a different vein. With the assistance of a qualified staff member, the IV drip should be turned off for at least 2 minutes and the first 5 mL of blood drawn must be discarded because it may be contaminated with IV fluid. A new syringe is then used for the specimen collection. If a coagulation test is ordered, an additional 5 mL of blood should be drawn prior to collecting the coagulation test specimen because IV lines are frequently flushed with heparin. This additional blood can be used for other tests, if they have been ordered. When blood is collected from an arm containing an IV drip, it must be noted on the requisition form.

USING CENTRAL VENOUS CATHETERS

Blood may also be obtained from **indwelling lines** called central venous catheters (**CVCs**). This procedure *must* be performed by personnel who have received training in these collection procedures, and physician authorization is required as well. Specific procedures must be followed for flushing the **catheters** with saline, and possibly heparin, when the blood collection is completed. Sterile technique procedures must be strictly adhered to when entering IV lines because they provide a direct path for infectious organisms to enter the patient's bloodstream.

Examples of CVCs include Hickman and Groshong catheters, which are surgically implanted; subcutaneous, jugular, and subclavian catheters; and more temporary devices such as Mediport and Port-a-Cath (Fig. 7–1). **Heparin locks** are inserted to provide a means for administering frequently required medications and for obtaining blood specimens. They do not contain an IV line, but techniques for using heparin locks for collecting blood specimens are similar to those for CVCs.

When IV fluids are being administered through the CVC, the flow should be stopped for 5 minutes prior to collecting the sample. Syringes larger than 20 mL should not be used because the high negative pressure produced may collapse the catheter walls. At all times, the first 5 mL of blood must be discarded and a new syringe must be used to collect the sample. Drawing coagulation tests from a venous catheter is not recommended, but if this is necessary, the tests should be collected after 20 mL of blood have been discarded or used for other tests.

The order of tube fill may vary slightly to accommodate the amount of blood that must be drawn prior to a coagulation test. As with other procedures, blood cultures are always collected first. If blood cultures are ordered, the draw will satisfy the additional discard needed for coagulation tests. Therefore, the order of draw or fill is as follows:

1 First syringe—5-mL discard
2 Second syringe—blood cultures
3 Third syringe—anticoagulated tubes (blue, lavender, green, and gray)
4 Clotted tubes (red and SST)

If blood cultures are not ordered, the coagulation tests (blue top tube) can be collected with a new syringe after the other specimens have been collected using the

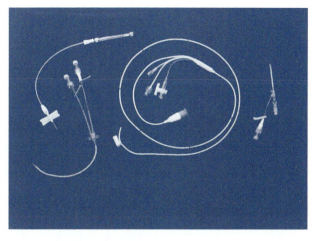

FIGURE 7–1   Examples of central venous catheters.

order just shown. PCTs are frequently responsible for assisting the person who is collecting blood from the CVC and should understand these specimen collection requirements. PCTs may also be trained to perform these collections. The source of the specimen should be noted on the requisition form.

Patients receiving renal dialysis have a permanent surgical fusion of an artery and a vein called a ***fistula*** in one arm, and this arm should be avoided for venipuncture because of the possibility of infection. The dialysis patient may also have a temporary connection between an artery and a vein formed by a ***cannula*** that contains a special T-tube connector with a diaphragm for drawing blood. Only specifically trained personnel are authorized to draw blood from a cannula.

Cleansing the Site

Certain procedures, primarily blood cultures and arterial blood gases, require that the site be cleansed with an antiseptic stronger than isopropyl alcohol (see Unit 8). The most frequently used solutions are povidone-iodine or chlorhexidine gluconate, which is used for persons allergic to iodine.

Alcohol should not be used to cleanse the site prior to drawing a blood alcohol level. Thoroughly cleansing the site with soap and water will ensure the least amount of interference, and some institutions find iodine to be acceptable.

Examination of Puncture Equipment

When using a syringe, the plunger is pulled back and pushed forward while the protective cap is still on the needle to ensure that it will move freely when the vein has been entered. The protective cap on the needle is then removed and the needle point examined for imperfections just prior to insertion.

Performing the Venipunctures

Although venipuncture is most frequently performed using an evacuated tube system, it may be necessary to use a syringe or a butterfly apparatus to better control the pressure applied to the delicate veins found in pediatric and elderly patients or when drawing from hand veins.

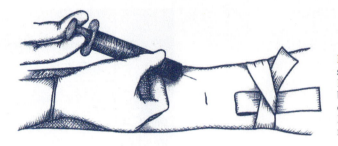

FIGURE 7–2   Venipuncture using a syringe. (From Strasinger, SK, and Di Lorenzo, MA: Phlebotomy Workbook for the Multiskilled Healthcare Professional. FA Davis, Philadelphia, 1996, p. 229, with permission.)

USING A SYRINGE

Except for a few minor differences, the procedure for drawing blood using a syringe is the same as when using an evacuated tube system. Blood is withdrawn from the vein by slowly pulling on the plunger of the syringe using the hand that is free after the vein is anchored, as shown in Figure 7–2. One advantage to using a syringe is that when the vein is entered, blood will appear in the hub of the needle and the plunger can then be pulled back at a speed that corresponds to the rate of blood flow into the syringe. Pulling the plunger back faster than the rate of blood flow may cause the walls of the vein to collapse (see Fig. 7–4*F*) and can cause hemolysis. Again, it is important to anchor the hand holding the syringe firmly on the patient's arm so that the needle will not move when the plunger is pulled.

Ideally, the size of the syringe used should correspond to the amount of blood needed; with small veins that collapse easily, however, it may be necessary to fill two or more smaller syringes. This will require assistance, because blood from the filled syringe must be transferred to the appropriate tubes while the second syringe is being filled. It is important that blood be added to anticoagulated tubes as soon as possible. Prior to exchanging syringes, gauze must be placed on the patient's arm under the needle because blood will leak from the hub of the needle during the exchange.

As discussed in Unit 5, blood is transferred from the syringe to evacuated tubes, following the prescribed order of fill, by puncturing the rubber tube stopper using a one-handed technique and allowing the blood to flow slowly into the tube. The entire assembly is then discarded into a sharps container.

USING A BUTTERFLY

All routine venipuncture procedures used with evacuated tubes and syringes also apply to blood collection using a butterfly. By folding the plastic needle attachments ("wings") upward while inserting the needle, the angle of insertion can be lowered to 10 to 15 degrees, thereby facilitating entry into small veins. Blood will appear in the tubing when the vein is entered. The needle can then be threaded securely into the vein and kept in place by holding the plastic wings against the patient's arm. It may be helpful to have a piece of tape available in case two hands are needed for the collection. Depending on the type of butterfly apparatus used, blood is collected into evacuated tubes or a syringe. To prevent hemolysis when using a small (23-gauge) needle, pediatric-size vacuum tubes should be used.

When disposing of the butterfly apparatus, use extreme care; many accidental sticks result from unexpected movement of the tubing. Accidents can be prevented by placing the needle into a sharps container prior to removing the vacuum tube adapter or the syringe and then allowing the tubing to fall into the container when the adapter or syringe is removed. Always hold a butterfly apparatus by the wings, not by the tubing. Use of an apparatus with automatic resheathing capability also prevents problems. Do not push the apparatus manually into a full sharps container.

The venipuncture procedure using a butterfly is shown in Figure 7–3.

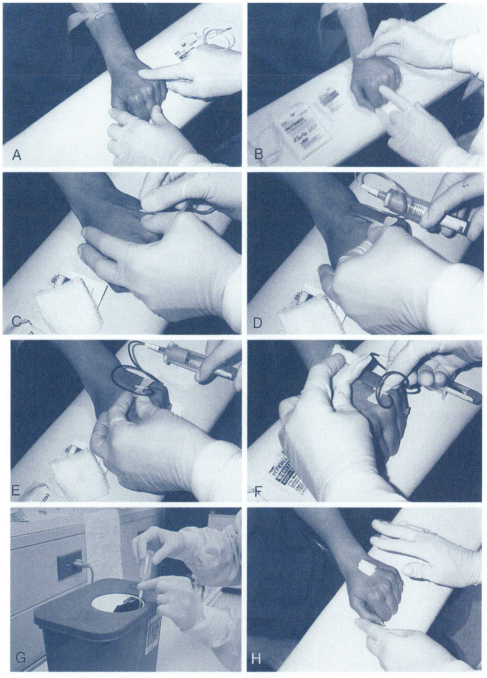

FIGURE 7–3   Venipuncture using a butterfly. *A*, Hand vein palpation. *B*, Cleansing the puncture site. *C*, Inserting the needle. *D*, Advancing an evacuated tube into the adapter. *E*, Blood flow through the butterfly apparatus. *F*, Removing the needle. *G*, Disposing of the butterfly apparatus. *H*, Patient's hand with pressure bandage. (From Strasinger, SK, and Di Lorenzo, MA: Phlebotomy Workbook for the Multiskilled Healthcare Professional. FA Davis, Philadelphia, 1996, p. 231, with permission.)

Complications

Not all venipunctures result in the immediate appearance of blood; in many instances, however, this is only a temporary setback that can be corrected by slight movement of the needle. As shown in Figure 7–4*B* and *C*, the bevel of the needle may be resting against the wall of the vein, and rotating the needle a quarter of a turn will allow blood

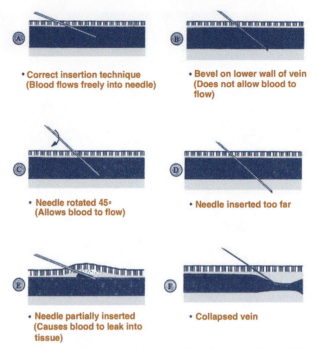

- Correct insertion technique
  (Blood flows freely into needle)

- Bevel on lower wall of vein
  (Does not allow blood to flow)

- Needle rotated 45°
  (Allows blood to flow)

- Needle inserted too far

- Needle partially inserted
  (Causes blood to leak into tissue)

- Collapsed vein

FIGURE 7–4 Possible reasons for failure to obtain blood. (From Strasinger, SK, and Di Lorenzo, MA: Phlebotomy Workbook for the Multiskilled Healthcare Professional. FA Davis, Philadelphia, 1996, p. 232, with permission.)

to flow freely. Pulling back a needle that has passed through a vein or slowly advancing a needle that is not fully in a vein also may correct the problem (Fig. 7–4D and E). Gentle touching of the area around the needle with a cleansed gloved finger may determine the positions of the vein and the needle and allow the needle to be redirected slightly. If the needle appears to be in the vein, a faulty vacuum tube may be the problem and a new tube should be used. The vein also may have collapsed (Fig. 7–4F) as a result of pressure from the vacuum tube, and use of a smaller vacuum tube may remedy the situation. If it does not help, another puncture must be performed, possibly using a syringe or a butterfly. It is important for PCTs to know these techniques; beginners have a tendency to remove the needle immediately when blood does not appear. The patient must then be stuck again when it may not have been necessary.

Movement of the needle should not include vigorous probing because this not only is painful to the patient but also enlarges the puncture site and blood may leak into the tissues and form a hematoma.

When blood is not obtained from the initial venipuncture, the PCT should select another site, either in the other arm or below the previous site, and repeat the procedure using a new needle. If the second puncture is not successful, another attempt should not be made by the same person. Another person from the unit staff or possibly a phlebotomist from the clinical laboratory should attempt to collect the specimen.

HEMOLYZED SPECIMENS

Hemolysis is detected by the presence of pink or red plasma or serum. Rupture of the red blood cell membrane releases cellular contents into the serum or plasma and produces interference with many test results, so that the specimen may need to be redrawn. Table 7–2 summarizes the major tests affected by hemolysis.

Errors in performance of the venipuncture account for the majority of hemolyzed specimens and include:

1 Using a needle with too small a diameter (above 23 gauge)
2 Using a small needle with a large vacuum tube

TABLE 7–2 **Laboratory Tests Affected by Hemolysis**

Seriously Affected	Noticeably Affected	Slightly Affected
Potassium (K)	Serum iron (Fe)	Phosphorus (P)
Lactic dehydrogenase (LD)	Alanine aminotransferase (ALT)	Total protein (TP)
Aspartate aminotransferase (AST)	Thyroxine (T_4)	Albumin
Complete blood count (CBC)		Magnesium (Mg)
		Calcium (Ca)
		Acid phosphatase

3 Using an improperly attached needle on a syringe so that frothing occurs as the blood enters the syringe
4 Pulling the plunger of a syringe back too fast
5 Drawing blood from a hematoma
6 Vigorously mixing tubes
7 Forcing blood from a syringe into a vacuum tube
8 Failing to allow the blood to run down the side of the tube when using a syringe to fill it
9 Collecting specimens from IV lines when not recommended by the manufacturer
10 Applying the tourniquet too close to the puncture site or for too long

Removal of the Needle

Improper technique when removing the needle is a frequent (although not the only) cause of the appearance of a hematoma on the patient's arm. Errors in technique that cause blood to leak or to be forced into the surrounding tissue and produce hematomas include the following:

1 Failing to remove the tourniquet prior to removing the needle
2 Applying inadequate pressure to the site after removal of the needle
3 Excessive probing to obtain blood
4 Failing to insert the needle far enough into the vein
5 Inserting the needle through the vein
6 Bending the arm while applying pressure

Under normal conditions the elasticity of the vein walls prevents the leakage of blood around the needle during venipuncture. A decrease in the elasticity of the vein walls in older patients causes them to be more prone to developing hematomas. Using small-bore needles and firmly anchoring the veins prior to needle insertion may prevent a hematoma.

Disposal of the Needle

There should be no deviations from the methods for needle disposal discussed in Unit 5.

Labeling the Tubes

Information contained on the labels of tubes from unidentified patients must follow the protocol used by the institution to provide a temporary but clear designation of the patient. When available, stickers from the patient's ID band should be attached to all specimens for the blood bank.

If preprinted labels are being used, it is important to double-check the name on the label while attaching it to the tube.

Bandaging the Patient's Arm

Patients receiving anticoagulant medications or large amounts of aspirin, or patients with coagulation disorders may continue to bleed after pressure has been applied for 5 minutes. The PCT should continue to apply pressure until the bleeding has stopped. The nurse should be notified in cases of excessive bleeding.

In the case of an accidental arterial puncture, which usually can be detected by the appearance of unusually red blood that spurts into the tube, the PCT, not the patient, should apply pressure to the site for 10 minutes. The fact that the specimen is arterial blood should be recorded on the requisition form, and a supervisor should be notified.

Some patients are allergic to adhesive bandages, and it may be necessary to wrap gauze around the arm prior to applying the adhesive tape. Omitting the bandage in these patients and those with hairy arms is another option, particularly if it is requested by the patient. Bandages are not recommended for children under 2 years old because children may put bandages in their mouths.

Leaving the Patient

Patients often request that the PCT change the position of their bed or provide them with a drink of water. This is acceptable only if the PCT is currently providing care for the patient and knows that the patient's condition will not be compromised. If you are unfamiliar with the patient, explain that you will inform the nursing station of the request and leave the room in the condition in which you found it (bed and bed rails in the same position).

Completing the Venipuncture

Specimens brought to the laboratory may be rejected if conditions are present that would affect the validity of the test results.

Major reasons for specimen rejection are as follows:

1 Unlabeled or mislabeled specimens
2 Inadequate volume
3 Collection in the wrong tube
4 Hemolysis
5 Clotted blood in an anticoagulant tube
6 Improper handling during transport, such as not chilling the specimen
7 Specimens without a requisition form
8 Obviously contaminated specimen containers

PCTs should make sure that none of these conditions exists for the specimens they deliver or send to the laboratory.

BIBLIOGRAPHY

National Committee for Clinical Laboratory Standards Approved Standard H3-A3: Procedures for the Collection of Diagnostic Blood Specimens by Venipuncture. NCCLS, Villanova, PA, 1991.

National Committee for Clinical Laboratory Standards Approved Guideline H18-A: Procedures for the Handling and Processing of Blood Specimens. NCCLS, Villanova, PA, 1990.

Read, DC, Viera, H, and Arkin, C: Effect of drawing blood specimens proximal to an in-place but discontinued intravenous solution. Am J Clin Pathol 90:702–706, 1988.

Statland, BE, and Per Winkle, MD: Preparing patients and specimens for laboratory testing. In Henry, JB (ed): Clinical Diagnosis and Management by Laboratory Methods. WB Saunders, Philadelphia, 1991.

STUDY QUESTIONS

1. How should a PCT greet an unconscious patient?

   _____

   _____

2. When should the needle be removed if the patient develops syncope?

   _____

3. Name a test that can be affected by each of the following patient activities:

   a. Strenuous exercise _____

   b. Smoking _____

   c. Posture _____

   d. Prolonged fasting _____

4. True or False. A patient can refuse to have blood drawn. _____

5. Why should extra evacuated tubes be available when performing a venipuncture?

   _____

6. When a blood pressure cuff is used as a tourniquet, how will inflation of the cuff to a pressure above the patient's systolic pressure affect blood flow?

   _____

   _____

7. List four test results that are affected by prolonged tourniquet application.

   a. _____

   b. _____

   c. _____

   d. _____

8. If a vein is not easily located in the patient's dominant arm, what is the first thing the PCT should do?

   _____

9. List four techniques to enhance the prominence of veins that are hard to find.

   a. _____

   b. _____

   c. _____

   d. _____

10. How does an occluded vein feel?

   _____

11. How does a mastectomy affect the adjacent blood supply?

_____

_____

12. Indicate whether each of the following is an acceptable or unacceptable venipuncture site by placing an "A" or a "U" in front of the statement. Explain all "U" answers, using "contamination," "infection," "hemolysis," or "decreased blood flow" in the appropriate space.

If U

a. _____ Antecubital area above an IV   _____
drip that has been discontinued
for 5 minutes

b. _____ Wrist below an antecubital   _____
hematoma

c. _____ Antecubital area containing   _____
a tattoo

d. _____ Vein surrounded by a   _____
hematoma

e. _____ Wrist below an IV drip that has   _____
been discontinued for 5 minutes

f. _____ Wrist containing scar tissue   _____

g. _____ Arm with a fistula   _____

h. _____ Right arm of a patient with a   _____
right mastectomy

i. _____ Veins on the back of the hand   _____

j. _____ Vein that feels hard   _____

13. What precaution must be taken when coagulation tests are drawn from an indwelling line?

_____

14. List three site-cleansing solutions other than isopropyl alcohol and state a reason for their use.

Solution   *Reason*

a. _____   _____

b. _____   _____

c. _____   _____

15. State two problems that may occur if the plunger of the syringe is pulled back too fast.

a. _____

b. _____

16. How can hemolysis be avoided when using a butterfly?

_____

_____

17. List three reasons why blood may not be obtained even though the needle is in the vein.

a. _____

b. _____

c. _____

18. List two tests that are seriously affected by hemolysis. Do the same for tests that are noticeably and slightly affected.

	Seriously	*Noticeably*	*Slightly*
a.	_____	_____	_____
b.	_____	_____	_____

19. List four causes of hematomas.

a. _____

b. _____

c. _____

d. _____

20. How can an arterial puncture be detected and what should the PCT do?

_____

_____

21. List six possible causes of specimen rejection and state a *specific* example of each.

a. _____

_____

b. _____

_____

c. _____

_____

d. _____

_____

e. _____

_____

f. _____

_____

VENIPUNCTURE
COMPLICATIONS EXERCISE

1. An unidentified patient in the emergency room requires a transfusion. What precautions must the PCT take?

   _____

   _____

   _____

2. The PCT has a requisition to collect a chemistry profile and a prothrombin time (PT). No blood is obtained from the left antecubital area. The PCT then moves to the right antecubital area and obtains a full SST tube but cannot fill the light-blue tube. What should the PCT do next?

   _____

   _____

3. A patient has an IV drip running in the left forearm. From the following sites, indicate your first choice with a "1," your second choice with a "2," and an unacceptable site with an "X."

   a. _____ left wrist

   b. _____ left antecubital area

   c. _____ right antecubital area

4. A PCT with a requisition for a PT, CBC, and glucose on a patient who is difficult to draw obtains 7 mL of blood using a syringe. Assuming the PCT has a 2.7-mL light-blue top tube, a 3-mL lavender top tube, and a 3-mL red top tube, how should the blood be distributed?

   _____

   _____

   _____

5. The PCT is assisting the nurse to collect a PT, a CBC, and a chemistry profile from an IV line.

   a. How many and what size syringes are needed, and what is done with the blood collected in each?

   _____

   _____

   _____

   b. What should the PCT write on the requisition form?

   _____

6. A PCT needs to collect 20 mL of blood for serum chemistry tests and selects two 10-mL red top tubes. A successful puncture is performed; however, blood stops flowing when the first tube is only half full.

   a. Assuming the problem does not lie with the equipment, what is a possible reason for this?

   _____

   b. State two methods the PCT could use to collect the required amount of blood.

   _____

   _____

7. When collecting a specimen from an elderly patient using routine evacuated tube equipment, the PCT notices that the puncture site is beginning to swell.

   a. Why is this happening?

   _____

   b. What should the PCT do?

   _____

   c. How can the specimen be collected?

   _____

8. While a CBC is being collected, the patient develops syncope and the PCT immediately removes the needle and lowers the patient's head. Once the patient has recovered, the PCT labels the lavender top tube, which fortunately contains enough blood, and delivers it to the clinical laboratory. Many results from this specimen are markedly lower than those from the patient's previous CBC.

   a. How could the quality of the specimen have caused this discrepancy?

   _____

   _____

   b. How could the venipuncture complication have contributed to this error?

   _____

   _____

   c. Could the PCT have done anything differently? Explain your answer.

   _____

   _____

9. A nurse from the cardiac care unit reports that she is observing hematomas on the patients whenever PCT "X" is assigned to the floor. Considering the condition and treatment of the patients in this unit, what is the most probable error being made by PCT "X"? Explain your answer.

   _____

   _____

   _____

10. A PCT sends a properly labeled specimen with sufficient volume collected in a red top tube to the clinical laboratory for a potassium determination. Fifteen minutes later the chemistry supervisor calls and asks that the specimen be redrawn.

a. Why did the chemistry section reject this specimen?

_____

b. What precautions should the PCT take with the second specimen?

_____

_____

_____

EVALUATION OF VENIPUNCTURE TECHNIQUE USING A SYRINGE

RATING SYSTEM   2 = Satisfactory   1 = Needs improvement   0 = Incorrect/did not perform

_____ **1.** Examines requisition form

_____ **2.** Greets patient, states procedure to be done

_____ **3.** Identifies patient verbally

_____ **4.** Examines patient's ID band

_____ **5.** Compares requisition information with ID band

_____ **6.** Puts on gloves

_____ **7.** Selects correct tubes and equipment for procedure

_____ **8.** Assembles and conveniently places equipment

_____ **9.** Positions patient's arm

_____ **10.** Applies tourniquet

_____ **11.** Identifies vein by palpation

_____ **12.** Releases tourniquet

_____ **13.** Cleanses site and allows it to air dry

_____ **14.** Checks plunger movement

_____ **15.** Reapplies tourniquet

_____ **16.** Does not touch puncture site with unclean finger

_____ **17.** Anchors vein below puncture site

_____ **18.** Smoothly enters vein at appropriate angle with bevel up

_____ **19.** Does not move needle when plunger is retracted

_____ **20.** Collects appropriate amount of blood

_____ **21.** Releases tourniquet

_____ **22.** Covers puncture site with gauze

_____ **23.** Removes the needle smoothly and applies pressure

_____ **24.** Uses correct and safe technique to fill tubes

_____ **25.** Fills tubes in correct order

_____ **26.** Mixes anticoagulated tubes promptly

_____ **27.** Disposes of the needle and syringe in sharps container

_____ **28.** Labels tubes

_____ **29.** Examines puncture site

_____ **30.** Applies bandage

_____ **31.** Disposes of used supplies

_____ **32.** Removes gloves and washes hands

_____ **33.** Thanks patient

_____ **34.** Converses appropriately with patient during procedure

Total points _____

Maximum points = 68

COMMENTS

EVALUATION OF VENIPUNCTURE TECHNIQUE USING A BUTTERFLY

RATING SYSTEM   2 = Satisfactory   1 = Needs improvement   0 = Incorrect/did not perform

_____ **1.** Examines requisition form

_____ **2.** Greets patient, states procedure to be done

_____ **3.** Identifies patient verbally

_____ **4.** Examines patient's ID band

_____ **5.** Compares requisition information with ID band

_____ **6.** Puts on gloves

_____ **7.** Selects correct tubes and equipment for procedure

_____ **8.** Assembles and conveniently places equipment

_____ **9.** Positions patient's hand

_____ **10.** Applies tourniquet

_____ **11.** Identifies vein by palpation

_____ **12.** Releases tourniquet

_____ **13.** Cleanses site and allows it to air dry

_____ **14.** Reapplies tourniquet

_____ **15.** Does not touch puncture site with unclean finger

_____ **16.** Anchors vein below puncture site

_____ **17.** Holds needle appropriately

_____ **18.** Smoothly enters vein at an appropriate angle with bevel up

_____ **19.** Maintains needle securely in vein

_____ **20.** Smoothly operates syringe or vacuum tube adapter

_____ **21.** Fills tubes in the correct order

_____ **22.** Mixes anticoagulated tubes promptly

_____ **23.** Collects appropriate amount of blood

_____ **24.** Releases tourniquet

_____ **25.** Covers puncture site with gauze

_____ **26.** Removes the needle smoothly and applies pressure

_____ **27.** Disposes of apparatus in sharps container

_____ **28.** Labels tubes

_____ **29.** Examines puncture site

_____ **30.** Applies bandage

_____ **31.** Disposes of used supplies

_____ **32.** Removes gloves and washes hands

_____ **33.** Thanks patient

_____ **34.** Converses appropriately with patient during procedure

Total points _____

Maximum points = 68

COMMENTS

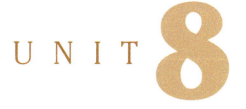

UNIT 8

SPECIAL VENIPUNCTURE COLLECTION

KEY TERMS

- *Aseptic* — Free of contamination by microorganisms
- *Basal state* — Metabolic condition after 12 hours of fasting and lack of exercise
- *Chain of custody* — Documentation of the collection and handling of forensic specimens
- *Diurnal* — Variations occurring during the day
- *Fasting* — Abstinence from food and liquids (except water) for a specified period
- *Lipemic* — Pertaining to turbidity from lipids
- *Peak level* — Specimen collected when a serum drug level is highest
- *Trough level* — Specimen collected when a serum drug level is lowest

Certain laboratory tests require the use of techniques that are not part of the routine venipuncture procedure. These special techniques may involve patient preparation, timing of specimen collection, venipuncture techniques, and specimen handling. PCTs must know when these techniques are required, how to perform them, and how specimen integrity is affected when they are not performed properly.

Fasting Specimens

Normal values (reference ranges) for laboratory tests are determined using specimens from a normal, representative sample of volunteers who usually have had nothing to eat or drink, except water (*fasting*), and who have refrained from strenuous exercise for 12 hours (*basal state*). Not all tests are affected by fasting and exercise, as evidenced by the collection and testing of specimens throughout the day. Many diagnostic results can be obtained at any time. However, the best comparison of patients' results with normal values can be made when the patients are in the basal state. This explains why PCTs frequently begin collecting blood specimens very early in the morning and why the majority of outpatients are told to arrive at collection areas as soon as they are open.

The test results most critically affected by nonfasting are those from glucose and triglyceride tests. When a fasting specimen is requested, it is the responsibility of the PCT to verify that the patient has been fasting for the required length of time. If the patient has not fasted, it must be reported to a supervisor and noted on the requisition form.

Serum or plasma collected from patients shortly after a meal may appear cloudy (*lipemic*) because of the presence of fatty compounds. Lipemia will interfere with many test results.

Timed Specimens

Blood collections are frequently requested for specific times. The reasons for timed specimens include the following:

1 Measurement of the body's ability to metabolize a particular substance
2 Monitoring of changes in a patient's condition (such as a steady decrease in hemoglobin)
3 Determination of blood levels of medications
4 Measurement of substances that exhibit *diurnal* variation (normal changes in blood levels at different times of the day)

PCTs should arrange their schedules to ensure that they are available at the specified time and should record the time of collection on the requisition and the specimen tube.

The most frequently encountered timed specimens are discussed in this unit. Other diagnostic procedures may also require timed specimens, and any request for a timed specimen should be strictly followed.

TWO-HOUR POSTPRANDIAL GLUCOSE

Comparison of a patient's fasting glucose level (**FBS**) with a glucose level 2 hours after eating a meal or ingesting a measured amount of glucose is used to evaluate diabetes mellitus. Ideally, the glucose level should return to the fasting level within 2 hours.

When caring for a patient for whom this procedure is ordered, the PCT must confirm that the patient has ingested a complete meal and must collect the **postprandial** (**pp**) specimen at the required time. When working with outpatients, the PCT must emphasize the importance of eating a full meal followed by fasting for 2 hours and the necessity of returning to the collection area in time to have the blood drawn exactly 2 hours after the meal is completed.

GLUCOSE TOLERANCE TEST

The glucose tolerance test (GTT) is a procedure performed for the diagnosis of diabetes mellitus (hyperglycemia) and for the evaluation of persons with symptoms associated with low blood glucose (**hypoglycemia**). PCTs may be responsible for the administration of this procedure, including instructing patients, administering the glucose solution, scheduling samples, and collecting and organizing samples that consist of timed blood collections and possibly urine collections. The procedure is scheduled for 3 hours to diagnose diabetes mellitus and 5 or 6 hours to evaluate hypoglycemia.

GTT procedures should be scheduled to begin between 0700 and 0900, because glucose levels exhibit a diurnal variation. The PCT draws a fasting glucose and may request that the patient collect a urine specimen. The fasting blood specimen is tested prior to continuing the procedure to determine whether the patient can safely be given a large amount of glucose. The PCT then asks the patient to drink a standardized amount of flavored glucose solution within a period of 5 minutes. Timing for the remaining GTT specimens begins when the patient finishes drinking the glucose. Sample schedules are shown in Table 8–1. Notice that all timing is based on completion of the glucose drink.

Outpatients are given a copy of the schedule and instructed to continue fasting, to drink water to facilitate urine collection, and to return to the drawing station at the scheduled times. Patients are usually instructed to remain in the outpatient area. Timing of inpatient collections is the responsibility of the PCT.

Corresponding labels containing routinely required information and specimen order in the test sequence, such as 1 hour, 2 hour, and so on, are placed on the specimens. Blood specimens that will not be tested until the end of the sequence should be collected in gray top tubes. Timing of specimen collection is critical because test results are related to the scheduled times; any discrepancies should be noted on the requisition. Consistency of venipuncture or dermal puncture must also be maintained, because glucose values differ between the two types of blood.

Some patients may not be able to tolerate the glucose solution and if vomiting occurs, the time of the vomiting must be reported to a supervisor and the physician must be contacted for a decision concerning whether to continue the test. Vomiting early in the procedure is considered to be the most critical. During scheduled sample collections, PCTs should also observe patients for any changes in their condition, such as dizziness, that might indicate a reaction to the glucose and should report any changes to a supervisor.

TABLE 8–1   **Sample Glucose Tolerance Test Schedule**

Test Procedure	3-Hour Test	6-Hour Test
Fasting blood	0700	0700
Patient finishes glucose	0800	0800
1/2-hour specimen	0830	0830
1-hour specimen	0900	0900
2-hour specimen	1000	1000
3-hour specimen	1100	1100
4-hour specimen		1200
5-hour specimen		1300
6-hour specimen		1400

DIURNAL VARIATION

The substances primarily affected by diurnal variation are corticosteroids, hormones, serum iron, and glucose. PCTs are often requested to draw specimens for these tests at specific times, usually corresponding to the peak diurnal level. Certain variations can be substantial. Plasma cortisol levels drawn between 0800 and 1000 will be twice as high as levels drawn at 1600, and serum iron levels drawn in the morning are one-third higher than those drawn in the evening. Consequently, requests for plasma cortisol levels frequently specify that the test be drawn between 0800 and 1000 or at 1600. If the specimen cannot be collected at the specified time, the physician should be notified and the test rescheduled for the next day.

THERAPEUTIC DRUG MONITORING (TDM)

The fact that medications affect all patients differently often results in the need to change dosages or medications. Some medications can reach toxic levels in patients who do not metabolize or excrete them within an expected time frame. Likewise, some patients metabolize and excrete medications at an increased rate. To ensure patient safety and medication effectiveness, the blood levels of many therapeutic drugs are monitored.

Examples of frequently monitored therapeutic drugs are digoxin, gentamicin, tobramycin, vancomycin, and theophylline. Random specimens are occasionally requested; the most beneficial levels, however, are those drawn before the next dose is given (***trough level***) and shortly after the medication is given (***peak level***). Trough levels are collected right before the drug is to be given and represent the lowest level in the blood. Ideally, trough levels should be tested prior to administering the next dose to ensure that the level is low enough for the patient to receive more medication safely. The time for collecting peak levels varies with the medication and the method of administration (IV, intramuscular, or oral). Information from the drug manufacturers provides the recommended times for collection of peak levels. To ensure correct documentation of the peak and trough levels, requisitions and specimen tube labels should include the time and method of administration of the last dose given, as well as the time that the specimen is drawn.

Blood Cultures

One of the most difficult phlebotomy procedures is collection of blood cultures. This is because of the strict ***aseptic*** technique required and the need to collect multiple specimens in special containers. Blood cultures are requested for patients when symptoms of fever and chills indicate a possible infection of the blood by pathogenic microorganisms (**septicemia**). The patient's initial diagnosis is often fever of unknown origin (**FUO**).

Blood cultures are usually ordered stat or as timed collections. Isolation of microorganisms from the blood is often difficult because of the small number of organisms needed to cause symptoms. Specimens are usually collected in sets of two or three drawn either 1 hour apart or just before the patient's temperature reaches its highest point (spike). The concentration of microorganisms fluctuates and is often highest just before the patient's temperature spikes. This explains why collections may be ordered at 1-hour intervals or ordered stat if a pattern has been observed in the patient's temperature chart. If antibiotics are to be started immediately, the sets are drawn at the same time from different sites. Specimens collected from multiple sites at the same time serve as controls for possible contamination and must be labeled as to the collection site, such as right arm antecubital vein, and their number in the series (#1,

#2, or #3). A known skin contaminant must be cultured from at least two of the sites for it to be considered a possible pathogen.

Blood for culture may be drawn directly into bottles containing culture media, transferred to the bottles from a syringe, or drawn into sterile tubes containing anticoagulant and transferred to culture media in the laboratory. Some institutions require that a new needle be placed on the syringe when transferring blood from a syringe to blood culture bottles. Because of the increased risk of contact with contaminated needles, this practice has been discontinued in many institutions. Studies have shown little difference in contamination rates when needles are not changed. An anticoagulant must be present in the tube or the medium to prevent microorganisms from being trapped within a clot, where they might be undetected. Blood culture bottles must therefore be mixed after the blood is added. The anticoagulant sodium polyanetholesulfonate (SPS) is used for blood cultures because it does not inhibit bacterial growth and may in fact enhance it by inhibiting the action of phagocytes, complement, and some antibiotics. Other anticoagulants should not be used. Some blood culture collection systems have antimicrobial removal devices (**ARDs**) containing a resin that inactivates antibiotics. As shown in Figure 8–1, a variety of blood culture collection systems are available.

Venipuncture technique for collecting blood cultures follows routine procedure with the exception of the increased requirements for asepsis. Cleansing of the venipuncture site begins by vigorous scrubbing of the site with alcohol, starting in the center and progressing outward in concentric circles. The alcohol is allowed to dry; then 2% iodine or povidone-iodine is applied in the same manner. The iodine must be allowed to dry for 1 minute. If the site must be touched after cleansing, the gloved palpating finger must be cleaned in the same manner. The tops of the collection containers are also cleaned with iodine at this time and then wiped with alcohol just prior to inoculation. To prevent irritation of the patient's arm, the iodine is removed with alcohol when the procedure is complete.

Two specimens are routinely collected for each blood culture set, one to be incubated aerobically and the other to be incubated anaerobically. When a syringe is used, the anaerobic bottle should be inoculated first to prevent possible exposure to air.

Because the number of microorganisms present in the blood is often small, the amount of blood inoculated into each container is critical. There should be at least a 1:10 ratio of blood to medium. PCTs should follow the instructions for the system being used. Pediatric patients usually have a higher concentration of microorganisms, so a smaller volume of blood can be used.

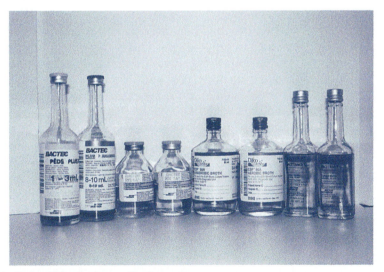

FIGURE 8–1 Types of blood culture collection systems.

Special Specimen Handling Procedures

COLD AGGLUTININS

Cold agglutinins are **autoantibodies** primarily produced by persons infected with *Mycoplasma pneumoniae* (atypical pneumonia). The autoantibodies react with red blood cells at temperatures below body temperature. Detection of a high titer of cold agglutinins in a patient's serum aids in the diagnosis of an *M. pneumoniae* infection.

Because the cold agglutinins in the serum attach to RBCs when the blood cools to below body temperature, the specimen must be kept warm until the serum can be separated from the cells. Specimens are collected in tubes that have been warmed in an incubator at 37°C for 30 minutes and that contain no additives or gels that could interfere with the test. The PCT can carry the warmed tube to the patient's room in a tightly closed fist or a prewarmed container, collect the specimen as quickly as possible, and immediately deliver the specimen to the laboratory in the same manner. Failure to keep a specimen warm prior to serum separation will produce falsely decreased test results.

CHILLED SPECIMENS

Specimens for arterial blood gases, ammonia, lactic acid, pyruvate, gastrin, ACTH, parathyroid hormone, and some coagulation studies must be chilled immediately after collection to prevent deterioration. For adequate chilling, the specimen must be placed in crushed ice or a mixture of ice and water at the bedside. Placing a specimen in or on ice cubes is not acceptable because uniform chilling will not occur. It is important that these specimens be immediately delivered to the laboratory for processing.

SPECIMENS SENSITIVE TO LIGHT

Exposure to light will decrease the concentration of bilirubin, beta carotene, vitamins A and B_6, and **porphyrins**. Specimens can be protected by wrapping the tubes in aluminum foil.

LEGAL (FORENSIC) SPECIMENS

When drawing specimens for test results that may be used as evidence in legal proceedings, extreme care must be taken to follow the stated policies exactly. Documentation of specimen handling, called the ***chain of custody***, is essential. It begins with patient identification and continues until testing is completed and results are reported. Special forms are provided for this documentation, and special containers and seals may be required (Fig. 8–2). Documentation must include the date, time, and identification of each person handling the specimen. Specimens should not be left sitting on a counter unattended. Patient identification and specimen collection should take place in the presence of a witness, often a law enforcement officer. Identification requires specific documents and may require photographs, fingerprints, or heel prints. The tests requested most frequently are alcohol and drug levels and DNA analysis.

As stated in Unit 7, when collecting blood alcohol levels, the site should be cleansed with soap and water or a nonalcoholic antiseptic solution. To prevent the escape of the volatile alcohol into the atmosphere, tubes should be filled completely and not left uncapped for longer than is necessary.

INSTRUCTIONS FOR SUBMITTING SAMPLES
Section A – Specimen Collection: Fill out section A1 and an AML Request Form completely. Label all specimen containers with the patient name, date of collection and a peel–off label from the AML request form. Place dated and initialed security seals over the openings of the containers. If possible, have a witness sign. Have the patient (donor) sign Section A2, line 1 Received From line. The collector must also date and sign the form on the Received By line.

Section B – Specimen Transfers: When transferring specimens(s) the collector must sign line B1. Each person receiving specimen(s) must sign on the Received By line. Indicate job title, and date and time received. The condition of the specimen(s) should be noted by checking the appropriate box. The condition of the specimen(s) may be unacceptable for the following reasons: broken container or substantial leakage, torn seal(s), improper collection or storage for requested tests.   Indicate under NOTE why the condition is unacceptable. The person that signs the Received By line is responsible for the security of the specimen(s) until the next person or secure area receives it. If the specimen(s) is being placed in a secure area, indicate location on the Received By line. Also indicate date and time.

A1. Patient Name _____   Age _____   Sex _____

   Client Name _____   Client Number_____

   Date_____Time of Collection _____   AML Peel Off Sticker # _____

   Type and Number of Specimens_____

   Collection Witness Signature (if applicable) _____

A 2   Received From: (Patient or Authorized Signature) _____

         Received By (Collector) _____Date/Time _____

B   1. Received From (Collector): _____ | Condition of Specimen
                                                                                  | Acceptable   ☐
        _____ | Unacceptable   ☐
        Received By   Title: Date/Time | NOTES: _____

B   2. Received From: _____ | Condition of Specimen
                                                                                  | Acceptable   ☐
        _____ | Unacceptable   ☐
        Received By   Title: Date/Time | NOTES: _____

B   3. Received From: _____ | Condition of Specimen
                                                                                  | Acceptable   ☐
        _____ | Unacceptable   ☐
        Received By   Title: Date/Time | NOTES: _____

B   4. Received From: _____ | Condition of Specimen
                                                                                  | Acceptable   ☐
        _____ | Unacceptable   ☐
        Received By   Title: Date/Time | NOTES: _____

B   5. Received From: _____ | Condition of Specimen
                                                                                  | Acceptable   ☐
        _____ | Unacceptable   ☐
        Received By   Title: Date/Time | NOTES: _____

COC–FORM
9/94

FIGURE 8–2   Sample chain-of-custody form. (Courtesy of Janet Beatey, American Medical Laboratories, Inc., Chantilly, VA.)

BIBLIOGRAPHY   Baron, EJ, Peterson, LR, and Finegold, SM: Diagnostic Microbiology. CV Mosby, St. Louis, 1994.
   National Committee for Clinical Laboratory Standards Approved Standard H3-A3: Procedures for the Collection of Diagnostic Blood Specimens by Venipuncture. NCCLS, Villanova, PA, 1991.
   National Committee for Clinical Laboratory Standards Approved Guideline H18-A: Procedures for the Handling and Processing of Blood Specimens. NCCLS, Villanova, PA, 1990.
   Kaplan, LA, and Pesce, AJ: Clinical Chemistry: Theory, Analysis, and Correlation, ed. 3. CV Mosby, St. Louis, 1996.

STUDY QUESTIONS

1. A possible reason for a lipemic serum is _____.

2. At 0730 the PCT receives requests for a cortisol level, an FBS, and a stat cross-match on three patients. In which order should these specimens be collected? Justify your answer.

   _____

   _____

   _____

3. Why should the fasting glucose specimen be tested prior to administering the glucose in a GTT?

   _____

   _____

4. Design a schedule for a 3-hour GTT, assuming the patient has a fasting specimen drawn at 0730 and completes drinking the glucose at 0745.

   _____

   _____

   _____

5. True or False. A PCT who cannot obtain the 1-hour sample in a GTT by venipuncture should perform a capillary puncture immediately. _____

6. When should trough and peak levels be drawn for TDM?

   a. Trough level _____

   b. Peak level _____

7. Which TDM level is used to determine whether the medication can safely be administered? _____

8. Give two reasons why blood cultures are frequently ordered stat.

   a. _____

   b. _____

9. The condition represented by a positive blood culture is called

   _____.

10. What is the purpose of inoculating two bottles of blood culture medium each time a specimen is drawn? Which bottle is inoculated first?

    _____

    _____

11. The major source of false-positive blood cultures is _____.

12. True or False. A specimen for cold agglutinins will have a falsely decreased value if it is chilled immediately after collection. _____ Why?

_____

_____

13. How will wrapping the collection tube in aluminum foil affect the results of a bilirubin test?

_____

14. How will the results of a serum gastrin test be affected if the specimen is held tightly in the PCT's fist when being delivered to the laboratory?

_____

15. How is documentation of patient identification, specimen collection, and specimen handling performed when forensic studies are requested?

_____

_____

_____

SPECIAL VENIPUNCTURE
COLLECTION EXERCISE

1. An outpatient comes to the collection station at 1300 with a requisition for a cardiac risk profile. Before collecting the specimen, what should the PCT ask the patient?

    _____

2. Requisitions are received requesting that specimens for hemoglobin and hematocrit be collected at 0800, 1200, 1600, and 2000 from a patient on a medical-surgical unit. Is there a reason for these requests and, if so, what is it?

    _____

    _____

3. An outpatient comes to the collection area with a requisition for an FBS and a 2-hour pp glucose. What should the PCT do?

    _____

    _____

    _____

4. A patient receiving a 3-hour GTT vomits 20 minutes before the 3-hour specimen is scheduled. What should the PCT do?

    _____

    _____

    _____

5. A patient is scheduled to have a cortisol level drawn and to go to physical therapy at 0900. How would the PCT handle this patient? Explain your answer.

    _____

    _____

    _____

6. Would it be unusual to receive requests to collect theophylline levels at 0800 and again at 1200? Explain your answer.

    _____

    _____

    _____

7. A PCT is requested to draw three blood cultures within 30 minutes from a patient in the ER. Is this a reasonable request? Why or why not?

    _____

    _____

    _____

8. A PCT collects two blood cultures in yellow top tubes and one in a lavender top tube and transfers each to bottles containing culture media. A known skin contaminant is cultured from two specimens.

   a. What errors in technique are indicated by this scenario?

   _____

   _____

   _____

   b. Why was one culture negative?

   _____

   _____

9. A PCT collects a stat ammonia level and is then asked to collect a cold agglutinin and a CBC from patients on opposite ends of the unit. The PCT sends the ammonia level to the laboratory in the pneumatic tube system, collects the cold agglutinin, goes to the other end of the unit and draws the CBC, and delivers both specimens to the laboratory. How will the quality of these test results be affected and why?

   _____

   _____

   _____

10. As the attorney for a defendant charged with having a blood alcohol level above the legal limit, you are questioning the PCT who collected the specimen.

    a. State three questions you would ask the PCT to try to discredit the test result.

    _____

    _____

    _____

    b. How should a competent PCT answer these questions?

    _____

    _____

    _____

EVALUATION OF BLOOD CULTURE COLLECTION TECHNIQUE

RATING SYSTEM   2 = Satisfactory   1 = Needs improvement   0 = Incorrect/did not perform

_____ **1.** Examines requisition form and identifies patient

_____ **2.** Correctly assembles equipment

_____ **3.** Applies tourniquet

_____ **4.** Selects puncture site

_____ **5.** Releases tourniquet

_____ **6.** Cleanses site with alcohol

_____ **7.** Cleanses site with iodine

_____ **8.** Puts on gloves

_____ **9.** Cleanses tops of blood culture containers

_____ **10.** Reapplies tourniquet

_____ **11.** Cleanses palpating finger if necessary

_____ **12.** Performs venipuncture

_____ **13.** Wipes tops of blood culture containers with alcohol

_____ **14.** Changes syringe needles if this is required

_____ **15.** Inoculates anaerobic container first

_____ **16.** Dispenses correct amount of blood into containers

_____ **17.** Mixes containers

_____ **18.** Disposes of used equipment and supplies

_____ **19.** Removes iodine from patient's arm

_____ **20.** Bandages patient's arm

_____ **21.** Correctly labels blood culture containers

_____ **22.** Observes overall aseptic technique

Total points _____

Maximum points = 44

COMMENTS

UNIT 9

DERMAL PUNCTURE

KEY TERMS

- *Calcaneus*   Heel bone
- *Dermal*   Pertaining to the skin
- *Ecchymosis*   Hemorrhagic discoloration
- *Microsample*   Sample of less than 1 mL
- *Neonatal*   Pertaining to the first 4 weeks after birth
- *Palmar*   Pertaining to the palm of the hand
- *Plantar*   Pertaining to the sole of the foot

Although venipuncture is the most frequently performed method of blood collection, it is not appropriate in all circumstances. Current laboratory instrumentation and procedures make it possible to perform a majority of laboratory tests on ***microsamples*** of blood obtained by ***dermal*** puncture on both pediatric and adult patients.

In most institutions, dermal puncture is the method of choice for collecting blood from infants and children under 2 years of age. Locating **superficial** veins large enough to accept even a small-gauge needle is difficult in these patients, and veins that are available may need to be reserved for IV therapy. Use of deep veins, such as the femoral vein, can be dangerous and may cause complications, including cardiac arrest, venous thrombosis, hemorrhage, damage to surrounding tissue and organs, infection, reflex **arteriospasm** (which can possibly result in gangrene), and injury caused by restraining the child. Drawing excessive amounts of blood from premature and small infants can rapidly cause anemia, because a 2-lb infant may have a total blood volume of only 150 mL.

In adults, dermal puncture may be required for a variety of reasons, including:

1 Burned or scarred patients
2 Patients receiving chemotherapy who require frequent tests and whose veins must be reserved for therapy
3 Patients with thrombotic tendencies
4 **Geriatric** or other patients with very fragile veins
5 Patients with inaccessible veins
6 Home glucose monitoring and point-of-care testing

It may not be possible to obtain a satisfactory specimen by dermal puncture from patients who are severely dehydrated or who have poor peripheral circulation.

Composition of Capillary Blood

Blood collected by dermal puncture comes from the capillaries, arterioles, and venules; it is therefore a mixture of arterial and venous blood and may also contain small amounts of tissue fluid. Because of arterial pressure, the composition of this blood more closely resembles arterial blood than venous blood. Warming the site prior to specimen collection increases blood flow as much as sevenfold, thereby producing a specimen that is very close to the composition of arterial blood.

With the exception of arterial blood gases, very few chemical differences exist between arterial and venous blood. The concentration of glucose is higher in blood obtained by dermal puncture than it is in blood obtained by venipuncture, and the concentrations of potassium, total protein, and calcium are lower. Therefore, when dermal punctures are performed, it should be noted on the requisition form. PCTs should not alternate between dermal puncture and venipuncture when results are to be compared.

Hemolysis is more frequently seen in specimens collected by dermal puncture than it is in those collected by venipuncture. Excessive squeezing of the puncture site to obtain enough blood is often the cause of hemolysis. However, newborns in general have increased numbers of RBCs and increased red cell fragility, which raises the possibility that hemolysis may occur even in properly collected samples. The presence of hemolysis may not be detected in specimens containing bilirubin, but it will interfere not only with the tests routinely affected by hemolysis, but also with the frequently requested ***neonatal*** bilirubin determination.

Dermal Puncture Equipment

In addition to the previously discussed venipuncture equipment, a phlebotomy collection tray or drawing station should contain lancets, microsample collection containers, glass slides, and possibly a heel warmer for use in performing dermal punctures.

SKIN PUNCTURE DEVICES

As shown in Figure 9–1, a variety of skin puncture devices are commercially available, including manual and automatic lancets with and without retractable blades. Many studies have compared the various devices with respect to efficiency of collection, specimen hemolysis, and the formation of bruising (**ecchymosis**) at the collection site. No single method appears to be superior.

To prevent contact with bone, the depth of the puncture is critical and should not exceed 2.4 mm. There is concern that even this may be too deep. The puncture depth is controlled by the length of manual lancets, the spring release mechanism, and the use of platforms in automatic devices. Punctures should never be performed using a surgical blade. Some companies provide separate devices designed for heel sticks or finger sticks on children and finger sticks on adults. The depth of the puncture can range from 0.85 mm in the Tenderfoot/Premi (Technidyne Corp., Edison, NJ) to 3.0 mm with the orange platform Autolet for adults (Ulster Scientific, New Paltz, NY).

To produce adequate blood flow, the depth of the puncture is actually much less important than is the width of the incision. This is because the major vascular area of the skin is located at the dermal-subcutaneous junction, which in a newborn is only 0.35 to 1.6 mm below the skin (Fig. 9–2). Therefore, any of the commercial lancets will reach the blood vessels, and the number of severed vessels depends on the incision width. Incision widths vary from needle stabs to 2.5 mm. Wider incisions should be avoided because they produce unnecessary damage to the heel or finger.

MICROSPECIMEN CONTAINERS

Figure 9–3 illustrates some of the major specimen containers available for collection of microsamples, including capillary tubes, micropipets, microcollection tubes, and micropipets with dilution systems. Some containers are designated for a specific test and others serve multiple purposes. The type of container chosen is usually related to institutional preference; advantages and disadvantages can be associated with each system.

CAPILLARY TUBES

Capillary tubes are small glass tubes used to collect approximately 50 to 75 mL of blood for the primary purpose of performing a microhematocrit test. They are frequently referred to as microhematocrit tubes. The tubes are designed to fit into a

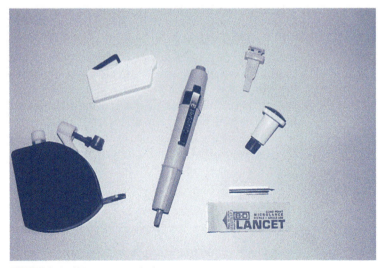

FIGURE 9–1   Skin puncture devices.

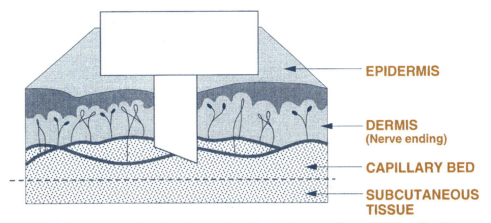

FIGURE 8–2   Vascular area of the skin. (Adapted from Product Literature, Becton Dickinson, Franklin Lakes, NJ.)

hematocrit centrifuge and its corresponding hematocrit reader. Tubes are available plain or coated with ammonium heparin and are color-coded with a red band for heparinized tubes and a blue band for plain tubes. Heparinized tubes should be used for hematocrits collected by dermal puncture and plain tubes are used when the test is being performed on previously anticoagulated blood. When sufficient blood has been collected, the end of the capillary tube that has not been used to collect the specimen is closed by embedding it in a clay sealant designated for use with the tubes. PCTs should use extreme care to prevent breakage when collecting specimens and sealing the microcapillary tubes. Tubes protected by plastic sleeves and self-sealing tubes have recently become available.

MICROPIPETS

Larger capillary tubes, called Caraway or Natelson pipets, are used when tests other than a microhematocrit are requested. The pipets have a tapered end for specimen collection and fill by capillary action. Pipet lengths vary from 75 mm for Caraway pipets to 150 mm for Natelson pipets. The capacity varies from 330 to 470 mL in Caraway pipets to 220 to 420 mL in Natelson pipets. Pipets are available plain or with ammonium heparin and are color-coded, respectively, with blue or red bands. After collection of the sample, the nontapered ends are sealed with specifically matched soft plastic caps or clay sealant.

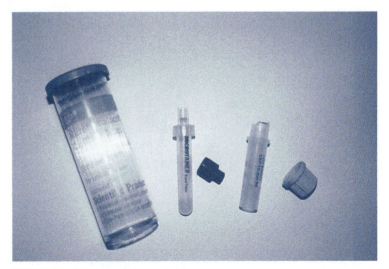

FIGURE 9–3   Microspecimen containers.

MICROCOLLECTION TUBES

Plastic collection tubes such as the Microtainer (Becton Dickinson, Franklin Lakes, NJ) provide a larger collection volume and present no danger from broken glass. A variety of anticoagulants and additives, including separator gel, are available, and the tubes are color-coded in the same way as vacuum tubes. As shown in Figure 9–3, the tubes are supplied with a capillary scoop collector top that is replaced by a color-coded plastic sealer top after the specimen is collected. Mixing of anticoagulated specimens is enhanced by the presence of small plastic beads in the collection tube. Microtainer tubes are designed to hold approximately 600 mL of blood, and separation is achieved by centrifugation in specifically designed centrifuges.

MICROPIPET AND DILUTION SYSTEM

The Unopette system (Becton Dickinson, Franklin Lakes, NJ) is designed for tests that can be performed on diluted whole blood, primarily hematology tests. The system con-

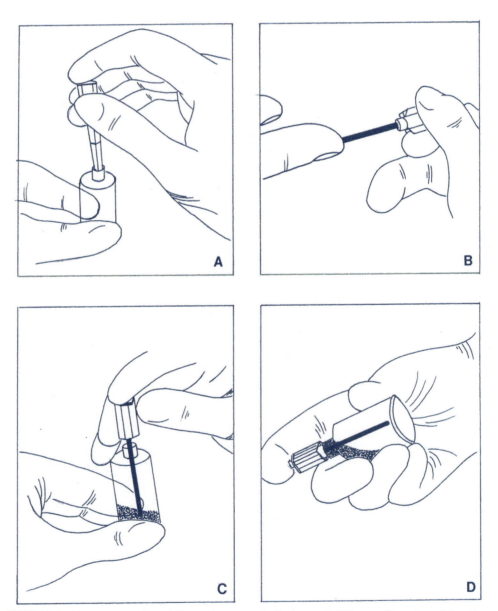

FIGURE 9–4   Unopette procedure. *A*, Puncturing reservoir diaphragm. *B*, Filling capillary pipet. *C*, Transferring specimen to reservoir. *D*, Mixing the reservoir. (From Wedding, ME, and Toenjes, SA: Medical Laboratory Procedures, ed 2, FA Davis, Philadelphia, 1997, p. 235, with permission.)

sists of a sealed plastic reservoir containing a measured amount of diluent, a calibrated glass capillary pipet in a plastic holder, and a plastic pipet shield. The amount and type of diluent and the size of the capillary pipet correspond to the specific test to be run. Pipets are designed to collect only the amount of blood for which they are calibrated.

The procedure for use of the Unopette system is shown in Figure 9–4A to D and includes:

1 Puncturing the diaphragm of the reservoir with the point of the pipet shield
2 Filling the capillary pipet and wiping excess blood from the outside
3 Slightly squeezing the reservoir
4 Placing the index finger over the opening in the pipet holder and inserting the pipet into the reservoir
5 Releasing pressure on the reservoir and removing the finger from the holder opening to cause blood to be drawn into the diluent
6 Carefully rinsing the pipet by squeezing the reservoir without overflowing the pipet
7 Placing the index finger over the opening and inverting the reservoir to mix

ADDITIONAL DERMAL PUNCTURE SUPPLIES

Alcohol pads, sterile gauze, and sharps containers are required for the dermal puncture just as they are for the venipuncture. Blood smears used for the white blood cell (WBC) differential and the examination of RBC morphology must be made during the dermal puncture procedure and require a supply of glass slides. PCTs prepare these slides using the procedure discussed in Unit 10.

As discussed earlier, warming the puncture site increases blood flow to the area. This can be accomplished by using warm washcloths or towels or a commercial heel warmer. A heel warmer is a packet containing sodium thiosulfate and glycerin that produces heat when the chemicals are mixed together by gentle squeezing of the packet. The packet should be wrapped in a towel and held away from the face during the initial activation.

Dermal Puncture Procedure

Many of the procedures associated with venipuncture also apply to dermal puncture; therefore, major emphasis in this unit is on the techniques and complications that are unique to dermal puncture.

PUNCTURE PREPARATION

Prior to performing a dermal puncture, the PCT must have a requisition form containing the information required for the venipuncture. When a specimen is collected by dermal puncture, it must be noted on the requisition form because, as discussed earlier, the concentration of some substances differs in venous and capillary blood.

Because of the variety of puncture devices and collection containers available for dermal puncture, PCTs should be certain that they have the appropriate equipment to collect all required specimens as well as the skin puncture device that corresponds to the age of the patient. Care should be taken to keep equipment out of the reach of pediatric patients.

PATIENT IDENTIFICATION AND PREPARATION

Patients for dermal puncture must be identified using the same procedures as those for venipuncture (requisition form, verbal identification, and ID band). In the nursery, an

ID band *must* be present on the infant and not just on the bassinet. Verbal identification of pediatric outpatients may have to be obtained from the parents.

Approaching pediatric patients can be difficult, and the PCT must present a friendly, confident appearance while explaining the procedure to the child and the parents. Do not say the procedure will not hurt, and explain the necessity of remaining very still.

Parents should be given the choice of staying with the child or leaving the room. If they choose to stay, they may be asked to assist in holding and comforting the child. Very agitated children may need to have their legs and free hand restrained. This can be accomplished by a parent or coworker or by confining the child in a blanket or commercially available papoose-style wrap. If a restraint is used, parental consent must be obtained and documented in the patient's medical record.

When necessary, the finger or heel from which the sample is to be taken may be warmed. This is most commonly required for patients with very cold fingers, for heel sticks to collect multiple samples, and for the collection of capillary blood gases. Warming is performed by moistening a towel with warm water (40°C) or by activating a commercial heel warmer and covering the site for 3 to 5 minutes.

SITE SELECTION

As mentioned in the discussion of skin puncture devices, a primary danger in dermal puncture is accidental contact with the bone, followed by infection (**osteomyelitis**). This can be avoided by selection of puncture sites that provide sufficient distance between the skin and the bone. The primary dermal puncture sites are the heel and the distal segments of the third and fourth fingers. The plantar surface of the large toe is also acceptable. Performing dermal punctures on earlobes is usually not recommended. The choice of a puncture area is based on the age and size of the patient.

Areas selected for dermal puncture should not be calloused, scarred, bruised, edematous, or infected. Punctures should *never* be made through previous puncture sites, because this can easily introduce microorganisms into the puncture and allow them to reach the bone.

HEEL PUNCTURE SITES

The heel is used for dermal punctures on infants less than 1 year of age because it contains more tissue than the fingers and has not yet become calloused from walking.

Acceptable areas for heel puncture are shown in Figure 9–5 and are described as the medial and lateral areas of the bottom (*plantar*) surface of the heel. These areas can be determined by drawing imaginary lines extending back from the middle of the large toe and from between the fourth and fifth toes. It is in these areas that the distance between the skin and the heel bone (*calcaneus*) is greatest. Notice the short distance between the back (posterior curvature) of the heel and the calcaneus (Fig. 9–5). This is the reason that this area is never acceptable for heel puncture.

Punctures should not be performed in other areas of the foot, and particularly not in the arch, where they may cause damage to nerves and tendons. In larger infants the plantar surface of the large toe may be used.

FINGER PUNCTURE SITES

Finger punctures are performed on adults and children over 1 year of age. Fingers of infants less than 1 year old may not contain enough tissue to prevent contact with the bone.

The fleshy areas located near the center of the third and fourth fingers on the *palmar* side are the sites of choice for finger puncture (Fig. 9–6). Because the tip and sides of the finger contain only about half the tissue mass of the central area, the possi-

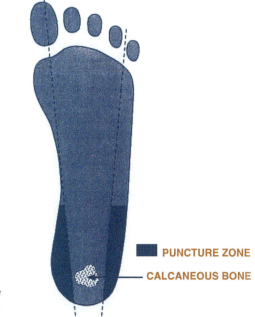

FIGURE 9–5   Acceptable heel puncture sites. (From Strasinger, SK, and Di Lorenzo, MA: Phlebotomy Workbook for the Multiskilled Healthcare Professional. FA Davis, Philadelphia, 1996, p. 268, with permission.)

bility of bone injury is increased in these areas. Problems associated with the use of the other fingers include possible calluses on the thumb, increased nerve endings in the index finger, and decreased tissue in the fifth finger. Patients who routinely perform home glucose monitoring may request a specific finger, and their wishes should be accommodated.

SUMMARY OF DERMAL PUNCTURE SITE SELECTION

1 Use the medial and lateral areas of the plantar surface of the heel.
2 Use the central fleshy area of the third or fourth fingers.
3 Do not use the back of the heel.

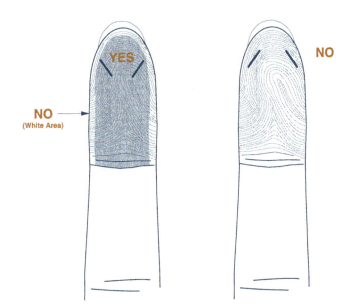

FIGURE 9–6   Acceptable finger puncture sites and correct puncture angle. (From Strasinger, SK, and Di Lorenzo, MA: Phlebotomy Workbook for the Multiskilled Healthcare Professional. FA Davis, Philadelphia, 1996, p. 269, with permission.)

4 Do not use the arch of the foot.
5 Do not puncture through old sites.
6 Do not use areas with visible damage.

CLEANSING THE SITE

The selected site is cleansed with 70% isopropyl alcohol using a circular motion. The alcohol should be allowed to dry on the skin for antiseptic action and the residue removed with a sterile gauze to prevent possible interference with test results. Failure to allow the alcohol to dry will:

1 Cause a stinging sensation for the patient
2 Contaminate the specimen
3 Hemolyze RBCs
4 Prevent formation of a rounded blood drop because blood will mix with the alcohol and run down the finger

Use of povidone-iodine is not recommended for dermal punctures because specimen contamination may elevate some test results, including bilirubin, phosphorus, and uric acid.

PERFORMING THE PUNCTURE

While the puncture is performed, the heel or finger should be well supported and held firmly, without squeezing the puncture area. Massaging the area before the puncture may increase blood flow to the area. The heel is held between the thumb and index finger of the nondominant hand (Fig. 9–7). The finger is held between the thumb and index finger with the palmar surface facing up and the finger pointing downward to increase blood flow.

Punctures performed with a manual lancet should be made with one continuous motion, and automatic devices should be placed firmly on the puncture site. Be sure the device chosen for the puncture corresponds to the size of the patient. As shown in Figure 9–6, the blade of the lancet should be aligned to cut across (perpendicular to) the grooves of the fingerprint or heel print. This aids in the formation of a rounded drop because the blood will not have a tendency to run into the grooves.

After completing the puncture, the lancet should be placed in an appropriate sharps container. A new puncture device must be used if an additional puncture is required.

SPECIMEN COLLECTION

Before beginning the collection, the first drop of blood must be wiped away with a sterile gauze. This will prevent contamination of the specimen with residual alcohol and tissue fluid released during the puncture. When collecting microspecimens it is important to understand that even a minute amount of contamination can severely affect the sample quality. Therefore, blood should be freely flowing from the puncture site as a result of firm pressure and should not be obtained by milking of the surrounding tissue, which will release tissue fluid. The most satisfactory blood flow is obtained by alternately applying and releasing pressure to the area. Tightly squeezing the area with no relaxation cuts off blood flow to the puncture site.

Because collection containers fill by capillary action, the collection tip can be lightly touched to the drop of blood and the blood will be drawn into the container. Collection devices should not touch the puncture site and should not be scraped over the skin because this will produce specimen contamination and hemolysis. Fingers

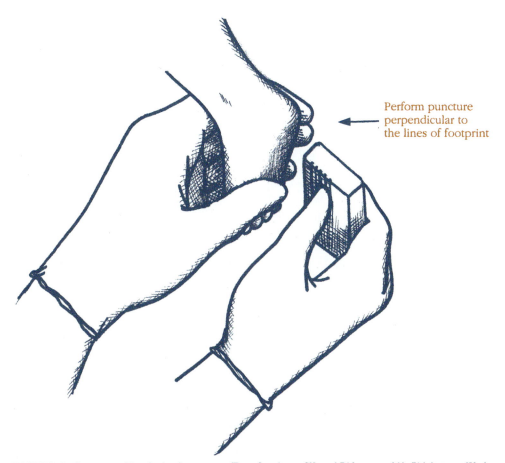

Perform puncture
perpendicular to
the lines of footprint

FIGURE 9–7   Correct position for heel puncture. (From Strasinger, SK, and Di Lorenzo, MA: Phlebotomy Workbook for the Multiskilled Healthcare Professional. FA Davis, Philadelphia, 1996, p. 270, with permission.)

are positioned slightly downward with the palmar surface facing up during the collection procedure (Fig. 9–8).

To prevent introduction of air bubbles, capillary tubes and micropipets are held horizontally while being filled. The presence of air bubbles limits the amount of blood that can be collected per tube and interferes with blood gas determinations and tests performed with Unopettes. When the tubes are filled, they are sealed with sealant clay or designated plastic caps.

Microcollection tubes are slanted down during the collection, and blood is allowed to run through the capillary collection scoop and down the side of the tube. Gently tapping the bottom of the tube may be necessary to force blood to the bottom.

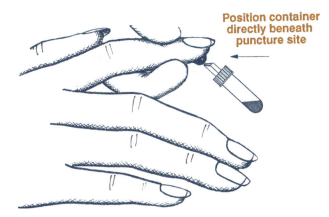

Position container
directly beneath
puncture site

FIGURE 9–8   Specimen collection from the finger. (From Strasinger, SK, and Di Lorenzo, MA: Phlebotomy Workbook for the Multiskilled Healthcare Professional. FA Davis, Philadelphia, 1996, p. 271, with permission.)

When a tube is filled, the scoop is removed and the color-coded top attached. Tubes with anticoagulants should be inverted 8 to 10 times. If blood flow is slow, it may be necessary to mix the tube while the collection is in progress.

Order of Draw

The order of draw for collecting multiple specimens from a dermal puncture is important because of the tendency of platelets to accumulate at the site of a wound. Tests for the evaluation of platelets, such as blood smear, platelet count, and CBC, must therefore be collected first. The blood smear should be made first, followed by the Unopette platelet system or the lavender top Microtainer, and then the specimens for other tests.

When sufficient blood has been collected, pressure is applied to the puncture site with a sterile gauze. The finger or heel is elevated and pressure is applied until the bleeding stops.

Bandages are not used for children under 2 years of age because they may remove the bandages, place them in their mouths, and possibly aspirate the bandage. The adhesive may also cause irritation to sensitive skin.

LABELING THE SPECIMEN

Microsamples must be labeled with the same information required for venipuncture specimens. Labels can be wrapped around microcollection tubes or groups of capillary pipets. For transport, capillary pipets are then placed in a large tube, because the outside of the capillary pipets may be contaminated with blood. This procedure also helps to prevent breakage.

COMPLETION OF THE PROCEDURE

The dermal puncture procedure is completed in the same manner as the venipuncture; this includes disposing of all used materials in appropriate containers, removing gloves, washing hands, and thanking the patient and/or the parents for their cooperation.

All special handling procedures associated with venipuncture specimens also apply to microspecimens. Microspecimens are frequently ordered stat.

To prevent excessive removal of blood from small infants, many nurseries have a log sheet for documenting the amount of blood collected each time a procedure is requested. The PCT should record the amount of blood collected on the log sheet after each collection.

If the PCT fails to collect a sufficient amount of blood after performing two punctures, another person should be asked to complete the procedure.

SUMMARY OF DERMAL PUNCTURE TECHNIQUE

1 Obtain and examine the requisition form.
2 Assemble equipment and supplies.
3 Greet the patient and/or the parents.
4 Identify the patient.
5 Position the patient and the parents.
6 Put on gloves.
7 Organize equipment and supplies.
8 Select the puncture site.
9 Warm the puncture site if necessary.
10 Cleanse and dry the puncture site.

11 Perform the puncture.
12 Wipe away the first drop of blood.
13 Make blood smears if requested.
14 Collect the hematology specimen and then other specimens.
15 Mix the specimens if necessary.
16 Apply pressure.
17 Dispose of the puncture device.
18 Label the specimens.
19 Perform appropriate specimen handling.
20 Thank the patient and/or the parents.
21 Dispose of used supplies.
22 Remove and dispose of gloves.
23 Wash hands.
24 Complete any required paperwork.
25 Deliver specimens to the appropriate locations.

BIBLIOGRAPHY   National Committee for Clinical Laboratory Standards Approved Standard H4-A3: Procedures for the Collection of Diagnostic Blood Specimens by Skin Puncture. NCCLS, Villanova, PA, 1991.
National Committee for Clinical Laboratory Standards Approved Guideline H14-A2: Devices for Collection of Skin Puncture Blood Specimens. NCCLS, Villanova, PA, 1990.

STUDY QUESTIONS

1. List six possible complications associated with femoral puncture in infants.

   a. _____

   b. _____

   c. _____

   d. _____

   e. _____

   f. _____

2. Daily collection of 3 mL of blood from a premature infant may produce

   _____.

3. Why are dermal punctures often performed on (a) patients receiving chemotherapy, (b) geriatric patients, and (c) diabetic patients?

   a. _____

   b. _____

   c. _____

4. State a major concern when collecting a specimen for potassium and bilirubin by dermal puncture.

   _____

5. Describe the composition of capillary blood.

   _____

   _____

6. Can dermal puncture and venipuncture collections be alternated on a patient receiving 4-hour hematocrit and hemoglobin (H & H) tests? Why?

   _____

   _____

7. The maximum length of a puncture device used on the heel is

   _____.

8. True or False. Surgical blades should be used when collecting more than 100 mL of blood. _____

9. Which is more important for producing adequate blood flow, the width or the depth of the puncture? _____

10. Collection of a microhematocrit by dermal puncture is performed using a tube that is color-coded (red) (blue). Circle one.

11. State a major safety concern when using capillary tubes.

_____

_____

12. A lavender top Microtainer contains _____.

13. What is the approximate temperature used for heel warming?

_____

14. List six visible reasons for avoiding a particular area as a skin puncture site.

a. _____

b. _____

c. _____

d. _____

e. _____

f. _____

15. Name two possible causes of osteomyelitis associated with dermal puncture.

a. _____

b. _____

16. Name two areas of the foot where dermal puncture should not be performed.

a. _____

b. _____

17. State a reason for not selecting each of the following as a puncture site:

a. Thumb _____

b. Index finger _____

c. Fifth finger _____

d. Tip of the finger _____

18. State four reasons for removing alcohol from the site prior to performing the puncture.

a. _____

b. _____

c. _____

d. _____

19. How should a dermal puncture be performed to encourage the formation of a rounded drop?

_____

20. List three sources of microspecimen contamination.

    a. _____

    b. _____

    c. _____

21. In what order should the following be collected: bilirubin, blood smear, and CBC?

    a. First: _____

    b. Second: _____

    c. Third: _____

22. State two reasons for not applying a bandage to the puncture site in a 1-year-old child.

    a. _____

    b. _____

23. What is the purpose of a collection volume log sheet in the nursery?

_____

_____

DERMAL PUNCTURE EXERCISE

1. A PCT must collect a CBC and a glucose from a diabetic patient with casts on both arms. How could these tests be collected?

   _____

   _____

2. The laboratory personnel notice that many of the specimens collected by the PCTs on the pediatric unit must be collected again because they are hemolyzed. What should the laboratory personnel stress when presenting a continuing education in-service to the PCTs?

   _____

   _____

   _____

3. A manual platelet count is requested on a patient receiving chemotherapy. What would be the most efficient method for collecting this specimen?

   _____

4. A very agitated 2-year-old child needing a CBC is carried into the outpatient draw-ing area by his equally agitated mother. How should the PCT handle this situation?

   _____

   _____

   _____

5. A PCT student is having difficulty obtaining rounded drops when performing der-mal punctures. What part of the student's technique should the instructor check?

   _____

   _____

6. After failing to collect a sufficient amount of blood from two dermal punctures, the PCT asks a coworker to complete the collection. What additional technique could the second PCT perform to obtain sufficient blood flow?

   _____

7. While selecting a site for a heel puncture, the PCT notices that a previous puncture has been performed on the back of the heel. What should the PCT do?

   _____

8. A PCT in the nursery examines a requisition for blood collection, checks the in-fant's name on the bassinet, selects an area on the plantar surface of the heel, cleanses the area with iodine, collects and labels the specimen, and bandages the heel. What is wrong with this scenario?

   _____

   _____

   _____

   _____

EVALUATION OF MICROTAINER COLLECTION BY HEEL STICK

RATING SYSTEM   2 = Satisfactory   1 = Needs improvement   0 = Incorrect/did not perform

_____ **1.** Examines requisition form and selects necessary equipment

_____ **2.** Assembles equipment and carries it to patient

_____ **3.** Identifies patient using arm/leg band

_____ **4.** Puts on gloves

_____ **5.** Warms heel

_____ **6.** Selects appropriate puncture site

_____ **7.** Cleanses puncture site with alcohol and allows it to air dry

_____ **8.** Does not contaminate puncture device

_____ **9.** Performs puncture smoothly

_____ **10.** Wipes away first drop of blood

_____ **11.** Collects rounded drops into lavender top Microtainer without scraping the skin

_____ **12.** Does not milk site

_____ **13.** Collects adequate amount of blood

_____ **14.** Mixes Microtainer

_____ **15.** Cleanses site and applies pressure until bleeding stops

_____ **16.** Removes all collection equipment from area

_____ **17.** Disposes of puncture device in sharps container

_____ **18.** Disposes of used supplies

_____ **19.** Labels tube

_____ **20.** Removes gloves and washes hands

_____ **21.** Completes nursery log sheet

Total points _____

Maximum points = 42

COMMENTS

EVALUATION OF FINGER STICK ON AN ADULT PATIENT

RATING SYSTEM   2 = Satisfactory   1 = Needs improvement   0 = Incorrect/did not perform

_____ **1.** Greets patient and explains procedure

_____ **2.** Examines requisition form

_____ **3.** Asks patient to state full name

_____ **4.** Compares requisition information and patient's statement

_____ **5.** Organizes and assembles equipment

_____ **6.** Selects appropriate finger

_____ **7.** Warms finger if necessary

_____ **8.** Puts on gloves

_____ **9.** Gently massages finger

_____ **10.** Cleanses site with alcohol and allows it to air dry

_____ **11.** Does not contaminate puncture device

_____ **12.** Smoothly performs puncture across fingerprint

_____ **13.** Wipes away first drop of blood

_____ **14.** Collects two microhematocrit tubes without air bubbles

_____ **15.** Seals tubes

_____ **16.** Cleanses site and asks patient to apply pressure

_____ **17.** Labels tubes

_____ **18.** Examines site and applies bandage

_____ **19.** Thanks patient

_____ **20.** Disposes of puncture device in sharps container

_____ **21.** Disposes of used supplies

_____ **22.** Removes gloves

_____ **23.** Washes hands

Total points _____

Maximum points = 46

COMMENTS

EVALUATION OF UNOPETTE COLLECTION ON A 2-YEAR-OLD CHILD

RATING SYSTEM   2 = Satisfactory   1 = Needs improvement   0 = Incorrect/did not perform

_____ **1.** Greets patient and parent(s)

_____ **2.** Examines requisition form

_____ **3.** Identifies patient using correct verbal identification procedure

_____ **4.** Explains procedure to patient and parent(s)

_____ **5.** Determines if parent(s) needs/wants to hold patient

_____ **6.** Puts on gloves

_____ **7.** Organizes equipment

_____ **8.** Removes pipet shield

_____ **9.** Punctures reservoir diaphragm

_____ **10.** Gently massages finger

_____ **11.** Cleanses site with alcohol and allows it to air dry

_____ **12.** Does not contaminate puncture device

_____ **13.** Smoothly performs puncture across fingerprint

_____ **14.** Wipes away first drop of blood

_____ **15.** Completely fills pipet with no air bubbles

_____ **16.** Wipes blood from outside of pipet without drawing blood out of the pipet

_____ **17.** Places index finger over opening in overflow chamber

_____ **18.** Squeezes reservoir

_____ **19.** Places pipet firmly into reservoir

_____ **20.** Removes index finger and releases reservoir

_____ **21.** Rinses pipet by squeezing reservoir

_____ **22.** Does not force fluid out of overflow chamber

_____ **23.** Places shield on overflow chamber

_____ **24.** Mixes container

_____ **25.** Cleanses site and applies pressure until bleeding stops

_____ **26.** Applies bandage

_____ **27.** Labels Unopette

_____ **28.** Disposes of puncture device in sharps container

_____ **29.** Disposes of used supplies

_____ **30.** Thanks patient and parent(s)

_____ **31.** Removes gloves and washes hands

Total points _____

Maximum points = 62

COMMENTS

UNIT 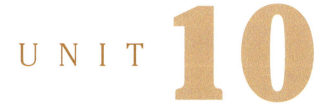10

SPECIAL DERMAL PUNCTURE

LEARNING OBJECTIVES

Upon completion of this unit, the reader will be able to:

1 Define the key terms associated with special dermal puncture.
2 Discuss the necessary precautions for collecting high-quality specimens for neonatal bilirubin tests.
3 Briefly discuss why and how neonatal filter paper screening tests are collected.
4 List six possible errors in technique that cause unacceptable blood smears.
5 Prepare an acceptable blood smear using the instructions provided.
6 State the purpose of the bleeding time (BT) and three reasons why it may be prolonged.
7 Discuss the standardization of the BT and errors in technique that affect test results.
8 Correctly perform a BT following the instructions provided in the text or by the manufacturer of the incision device.

KEY TERMS

■ *Exchange transfusion*	Removal of blood and replacement with an equal volume of donor blood
■ *Feathered edge*	Area of the blood smear at which the microscopic examination is performed
■ *Phenylketonuria*	Presence of abnormal phenylalanine metabolites in the urine
■ **Plasmodium**	Genus of malarial parasites
■ *Platelet plug*	Initial blockage of a vascular puncture by platelets
■ *Volar*	Pertaining to the palm side of the forearm

Several of the special collection techniques discussed in Unit 8 also apply to specimens collected by dermal puncture. These include:

1 Fasting specimens
2 Specimens for glucose tolerance tests (GTT)

3 Timed specimens for postprandial (pp) glucose (it is recommended that sodium fluoride be used when collecting neonatal glucose tests because the normally high RBC count increases glycolysis)
4 Specimens for therapeutic drug monitoring (TDM)
5 Specimens affected by diurnal variation
6 Specimens that must be warmed or chilled during transport
7 Forensic specimens

Procedures primarily associated with dermal punctures are as follows:

1 Collection of neonatal bilirubins
2 Collection of neonatal filter paper screening tests
3 Preparation of blood smears
4 Bleeding time (BT) tests
5 Point-of-care testing (POCT)

Collection of Neonatal Bilirubins

One of the most frequently performed tests on newborns measures **bilirubin** levels, and specimens for this determination are often collected at timed intervals over several days. Bilirubin is a very light-sensitive chemical and is rapidly destroyed when exposed to light.

Increased serum bilirubin in newborns may be caused by the presence of hemolytic disease of the newborn (HDN), or it may simply be due to the fact that the liver of newborns (particularly premature infants) is often not developed enough to process the bilirubin produced from the normal breakdown of RBCs. Bilirubin test results are critical to infant survival and to mental health because the blood-brain barrier is not fully developed in neonates, a condition that allows bilirubin to accumulate in the brain and cause permanent or lethal damage. Bilirubin levels reaching 18 mg/dL or rising at a rate of 0.5 mg/dL per hour indicate the need for an *exchange transfusion*.

Phlebotomy technique is critical to the determination of accurate bilirubin results, and specimens must be protected from excess light during and after the collection. Infants that appear **jaundiced** are frequently placed under an ultraviolet light (bili light) to lower the level of circulating bilirubin. This light must be turned off during specimen collection. Amber-colored Microtainer tubes are available for collecting bilirubins or, if multiple capillary pipets are used, the filled tubes should be shielded from light. Hemolysis must be avoided; it will falsely lower bilirubin results in some procedures and must be corrected for in others. Also, specimens must be collected at the specified time so that the rate of bilirubin increase can be determined.

Neonatal Screening

Screening of newborns for 50 inherited **metabolic** disorders can currently be performed from blood collected by heel stick and placed on specially designed filter paper. Most states have laws requiring the screening of newborns for the presence of the most prevalent disorders: *phenylketonuria* **(PKU)**, which is caused by a lack of the enzyme needed to metabolize **phenylalanine**, and **hypothyroidism**. Both disorders produce severe mental retardation, but retardation can be avoided by changes in diet and the use of medication if these disorders are detected within the first few weeks after birth. Routine screening is not usually performed for other disorders, but the screening may be requested when symptoms or family history indicates a need or when state law requires a more extensive battery of neonatal tests.

The filter paper blood screening test for PKU uses bacterial growth to determine the presence or absence of phenylalanine in the blood. The blood-impregnated filter

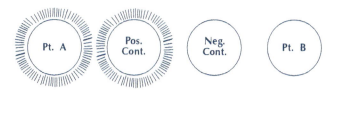

FIGURE 10–1   Sample bacterial inhibition test. (From Strasinger, SK: Urinalysis and Body Fluids, ed. 3. FA Davis, Philadelphia, 1994, p. 119, with permission.)

paper disks are placed on culture media containing bacteria, and the media are then observed for bacterial growth, as shown in Figure 10–1. Hypothyroidism is detected by performing immunochemical analysis of the dried blood.

It can be understood from this brief explanation of the bacterial testing procedure that correct collection of the blood specimen is critical for accurate test results. Special collection kits are used, consisting of a patient information form attached to specifically designed filter paper that has been preprinted with an appropriate number of 1/2-inch diameter circles. The filter paper and the ink must be biologically inactive and approved by the Food and Drug Administration. The PCT must be careful not to touch or contaminate the area inside the circles or to touch the dried blood spots.

The heel stick is performed in the routine manner, and the first drop of blood is wiped away. A large drop of blood is then applied directly into a filter paper circle. To obtain an even layer of blood, only one drop should be used to fill a circle. Blood is applied to only one side of the filter paper, and there must be enough to soak through the paper and be visible on the other side. As shown in Figure 10–2, if a circle is not evenly or completely filled, a new circle and a larger drop of blood should be used. The collected specimen must be allowed to air dry in a suspended horizontal position, at room temperature, and away from direct sunlight. To prevent cross-contamination, specimens should not be stacked during or after the drying process.

Collection of blood in heparinized capillary pipets followed by its immediate transfer to the filter paper circles is an acceptable but not recommended technique. Each circle requires 100 μL of blood, which must be added without scratching or denting the filter paper with the capillary tip.

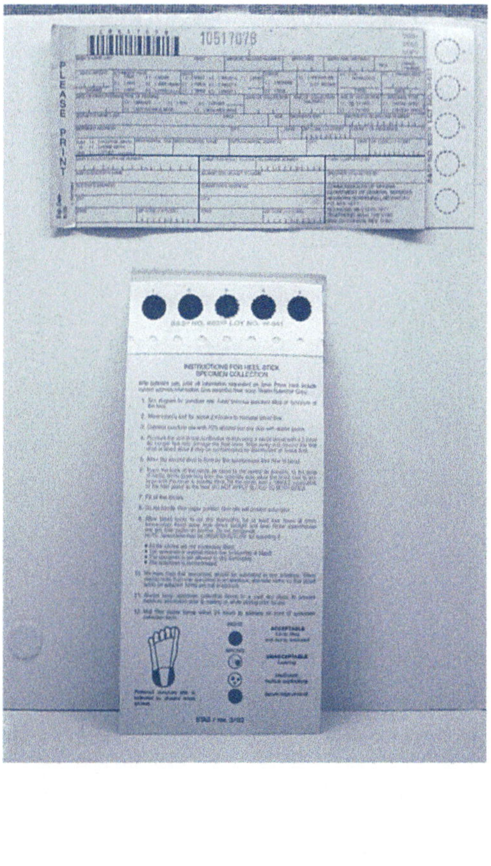

FIGURE 10–2   Collection kit for neonatal screening tests. (Notice the acceptable and unacceptable collection examples.)

Preparation of Blood Smears

Blood smears are needed for the microscopic examination of blood cells, for special staining procedures, and for nonautomated **reticulocyte** counts. PCTs must make smears when one of these tests is ordered and a dermal puncture is performed. When specimens are collected by venipuncture, the smear is usually made in the laboratory from the EDTA tube. Performing smears at the bedside following a venipuncture may sometimes be necessary to ensure a fresh smear. This can be dangerous, however, because blood must be forced from the needle onto the slide, and the needle cannot be disposed of until the smear has been made. In addition, blood smears must be considered infectious until they have been fixed with alcohol in the laboratory, and gloves must be worn when handling them.

BLOOD SMEAR PREP

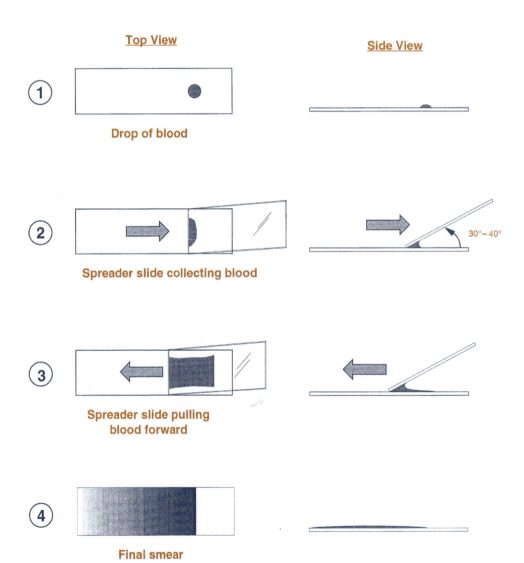

FIGURE 10–3   Preparation of a blood smear. (Adapted from Strasinger, SK, and Di Lorenzo, MA: Phlebotomy Workbook for the Multiskilled Healthcare Professional. FA Davis, Philadelphia, 1996, p. 290.)

Learning to prepare an acceptable blood smear requires considerable practice and can be a source of frustration for beginners. Once the technique is mastered, however, it is seldom that an acceptable smear is not achieved on the first attempt. The technique for preparing a blood smear is described below and illustrated in Figures 10–3 and 10–4:

1 Obtain three clean glass slides and perform the dermal puncture in the manner discussed in Unit 9. Be certain to wipe away the first drop of blood.

2 Place the second drop of blood in the center of a glass slide approximately 1/2 to 1 inch from the end, or just below the frosted end, by lightly touching the drop with the slide. The drop should be 1 to 2 mm in diameter.

3 Immediately place the slide in one of the positions shown in Figure 10–4. Choose the one that works best for you.

4 Place a second slide (spreader slide) with a clean smooth edge in front of the drop at a 30- to 40-degree angle inclined over the blood.

5 Draw the spreader slide back to the edge of the drop of blood, allowing the blood to spread across the end.

6 When blood is evenly distributed across the spreader slide, lightly push the spreader slide forward with a continuous movement all the way past the end of the smear slide. Be certain to maintain the 30- to 40-degree angle and do not apply pressure to the spreader slide.

7 Place the slide in an area in which it can dry undisturbed and repeat the procedure for the second smear.

8 Smears collected on slides with frosted ends are labeled by writing the patient information on the frosted area with a pencil. Labels containing the appropriate information are attached to the thick end of smear slides that do not have frosted ends.

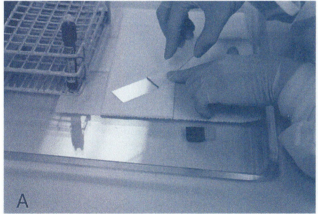

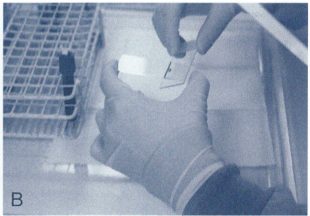

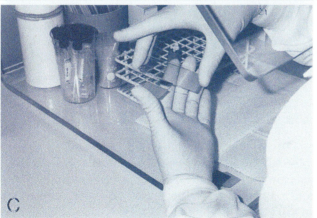

FIGURE 10–4   Examples of slide positioning for blood smear preparation. (From Strasinger, SK, and Di Lorenzo, MA: Phlebotomy Workbook for the Multiskilled Healthcare Professional. FA Davis, Philadelphia, 1996, p. 291, with permission.)

TABLE 10–1 **Effect of Technical Errors on Blood Smears**

Discrepancy	Possible Cause
Uneven distribution of blood (ridges)	Pressure on the spreader slide
	Movement of the spreader slide not continuous
	Delay in making slide after drop is placed on slide
Holes in the smear	Dirty slide
No feathered edge	Spreader slide not pushed the entire length of the smear slide
Streaks in the feathered edge	Chipped or dirty spreader slide
	Spreader slide not placed flush against the smear slide
	Pulling the spreader slide into the drop of blood so that the blood is pushed instead of pulled
Smear too thick and short	Drop of blood is too big
	Angle of spreader slide is greater than 40°
Smear too thin and long	Drop of blood is too small
	Angle of spreader slide is less than 30°

A properly prepared blood smear has a smooth film of blood that covers approximately one half to two thirds of the slide, does not contain ridges or holes, and has a lightly *feathered edge* without streaks. The microscopic examination is performed in the area of the feathered edge because the cells have been spread into a single layer. An uneven smear indicates that the cells are not evenly distributed; therefore, test results will not be truly representative of the patient's blood. Errors in technique that result in an unacceptable specimen are summarized in Table 10–1.

Blood Smears for Malaria

The parasites (*Plasmodium* species) that cause malaria invade RBCs, and their presence is detected by microscopic examination of thick and thin blood smears. Patients with malaria exhibit periodic episodes of fever and chills related to the multiplication of the parasites within the RBCs. Therefore, specimen collection is frequently requested on a stat or timed basis similar to that of blood cultures. Smears are usually prepared in the laboratory from EDTA anticoagulated blood, unless a dermal puncture must be performed.

Thin smears (two or three) are prepared in the manner previously described. Thick smears are made by placing a large drop of blood in the center of a glass slide and then using the corner of another glass slide to spread the blood into a circle about the size of a dime. The smear must be allowed to dry for at least 2 hours prior to staining. Thick smears concentrate the specimen for detection of the parasites and thin smears are then examined for parasitic morphology and identification.

Bleeding Time

The bleeding time (BT) is performed to measure the time required for platelets to form a plug strong enough to stop bleeding from an incision. The length of the BT is increased when the platelet count is low, when platelet disorders affect the ability of the platelets to stick to each other and to the incision to form a plug, and when people are taking medications that contain aspirin. Test results can also be affected by the type and condition of the patient's skin, vascularity, temperature, and the PCT's technique.

Therefore, the BT is considered a screening test, and abnormal results are followed by additional testing. BTs are frequently ordered as part of a presurgical workup.

Measurement of the BT was first introduced by Duke in 1910 and was performed by timing the length of bleeding from a lancet puncture of the earlobe. The Duke method is not as well-standardized as current methods are; however, it may occasionally be requested in special situations.

Standardization of the BT began in 1941 when Ivy modified the Duke method by performing the incision on the *volar* surface of the forearm and inflating a blood pressure cuff to 40 mm Hg to control blood flow to the area. These modifications are still a part of the BT procedure. In 1969 Mielke introduced a plastic template, used with a surgical blade rather than a lancet, to control the length and depth of the incision. Automated disposable incision devices such as the Simplate and Simplate-II (Organon Teknika Corp., Durham, NC) and Surgicutt (International Technidyne, Edison, NJ) that produce standardized incisions of 1 mm in depth and 5 mm in length have now replaced the original template method (Fig. 10–5).

Steps in performing the BT using an automated device are as follows:

1 Identify the patient following routine protocol.
2 Explain the procedure to the patient, including the possibility of leaving a small scar, and obtain information about any prescribed or over-the-counter medications, particularly aspirin, that may have been taken in the last 7 to 10 days. Many medications contain salicylate (aspirin); therefore, the contents of any medication mentioned by the patient should be checked prior to performing the test and, if salicylate has been taken, the physician should be notified.
3 Place the patient's arm on a steady surface with the volar side up.
4 Select an area approximately 5 cm below the antecubital crease and in the middle of the arm that is free of surface veins, scars, bruises, and edema.
5 Cleanse the area with alcohol and allow it to air dry.
6 Assemble required materials, filter paper, stopwatch, and bandages.
7 Place a blood pressure cuff on the upper arm.
8 Remove the incision device from its package and release the safety lock, being careful not to touch the blade area.
9 Inflate the blood pressure cuff to 40 mm Hg. This pressure must be maintained throughout the procedure.
10 Place the incision device firmly, but without making an indentation, on the arm and position it so that the incision will be horizontal (parallel to the antecubital crease) (Fig. 10–5). In adults, horizontal incisions are slightly more sensitive to hemorrhagic disorders and are less likely to leave a scar, whereas in newborns a vertical incision is preferable for the same reasons.
11 Depress the trigger and simultaneously start a stopwatch and then remove the incision device.
12 After 30 seconds remove the blood that has accumulated on the incision by gently "wicking" it onto a circle of Whatman No. 1 filter paper or Surgicutt Bleeding Time Blotting Paper (International Technidyne, Edison, NJ) (Fig. 10–6). Do not touch the incision because it will disturb formation of the *platelet plug* and prolong the BT.
13 Continue to remove blood from the incision every 30 seconds in the manner described previously until the bleeding stops.
14 Record the time on the stopwatch to the nearest 30 seconds.
15 Deflate and remove the blood pressure cuff.
16 Clean the patient's arm and apply a butterfly bandage to tightly hold the edges of the incision together. Cover this bandage with a regular bandage. Instruct the patient to leave the bandages on for 24 hours.
17 Depending on the method and device used, normal BTs range from 2 to 10 minutes. The test can be discontinued after 20 minutes and reported as greater than 20 minutes to a supervisor.

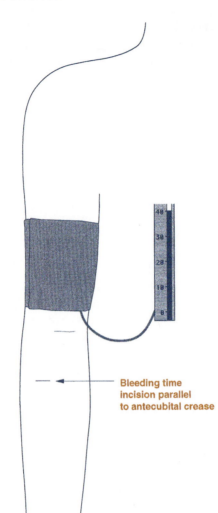

Bleeding time incision parallel to antecubital crease

FIGURE 10–5 Template bleeding time procedure. (From Strasinger, SK, and Di Lorenzo, MA: Phlebotomy Workbook for the Multiskilled Healthcare Professional. FA Davis, Philadelphia, 1996, p. 293, with permission.)

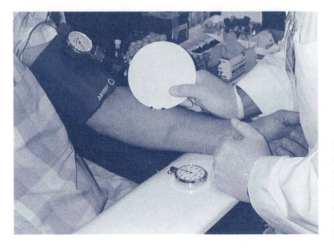

FIGURE 10–6 Wicking of blood during the bleeding time procedure. (From Strasinger, SK, and Di Lorenzo, MA: Phlebotomy Workbook for the Multiskilled Healthcare Professional. FA Davis, Philadelphia, 1996, p. 294, with permission.)

Point-of-Care Testing

The development of portable handheld instruments capable of performing a variety of routine laboratory procedures has contributed greatly to the concept of patient-focused care. Specimens can be collected by dermal puncture and tested by the PCT in the patient area. Test results are quickly available and transportation of specimens to the laboratory is avoided. Dermal punctures are performed following the procedure detailed in Unit 9. However, instrumentation manufacturers may recommend some modifications. All manufacturer recommendations should be followed by PCTs performing point of care testing. The most routinely performed point-of-care tests are discussed in Unit 12.

BIBLIOGRAPHY

Brown, BA: Hematology: Principles and Procedures, ed. 6. Lea & Febiger, Philadelphia, 1995.
Buchanan, GR, and Holtkamp, CA: A comparative study of variables affecting the bleeding time using two disposable devices. Am J Clin Pathol 9(1), 1989.
Henry, JB: Clinical Diagnosis and Management by Laboratory Methods. WB Saunders, Philadelphia, 1996.
Koepke, JA: Bleeding time test (Tips on Technology). Medical Laboratory Observer 25(7), 1993.
National Committee for Clinical Laboratory Standards Approved Standard LA4-A2: Blood Collection on Filter Paper for Neonatal Screening Programs. NCCLS, Villanova, PA, 1992.

STUDY QUESTIONS

1. List two reasons for elevated neonatal bilirubins.

    a. _____

    b. _____

2. Why are neonatal bilirubins frequently ordered as timed tests?

    _____

    _____

3. A neonatal bilirubin collected at 0600 is 10.0 mg/dL, the specimen collected at 1800 reads 12.0 mg/dL, and the specimen collected the next morning at 0600 has a value of 5.0 mg/dL.

    a. State an error in phlebotomy technique that could cause the last result.

    _____

    b. State a specimen characteristic that could cause the last result.

    _____

4. Name two disorders in which neonatal filter paper tests are frequently used for screening.

    a. _____

    b. _____

5. How should blood collected on a filter paper disk appear?

    _____

    _____

6. State a reason why collecting blood for filter paper testing with a capillary pipet may not be recommended.

    _____

7. Name two tests that require a blood smear.

    a. _____

    b. _____

8. True or False. Unfixed blood smears are a biological hazard. _____

9. The proper angle of the spreader slide when preparing a blood smear is

    _____ .

10. If the angle of the spreader slide is too large, the blood smear will be too

    _____ and _____ .

11. What is the purpose of the feathered edge on a blood smear?

_____

_____

12. A chipped spreader slide will cause _____.

13. Why is a blood smear containing ridges or holes considered unacceptable?

_____

_____

14. List three reasons for a BT to be prolonged.

a. _____

b. _____

c. _____

15. State the basic principle of the BT.

_____

_____

_____

16. True or False. To obtain an accurate BT result, the patient must be given aspirin prior to having the test performed. _____

17. What is the purpose of "wicking"?

_____

_____

18. In adults the BT incision is made (horizontal) (vertical) to the antecubital crease. (Circle one.) Why?

_____

_____

19. The normal BT is approximately _____.

SPECIAL DERMAL PUNCTURE EXERCISE

1. The laboratory supervisor is asked to present an in-service to the PCTs who collect neonatal bilirubins on the night shift. Specimens are not hemolyzed. However, test results are consistently lower than those of tests collected on the morning and evening shifts. What should the supervisor stress?

   _____

2. A PCT collects three Caraway micropipets for a bilirubin, labels a large tube, places the sealed tubes into it, delivers it to the laboratory, and leaves the tube on the counter in Chemistry while everyone is at lunch. The Chemistry supervisor rejects the specimen. Why? How could this have been avoided?

   _____

   _____

   _____

3. In what circumstance might a PCT deliver a blood smear without a feathered edge to the laboratory?

   _____

4. BTs performed by a new employee are consistently prolonged. What part of the employee's technique should the supervisor observe most closely? Why?

   _____

   _____

   _____

5. A PCT with a requisition for a BT identifies the patient, checks on medications, selects and chooses an appropriate site, inflates the blood pressure cuff to halfway between the systolic and diastolic pressures, performs the puncture, wipes away the first drop of blood, starts the stopwatch, blots the area with gauze every 30 seconds until the bleeding stops, records the time, and completes the procedure. What is wrong with this scenario?

   _____

   _____

   _____

   _____

6. How could failure to wipe away the first drop of blood affect the results of a filter paper PKU?

   _____

   _____

7. A PCT has requisitions for a blood smear and a BT. Can this be accomplished with one puncture? Why or why not?

_____

_____

EVALUATION OF NEONATAL FILTER PAPER COLLECTION

RATING SYSTEM   2 = Satisfactory   1 = Needs improvement   0 = Incorrect/did not perform

_____ **1.** Examines requisition form

_____ **2.** Assembles equipment

_____ **3.** Identifies patient

_____ **4.** Puts on gloves

_____ **5.** Selects appropriate heel site

_____ **6.** Cleanses site and allows it to air dry

_____ **7.** Performs the puncture

_____ **8.** Wipes away first drop of blood

_____ **9.** Evenly fills a circle with one drop of blood

_____ **10.** Fills all required circles

_____ **11.** Does not touch inside of circles or blood spots

_____ **12.** Places filter paper in appropriate transport position

_____ **13.** Applies pressure until bleeding stops

_____ **14.** Disposes of equipment and supplies

_____ **15.** Correctly completes all required paperwork

_____ **16.** Removes gown and gloves

_____ **17.** Washes hands

Total points _____

Maximum points = 34

COMMENTS

EVALUATION OF BLOOD SMEAR PREPARATION

RATING SYSTEM   2 = Satisfactory   1 = Needs improvement   0 = Incorrect/did not perform

_____ **1.** Examines requisition form

_____ **2.** Obtains three clean glass slides

_____ **3.** Identifies patient

_____ **4.** Puts on gloves

_____ **5.** Selects and cleanses an appropriate site and allows it to air dry

_____ **6.** Performs puncture

_____ **7.** Wipes away first drop of blood

_____ **8.** Puts correct-sized drop on appropriate area of slide

_____ **9.** Positions slide

_____ **10.** Places spreader slide at correct angle

_____ **11.** Pulls spreader slide back to blood drop

_____ **12.** Allows blood to spread across spreader slide

_____ **13.** Pushes spreader slide evenly forward

_____ **14.** Places smear to dry

_____ **15.** Collects second smear using correct technique

_____ **16.** Labels smears

_____ **17.** Smear has feathered edge with no streaks

_____ **18.** Blood is evenly distributed

_____ **19.** Smear does not have holes

_____ **20.** Smear is not too long or too thick

_____ **21.** Smear is not too short or too thin

_____ **22.** Disposes of equipment and supplies

_____ **23.** Removes gloves and washes hands

Total points _____

Maximum points = 46

COMMENTS

EVALUATION OF BLEEDING TIME TECHNIQUE

RATING SYSTEM   2 = Satisfactory   1 = Needs improvement   0 = Incorrect/did not perform

_____ **1.** Examines requisition form

_____ **2.** Identifies patient

_____ **3.** Explains procedure to patient

_____ **4.** Asks patient about medications

_____ **5.** Assembles equipment

_____ **6.** Puts on gloves

_____ **7.** Positions patient's arm

_____ **8.** Selects appropriate site

_____ **9.** Cleanses site and allows it to air dry

_____ **10.** Puts blood pressure cuff on upper arm

_____ **11.** Opens and does not contaminate puncture device

_____ **12.** Inflates blood pressure cuff to 40 mm Hg

_____ **13.** Correctly aligns puncture device on patient's arm

_____ **14.** Simultaneously punctures and starts stopwatch

_____ **15.** Quickly removes puncture device

_____ **16.** Correctly wicks blood after 30 seconds

_____ **17.** Continues wicking every 30 seconds

_____ **18.** Recognizes end point and discontinues timing

_____ **19.** Records stopwatch time

_____ **20.** Deflates and removes blood pressure cuff

_____ **21.** Cleans patient's arm

_____ **22.** Applies butterfly bandage

_____ **23.** Applies regular bandage

_____ **24.** Instructs patient when to remove bandages

_____ **25.** Disposes of equipment and supplies

_____ **26.** Removes gloves and washes hands

Total points _____

Maximum points = 52

COMMENTS

ADDITIONAL SPECIMEN COLLECTION, PROCESSING, AND RELATED DUTIES

KEY TERMS

- *Aliquot* — Portion of a sample
- *Anaerobic* — Unable to survive in oxygen
- *Antibiotic susceptibility* — Procedure to determine the effectiveness of antibiotics against microorganisms
- *Bar code* — Computerized identification system

- ■ *Centrifuge*   Instrument that spins test tubes at high speeds to separate the cellular and liquid portions of blood
- ■ *Hardware*   Solid components of a computer system
- ■ *Iontophoresis*   Electrical stimulation of soluble salt ions used in collection of sweat electrolyte specimens
- ■ *Occult*   Hidden (not visible)
- ■ *Pilocarpine*   Sweat-inducing chemical
- ■ *Pneumatic tube system*   Air-driven transport system
- ■ *Software*   Computer application programs
- ■ *Urinalysis*   Physical, chemical, and microscopic analysis of urine

The extent to which PCTs perform collection of nonblood clinical specimens, basic specimen processing, specimen testing (discussed in Unit 12), and computer data entry and recovery varies greatly among healthcare institutions. Examples of this variation in duties include the following:

1 Hospital-based PCTs perform very little specimen processing because they can deliver specimens to the clinical laboratory immediately. PCTs working in outpatient facilities, however, may be required to preserve specimens, separate blood specimens by centrifugation, and package specimens for transportation to a laboratory.
2 PCTs employed in outpatient facilities must be able to clearly explain patient preparation and specimen collection instructions to their patients, whereas PCTs serving as primary caregivers are often present during the specimen collection activities and are able to assist the patient if necessary.
3 The sophistication of the computer equipment present in the facility will determine the duties of the PCT, such as the automatic transfer of data between departments versus the manual entry of reports received by telephone, for example.

This unit is designed to provide basic information on the most frequently performed miscellaneous PCT duties.

Patient Instruction

As primary caregivers, PCTs are often required to provide instructions to patients regarding the activities of the PCT and/or the patient before, during, and after diagnostic testing. To provide accurate instructions or to perform a procedure correctly, the PCT must be thoroughly familiar with the instructions and be able to answer any questions asked by the patients. If PCTs are unsure of a particular instruction, they should refer to the **procedure manuals** available at their stations or consult a supervisor. Remember to observe the rules for effective communication discussed in Unit 1 when providing patient instructions.

In the outpatient setting, the patient may be collecting the specimen while at the facility or collecting the specimen at home and returning it to the facility at a later time. When patients are collecting specimens at home, it is extremely important that they understand the procedure and the necessity of observing special precautions, such as the necessary time frame for returning the specimen or the need for refrigeration. Areas designated for specimen collection at the facility should be conveniently located and should contain the appropriate materials for satisfactory specimen collection.

Urine Specimen Collection

Frequently collected urine specimens include random, first-morning, midstream clean-catch, and 24-hour (timed) specimens. PCTs should understand that the composition of urine changes quickly, and specimens should be delivered to the laboratory promptly or refrigerated.

Random specimens may be collected at any time without prior patient preparation. They are used primarily for routine ***urinalysis***, which is discussed in Unit 12.

A first-morning specimen is the specimen of choice for urinalysis because it is more concentrated and may be used to confirm results obtained from random specimens. Patients are provided with a container and instructed to collect the specimen immediately after arising and deliver the specimen to the laboratory within 1 hour or refrigerate it.

Midstream clean-catch specimens are used for urine cultures. Patients are provided with sterile containers and antiseptic materials for cleansing the **genitalia**. Sterile soapy gauze pads followed by gauze pads soaked in sterile water or mild antiseptic towelettes followed by sterile water-soaked gauze pads may be used. Women should be instructed to spread the **labia** and cleanse from the front to back using a new pad for each cleansing stroke (three strokes: right, left, and center are recommended). Men should clean the tip of the penis; the cleansing should include retraction of the foreskin if the man is uncircumcised. Patients are instructed to begin voiding into the toilet, then collect the specimen without touching the inside of the container, and finish voiding into the toilet. The PCT should be prepared to assist the patient with this procedure, if necessary.

Timed or 24-hour specimens require larger containers that may contain a preservative specific for a particular substance to be quantitatively measured (Fig. 11–1). To obtain an accurate timed specimen, it is necessary for the patient to begin and end the collection period with an empty bladder.

EXAMPLE: Day 1–0700: Patient voids and *discards* urine, then collects all urine for 24 hours. Day 2–0700: Patient voids and *adds* this urine to the previously collected urine.

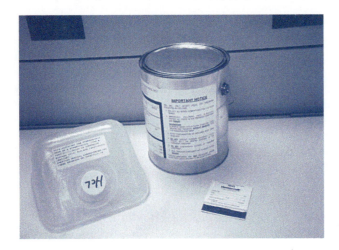

FIGURE 11–1 Containers for urine and fecal specimens. (From Strasinger, SK, and Di Lorenzo, MA: Phlebotomy Workbook for the Multiskilled Healthcare Professional. FA Davis, Philadelphia, 1996, p. 335, with permission.)

When collecting timed specimens from catheterized patients, PCTs are responsible for performing the previous procedure. To preserve the integrity of the test substance, it may be necessary to empty the contents of the catheter bag into an appropriate container at periodic intervals. Certain tests may require placing the catheter bag on ice during the collection period. Of primary importance in any timed collection is ensuring that all of the urine passed during the collection period is included in the final specimen. Failure to do so will cause an abnormal test result, which at the very least will require the collection to be repeated.

Fecal Specimen Collection

Fecal specimens are collected for a variety of diagnostic tests, including cultures for pathogenic microorganisms, detection of ova and parasites, microscopic examination for the presence of white blood cells (WBCs) and undigested fibers and fats, the detection of *occult* blood, and the quantitative measurement of fecal fats. Random specimens can be collected and delivered to the laboratory in plastic containers or cardboard containers with wax-coated interiors. Specimens for the detection of ova and parasites may be collected in containers with a preservative. Large paint can–style containers are used for collection of 72-hour specimens for quantitative fecal fat. Kits containing reagent-impregnated filter paper are available to screen for the presence of occult blood. Figure 11–1 shows a variety of fecal specimen containers. Patients can use these kits to collect specimens at home and mail or deliver them to the testing center. As discussed in Unit 12, these kits are used by PCTs when performing point-of-care testing (POCT).

Certain procedures require that patients be instructed to avoid contaminating the specimen with urine or toilet water containing disinfectants. It may be necessary to collect the specimen in a bedpan or to place a plastic hat strainer in the toilet and then transfer the specimen to the appropriate container. Specific instructions are required for the collection of specimens for occult blood testing, and these are discussed in Unit 12. Specimens should be delivered to the laboratory as soon as possible for the detection of parasites and microbiological cultures.

Cerebrospinal Fluid Collection

PCTs may assist a physician in the collection of **cerebrospinal fluid (CSF)** by **lumbar puncture**. Specimens are collected not only for culture but also for cell counts and chemical analysis. Fluid from the puncture is collected directly into sterile tubes. It is critical that the tubes be numbered in the order in which they are collected to avoid interference with laboratory tests. For example, the first tube collected is the most likely to contain contamination from blood cells resulting from the puncture or microorganisms from the skin and should not be used for cell counts or cultures.

The most commonly used order of tube distribution is Tube #1 to Chemistry, Tube #2 to Microbiology, and Tube #3 to Hematology.

Semen Analysis

Patients required to collect a specimen for semen analysis should be instructed to abstain from sexual activity for 3 days prior to collecting the specimen. Ideally, the specimen should then be collected at the laboratory in a sterile container. The specimen must not be collected in a condom because they frequently contain spermicidal agents. If the specimen is collected at home, it must be kept warm and delivered to the laboratory within 1 hour. When accepting a semen specimen, it is essential that the PCT record the time of specimen collection, not the time of specimen receipt, and provide this information to the laboratory, because certain parameters of the semen analysis are based on specimen life span.

Sweat Electrolyte Collection

Measurement of the sweat electrolytes sodium (**Na**) and chloride (**Cl**) is performed to confirm the diagnosis of cystic fibrosis, a genetic disorder of the mucous-secreting glands. Because cystic fibrosis involves multiple organs, many clinical symptoms can lead the physician to suspect its presence. Symptoms usually appear early in life; therefore, sweat electrolytes are frequently collected from infants.

Specimen collection is time consuming and must be performed under very controlled conditions to ensure that the small amount of sample collected is not altered by contamination or evaporation.

Patients are induced to sweat using a technique called ***pilocarpine iontophoresis***, which is illustrated in Figure 11–2. Pilocarpine, a sweat-inducing chemical, is applied to an area of the forearm or leg that has been previously cleansed with deionized water. The pilocarpine is then introduced into the skin by the application of a mild electric current (iontophoresis) provided by a device designed for pilocarpine iontophoresis. Following iontophoresis, the area exposed to the pilocarpine is again thoroughly cleansed with deionized water.

Several methods are available for collection of sweat for electrolyte analysis, including the use of preweighed gauze or filter paper pads or coil collectors. The collection apparatus is placed on the stimulated area, covered securely with plastic if the collection material is gauze or filter paper, and allowed to remain for a specified length of time, usually 30 minutes.

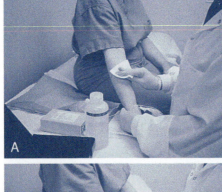
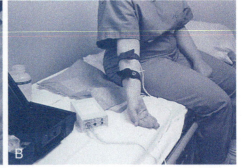
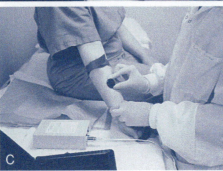

FIGURE 11–2   Sweat collection by means of pilocarpine iontophoresis. *A*, Cleansing the collection site with distilled water. *B*, Performing iontophoresis sweat stimulation. *C*, Applying the sweat collection container. (From Strasinger, SK, and Di Lorenzo, MA: Phlebotomy Workbook for the Multiskilled Healthcare Professional. FA Davis, Philadelphia, 1996, p. 340, with permission.)

Regardless of the collection method used, it is essential that:

1 The collection apparatus be handled only with sterile forceps or powder-free gloves and not contaminated by use of the fingers
2 The collection apparatus be tightly sealed during the collection period to prevent evaporation of the collected sweat
3 The collected sweat be tightly sealed during transportation to the laboratory to prevent evaporation

PCTs may be involved in scheduling, assisting with specimen collection, or performing the collection of sweat electrolytes. Most laboratories require that the test be scheduled with the particular laboratory and that they provide the collection materials.

Culture Specimen Collection

As discussed previously, urinary and fecal specimens are often collected for the purpose of microbial culture; however, any area of the body can be infected by pathogenic microorganisms. A common duty of the PCT is to collect specimens from the infected areas for the identification of the responsible microorganisms and the determination of their *antibiotic susceptibility* (C & S). The specimens collected are usually either body fluids such as urine, feces, sputum, and CSF collected in sterile containers or swabs collected from intact areas of the body such as the throat, the vagina, or a wound.

When collecting specimens for culture, some basic rules must be followed to ensure that the cause of the infection is correctly identified:

1 Specimens must be collected using sterile technique to prevent contamination by organisms that are not the cause of the infection.
2 The specimen must come directly from the infected area and must not include material from surrounding tissue. Whenever possible, the swab should be rotated to expose as much of it as possible to the infectious material.
3 Specimens must be placed in appropriate containers and delivered to the testing area as soon as possible to ensure the presence of viable organisms. Swabs for specimen collection are usually part of a collection system containing a small amount of transport culture medium (Fig. 11–3).
4 Specimens must be correctly labeled, including the type of specimen and the time of collection.

Considering the numerous body sites available for culturing, many special requirements exist. The most frequently collected specimens are discussed briefly in this

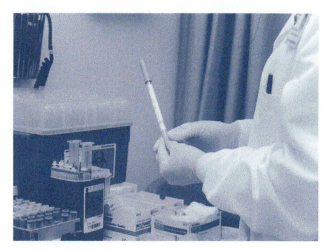

FIGURE 11–3 PCT crushing ampule of transport medium following specimen collection.

unit. PCTs should consult the procedure manuals provided by their laboratories before collecting any specimens.

THROAT CULTURES

PCTs will frequently be requested to collect throat culture specimens. They are performed primarily for the detection of the streptococcal infection "strep throat." Specimens may be collected for the purpose of performing a culture or a rapid immunologic group A streptococcus (strep) test (Unit 12).

Materials needed to collect a throat culture include a tongue depressor, a collection swab in a sterile tube containing transport medium, and possibly a flashlight.

To obtain the specimen (Fig. 11–4):

1 Have the patient tilt the head back and open the mouth wide.
2 Remove the cap with its attached swab from the holder using aseptic technique.
3 Gently depress the tongue with the tongue depressor.
4 Being careful not to touch the cheeks, tongue, or lips, swab the area in the back of the throat, including the tonsils and any inflamed or ulcerated areas.
5 Return the swab to the holder tube without touching the outside of the holder.
6 Crush the ampule of transport medium, making certain the released medium is in contact with the swab if a culture is to be performed.
7 Label the specimen and deliver it to the laboratory or perform a rapid immunologic test.

SPUTUM CULTURES

The primary concern when collecting a **sputum** culture is ensuring that the specimen is actually sputum and not saliva. Patients must be instructed to expectorate the specimen after a deep cough. PCTs should arrange for first-morning specimens to be collected whenever possible. Specimens that do not meet the criteria for a sputum culture will be rejected by the laboratory and must be re-collected.

WOUND CULTURES

Wound cultures are frequently collected and transported under **anaerobic** conditions. When collecting wound cultures, it is important that the specimen not be con-

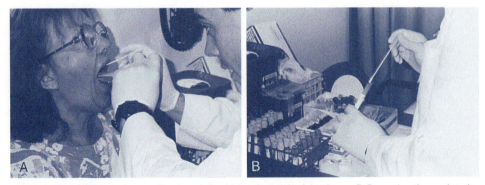

FIGURE 11–4   Throat culture collection. *A*, Swabbing the back of the throat. *B*, Returning the swab to its sterile container. (From Strasinger, SK, and Di Lorenzo, MA: Phlebotomy Workbook for the Multiskilled Healthcare Professional. FA Davis, Philadelphia, 1996, p. 337, with permission.)

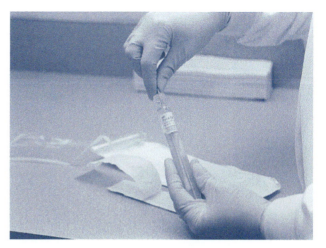

FIGURE 11–5 Swab being placed into anaerobic transport medium.

taminated with organisms from the surrounding tissue. The PCT may be asked to cleanse the area around the wound prior to specimen collection. When assisting with the collection of anaerobic specimens, the PCT must be certain that the appropriate materials are available for specimens collected either by needle and syringe aspiration or by swab. When material is collected in a syringe, any air present in the syringe should be expelled and then the material inoculated into an anaerobic transport vial.

Swabs are immediately placed into anaerobic transport systems (Fig. 11–5). Specimens should be delivered to the laboratory as soon as possible.

GENITAL CULTURES

When specimens are obtained to detect the presence of *Neisseria gonorrhoeae* from a urethral discharge or the vagina, it is usually necessary for the PCT to inoculate the specimen directly to culture medium prior to delivery to the laboratory. Several varieties of media transport systems are available, and PCTs should become familiar with the requirements of the system used in their facility (Fig. 11–6).

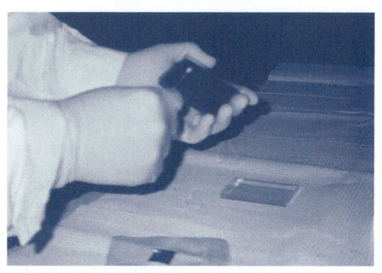

FIGURE 11–6 Plating a genital culture.

Specimen Handling

Depending on the type of facility, the responsibilities of a PCT with regard to the transport of specimens to the laboratory and the processing of these specimens prior to transportation will vary greatly. Of primary importance is the proper labeling of specimens, transporting the specimens as quickly as possible, and adhering to the specific handling instructions discussed previously in this unit and in Units 8 and 10. It may be necessary to time-stamp requisition forms delivered to the laboratory (Fig. 11–7).

SPECIMEN LABELING

One of the most frequent causes of specimen rejection by a laboratory is an unlabeled or improperly labeled specimen. The rules for proper labeling of phlebotomy specimens apply to all specimens. Just as two unidentified lavender top tubes with blood specimens cannot be matched with their appropriate patients, neither can two throat swabs or two urine specimens. Following institutional protocol, specimens should be labeled with the patient's name and ID number, the date, and other required information before leaving the patient. Requests for specimens for cultures must also contain the location from which the specimen was taken. An improperly labeled specimen indicates the possibility of a distraction from routine procedure that could compromise the proper identification of the patient and/or the specimen.

Specimen labeling is facilitated by the use of preprinted computer-generated labels. The labels must be taken with the equipment to the patient when the specimen is collected and must be applied before leaving the area. Allowing unlabeled specimens

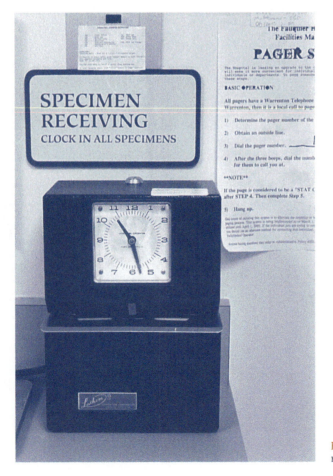

FIGURE 11–7   Clock for stamping requisitions.

to sit on a counter while a label is being printed is a major cause of misidentification because PCTs cannot predict when they will be interrupted by a patient or an emergency.

An additional aid in specimen identification is the use of **bar code** labeling. Information obtained from a bar code may be only the patient's name and ID number or may include the tests to be performed on the specimen. In some institutions bar codes are generated in the laboratory, but in other institutions bar codes are a part of the computer-generated labels printed when a request for a particular test is entered into the computer. Many laboratory instruments are capable of scanning the bar code on a tube of blood, performing the tests requested, and printing out a report with the patient's name, ID number, and requested test results. Bar coding also aids in identifying mislabeled specimens. For example, the receipt of a culture swab with a bar code for a midstream clean-catch urine culture immediately results in specimen rejection. Likewise, a lavender top tube of blood with a bar code for a prothrombin time will be rejected.

SPECIMEN TRANSPORT

Once the specimen has been properly labeled, it must be delivered to the laboratory. In facilities with on-site laboratories, PCTs may deliver specimens to the laboratory, arrange for designated transporters to pick up the specimens, or pack specimens for delivery through a **pneumatic tube system**. Allowing specimens to sit for extended periods prior to delivery is detrimental to both the quality of patient care that depends on the test results and the integrity of the specimens. Delivery of specimens via a pneumatic tube system is one of the most efficient methods because both personnel time and delivery time are saved. Care must be taken when loading specimens into the pneumatic tube capsule to ensure they are properly cushioned against breakage and enclosed in leakproof containers (Fig. 11–8). Specimens requiring consistent cooling or warming after collection cannot be transported via a pneumatic tube system. All specimens contain potentially infectious material, and Standard (Universal) Precautions must be followed during specimen transport. Containers contaminated on the outside are not accepted by laboratories.

Facilities that do not have on-site laboratories often have a contract with a particular laboratory that picks up specimens on a daily basis or provides specific packaging materials and mailing instructions. PCTs must be sure to include all necessary labels, requisition forms, and patient or specimen information in the package.

Specimens vary as to their storage requirements (refrigeration, freezing, and so on). Specimens requiring refrigeration can be transported in Styrofoam containers with refrigerant packs or ice enclosed in leakproof bags. Specimens that must remain frozen are packaged in containers with dry ice.

SPECIMEN PROCESSING

PCTs employed in facilities that do not have on-site laboratories may be required to perform additional procedures to preserve specimen integrity. This can include separating blood specimens and preparing **aliquots** of specimens, in addition to providing special packaging of specimens for transport.

Separation of blood specimens is performed by centrifugation and is needed for laboratory tests performed on plasma or serum. Plasma is obtained by centrifugation of anticoagulated blood, and serum is similarly obtained from clotted blood. To prevent contamination of plasma and serum by cellular constituents, it is recommended that specimens be separated within 2 hours.

Anticoagulated specimens can be centrifuged immediately after collection and the plasma removed. Specimens collected without anticoagulant must be fully clotted

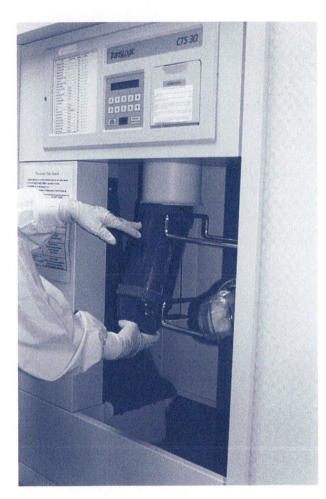

FIGURE 11–8   Loading specimens into a pneumatic tube system.

prior to centrifugation. Clotting time can vary from 5 minutes, when clot activators are present, to 1 hour for specimens from patients receiving anticoagulant therapy. When collection tubes containing gel separators (SST and PST) are used, it is not necessary to transfer the serum or the plasma to a separate tube because the gel prevents contamination by the blood cells.

There are many types of ***centrifuges***, ranging from small tabletop models to large refrigerated floor models. PCTs most frequently work with tabletop models, often supplied by the laboratory that performs the testing for their facility. These models are usually preset to rotate at the speed necessary for blood separation. The PCT places the tubes in the centrifuge and sets the time of centrifugation (usually 5 to 10 minutes). Improper use of the centrifuge can be dangerous, and the following rules of operation must be observed:

1 Tubes placed in the cups of the **rotor head** must be equally balanced. This is accomplished by placing tubes of equal size and volume directly across from each other. Matching tubes containing water should be used whenever necessary to achieve proper balance. Failure to do this will cause the centrifuge to vibrate and possibly break the tubes. A final check for balancing should be made just prior to closing the centrifuge lid (Fig. 11–9).

2 A centrifuge should never be operated until the top has been firmly fastened down and the top should never be opened until the rotor head has come to a complete stop. Should a tube break during centrifugation, pieces of glass and biohazardous aerosols can be sprayed from an uncovered centrifuge.

3 Do not walk away from a centrifuge until it has reached its designated rotational speed and does not have excessive vibration.

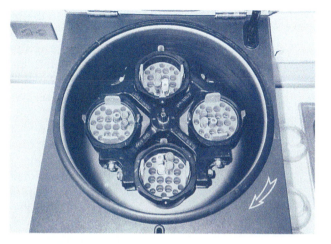

FIGURE 11–9 A properly balanced centrifuge. (From Strasinger, SK, and Di Lorenzo, MA: Phlebotomy Workbook for the Multiskilled Healthcare Professional. FA Davis, Philadelphia, 1996, p. 342, with permission.)

4 If a tube breaks in the centrifuge, the cup containing the broken glass must be completely emptied into a sharps container and disinfected. The inside of the centrifuge must also be cleaned of broken glass and disinfected. Puncture-resistant gloves should be worn for the cleanup.

When transferring specimens to another container, Standard Precautions must be strictly followed. Gloves, fluid-resistant coats that are completely closed, and face shields should be worn. Care must be taken to prevent the formation of **aerosols** when stoppers are removed from evacuated tubes. As discussed in Unit 5, stoppers should be covered with gauze and twisted rather than "popped" off. Specimens should not be poured from one container to another, because this can result in splashing of infectious material. Containers into which specimens are transferred must be labeled with the same information as that on the original collection container.

Laboratories provide instructions regarding specimen stability and the volume and type of specimen required, and this information should be consulted when specimens are prepared for transport. PCTs may be required to measure large-volume specimens, such as 24-hour urine specimens; record the volume; and send only an aliquot to the laboratory. Particular care should be paid to the specific preservation requirements of various specimens. All required information must be included with the specimen when it is shipped.

Use of the Computer

Computers have become an essential part of the healthcare delivery system. PCTs may use computers to generate requisitions and specimen labels, request and schedule diagnostic procedures, record patient information, access test results, and enter billing information. They should understand the basic components of computer systems, be able to enter and retrieve data, be willing to learn new applications as the computer system expands, and realize that computers are intended to increase the efficiency and accuracy of patient care.

Most people have some experience using microcomputers or personal computers in school, in the workplace, or at home. The differences between these computers and computers in healthcare institutions are, primarily, the amount of information that can be processed, the speed of processing, and the ability to transfer information to other computers. The actual computer operated by a PCT may appear to be no different from a familiar school or home model, although it may be connected to a higher-powered minicomputer or mainframe computer for transfer and storage of data.

Knowledge of the basic computer terminology needed to effectively operate the computer begins with the terms *hardware* and *software*.

Hardware refers to the solid components of the computer, including the central processing unit (**CPU**), workstation, printer, and storage disks. The CPU contains the power supply, integrating circuits, processing chips, and random access memory (**RAM**) chips. RAM determines the amount of data that can be newly entered into or retrieved from the CPU during operation. The data must be saved prior to shutting off the computer. The workstation consists of the keyboard for data input and the monitor that displays the entered data. The printer provides output of data, and there are many types of printers that vary in speed and quality of print. Depending on the computer system, data may be stored on removable "floppy disks" or hard disks or in central computer system storage devices.

Software refers to the instructions provided to the computer and consists of an operating system that is specific for the particular brand of computer because of the read-only memory (**ROM**) installed by the manufacturer. The application programs such as word processing, spreadsheets, and data management must be compatible with the hardware that is being used.

Many application programs for healthcare use are available, and the decision to use a particular program is determined by the requirements of the facility. In a small urgent care facility or a physician's office, a program may be needed only for billing purposes and word processing. In a large acute-care facility, however, the computer system may be connected to all departments.

PCTs required to input or retrieve data on the computer are assigned a password that allows them to use the computer. The purpose of the password is to provide computer security so that patient data will be available only to authorized personnel. PCTs should understand that any computer transaction performed when their password has been used to access the computer can be traced back to them. The password should never be given to other persons or used to retrieve data on persons who are not their patients. Often, the most difficult task when beginning a job in a new facility is learning how to use the new computer system.

BIBLIOGRAPHY

Henry, JB: Clinical Diagnosis and Management by Laboratory Methods, ed. 19. WB Saunders, Philadelphia, 1996.

Strasinger, SK: Urinalysis and Body Fluids, ed. 3. FA Davis, Philadelphia, 1994.

Strasinger, SK, and Di Lorenzo, MA: Phlebotomy Workbook for the Multiskilled Healthcare Professional. FA Davis, Philadelphia, 1996.

STUDY QUESTIONS

1. If a urine specimen cannot be delivered to the laboratory within 1 hour, how should the specimen be stored?

   _____

2. State the specific type of specimen a patient should be instructed to collect for the following tests:

   a. Urine culture _____

   b. Quantitative fecal fat _____

   c. Routine urinalysis _____

   d. Ova and parasites _____

   e. Follow-up urinalysis _____

   f. Quantitative urine creatinine _____

3. Why should a patient begin and end a timed urine collection period with an empty bladder?

   _____

   _____

4. Name a specimen and test that patients can mail to the laboratory.

   _____

5. State the most common order of CSF tube distribution.

   a. #1 _____

   b. #2 _____

   c. #3 _____

6. True or False. A patient delivers a semen specimen to the laboratory in a condom for fertility studies. He should be given a sterile container and told to collect another specimen in 3 days. _____ Explain your answer.

   _____

   _____

7. What information (other than patient ID) must be placed on the requisition that accompanies a semen specimen?

   _____

8. Sweat electrolytes are collected to confirm the diagnosis of

   _____.

9. List three collection errors that could produce falsely elevated sweat electrolytes.

a. _____

b. _____

c. _____

10. The name of the technique used for collection of sweat electrolytes is

_____.

11. Describe the areas that should be swabbed when collecting a throat specimen.

_____

_____

12. Name three areas that should be avoided when collecting a throat specimen.

a. _____

b. _____

c. _____

13. Name a cause for laboratory rejection of a properly labeled sputum culture.

_____

14. What type of culture specimens are frequently collected and transported using anaerobic conditions?

_____

15. Genital cultures may be streaked directly onto culture media when the presence

of _____ is suspected.

16. List three reasons why a specimen delivered to the laboratory area would be unacceptable.

a. _____

b. _____

c. _____

17. What protective apparel must be worn when processing blood specimens?

_____

_____

_____

18. True or False. Specimens collected in light-blue top tubes must be allowed to sit for 30 minutes prior to centrifugation. _____ Explain your answer.

_____

_____

19. Given the following tubes and spaces in a centrifuge rotor head, show how you would balance the centrifuge by placing the numbers of the appropriate tubes in the spaces on the rotor head.

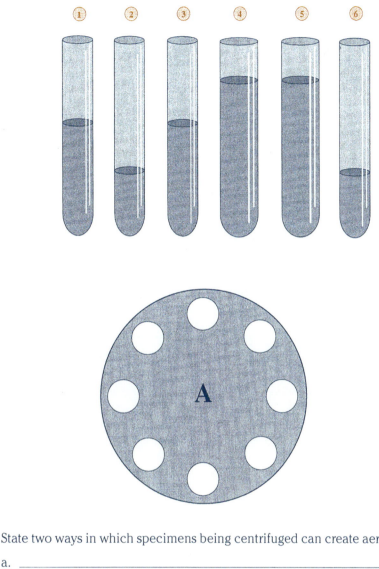

20. State two ways in which specimens being centrifuged can create aerosols.

a. _____

b. _____

21. State two ways by which an aerosol can be produced when processing blood specimens after centrifugation.

a. _____

b. _____

22. When might a PCT be required to make an aliquot of a specimen?

_____

_____

23. Match the following terms or statements with the appropriate computer component:

Term/Statement

a. _____ Billing program

b. _____ Floppy disk

c. _____ RAM

d. _____ Word processing

e. _____ Output device

f. _____ Input device

g. _____ Power supply

h. _____ Keyboard

i. _____ Monitor

j. _____ Hard disk

Component

1. CPU

2. Workstation

3. Printer

4. Storage device

5. Software

24. A PCT is counseled by the supervisor because two computer entry errors on the previous day were traced back to the PCT. The PCT states that he or she did not use the computer on that day. Explain how this could occur and how it could be avoided.

_____

_____

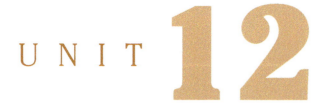

UNIT 12

POINT-OF-CARE TESTING

KEY TERMS

- ■ *Calibration* — Standardization of an instrument used to perform diagnostic tests

- ■ *Control* — Substance of known concentration used to monitor the accuracy of test results

- ■ *Documentation* — Recording of pertinent information such as test results, quality control, and observations

- ■ *Enzyme* — Protein capable of producing a chemical reaction with a specific substance (substrate)

- ■ *Immunoassay* — Testing procedure using specific antibodies to detect the presence of an antigen in a patient specimen

- ■ *Package insert* — Testing procedure information provided by the manufacturer of the testing materials

- ■ *Panic value* — Critically abnormal patient test result

- ■ *Point-of-care testing* — Laboratory tests performed in the patient care area

- ■ *Proficiency testing* — Performance of tests on specimens provided by an external monitoring agency

- ■ *Quality control* — Methods used to monitor the accuracy of procedures

- ■ *Reagent* — Substance used to produce a chemical reaction

Point-of-care testing **(POCT)** refers to laboratory testing procedures performed in the area where a patient is located, instead of in the traditional clinical laboratory. POCT is frequently performed at the bedside of a hospitalized patient and is particularly beneficial to patient care in the intensive care unit and the operating room. POCT is also performed in outpatient facilities such as HMOs, physicians' offices, clinics, dialysis centers, and home healthcare settings. Factors that have contributed to the increased practice of POCT include the increased acuteness of inpatient illnesses, requiring faster turnaround time of results; decreased length of hospital stays; and increased performance of procedures and care on an outpatient basis.

POCT is well suited to the concept of patient-focused care, because testing is not dependent on sources outside the nursing unit. The immediate availability of results provides convenience to both the patient and the healthcare providers by decreasing the time required for diagnosis and treatment, resulting in faster patient recovery.

The growing popularity and scope of POCT is due in large part to advances in technology. Small, handheld instruments and analyzers located in patient-care areas provide mobility, low maintenance, ease of use, cost effectiveness, and, most important, reliable test results when properly used.

There are many tests available from a variety of reputable manufacturers, and new POCT procedures are continuously being developed. The instrumentation and kit test procedures discussed in this unit were selected solely because of availability to the author. The importance of proper instrument maintenance and ***calibration***, quality control, and ***documentation***, however, is the same for all procedures.

Regulation of Point-of-Care Testing

The Clinical Laboratory Improvement Act of 1988 (**CLIA '88**) defined categories of diagnostic laboratory tests and specified the training and educational levels required of personnel performing the tests. Tests are assigned to the following categories: waived, moderate complexity, and high complexity.

Waived tests are considered easy to perform and interpret, require no special training or educational background, and require only a minimum of standardization and quality control. Many waived tests, such as glucose monitoring and pregnancy tests, are available over the counter to all consumers.

Moderate-complexity tests are more difficult to perform than are waived tests and require documentation of training in testing principles, instrument calibration, and quality control. Facilities performing moderate-complexity tests may be subject to periodic ***proficiency testing*** and on-site inspections. In the hospital setting, even waived tests must adhere to the moderate-complexity test standards. PCTs performing POCT should be thoroughly familiar with the regulations governing the tests they are performing and the documentation needed to demonstrate compliance. In most institutions, training, proficiency testing, and monitoring of quality control are administered by the clinical laboratory. Persons performing POCT may be required to demonstrate testing competency on a periodic basis.

High-complexity tests require sophisticated instrumentation and a high degree of interpretation by the testing personnel. They are not performed as POCTs.

Quality Control

Quality control (QC) of testing procedures is part of a much larger system referred to as quality assurance (QA), the purpose of which is to provide quality patient care. QC procedures are performed to ensure that acceptable standards are being met during the process of patient testing. Performance and monitoring of QC is a major part of

POCT. It is performed to ensure that instrumentation is functioning properly and has been accurately calibrated, that **reagents** are reacting appropriately, and that the testing is being performed correctly. QC does not verify the integrity of the specimen. Collection procedures discussed in previous units must be followed.

QC is performed at scheduled times, such as at the beginning of each shift and prior to testing patient samples, and it must always be performed if an instrument is dropped or if test results are questioned by the physician. **Controls** are manufactured specimens with known values, and these are usually available in several strengths, such as low, normal, and high ranges, for a particular test.

Documentation of QC includes dating and initialing the material when it is first opened and recording the manufacturer's lot number and the expiration date each time a control is run and the test result obtained. The person performing patient testing must also be the person performing the QC. All QC results are reviewed by a designated supervisor.

Procedures

Equipment, reagents, and controls for POCT are well-supported by the manufacturers, who supply detailed information in the form of **package inserts**. The information in package inserts includes safety precautions regarding biologic, chemical, electrical, and mechanical hazards; instrument maintenance and calibration; reagent storage requirements; acceptable control ranges; specimen requirements; procedural steps; interpretation of results and normal values; and sources of error. Manufacturers also provide training materials and assistance in troubleshooting technical problems.

Areas in which POCT is performed are required to maintain a procedure manual that is readily available to all testing personnel. The procedure manual contains the information provided in the package inserts from the instrumentation, reagents, and controls for each procedure. It also contains site-specific information, such as the location of supplies, instructions for reporting and recording results, and the protocol to follow when critically low or high test results (**panic values**) are encountered. Training for personnel performing POCT includes reading both the package inserts and the procedure manual thoroughly and demonstrating an understanding of the information they contain. It is important to understand that POCT procedures vary among manufacturers; therefore, package inserts and procedures in the procedure manual are not interchangeable.

This unit provides a general overview of some of the most commonly performed POCT procedures and does not include all of the material that would be found in the package inserts or a procedure manual. It also does not include all of the currently available tests.

BLOOD GLUCOSE

Measurement of blood glucose is performed as a POCT primarily to monitor persons with diabetes mellitus to determine whether their diet and insulin dosage is maintaining an acceptable level of glucose in the body. Testing may also be performed in an outpatient setting to screen persons for the presence of diabetes mellitus. Normal values for blood glucose vary slightly among testing procedures and are higher when serum or plasma, instead of whole blood, is tested in the clinical laboratory. Keep in mind that all POCT is performed on whole blood. POCT glucose normal values are approximately 60 to 115 mg/dL in a fasting blood sugar. Levels below 60 mg/dL are termed hypoglycemic, and increased levels are termed hyperglycemic. The PCT should be aware of the established panic value levels for blood glucose and notify the appropriate personnel immediately when they are encountered.

Many varieties of blood glucose POCT instrumentation are available. Older instruments work on the principle of reflectance of color intensity resulting from the reaction of chemicals on a reagent pad with blood glucose. In these instruments, the blood comes in direct contact with the instrument's detecting system, thereby requiring more frequent cleaning of the lenses.

Two newer instruments, the Ames Glucometer Elite (Bayer Diagnostics, Elkhart, IN) and Boehringer Mannheim Accu-Chek Advantage (Boehringer Mannheim Corporation, Indianapolis, IN) (Figs. 12–1 and 12–2), both work on the principle of the measurement of electrical potential caused by the reaction of glucose with reagents on the electrode of the testing strip. This type of instrumentation is advantageous in a POCT setting because the blood sample does not come in direct contact with the instrument, thus requiring a minimum of instrument cleaning.

Test Procedure (Boehringer Mannheim Accu-Chek Advantage)

Materials Required

1 Battery-operated testing instrument.
2 Electronic check strip (included with the monitor). When the check strip is acceptable, the monitor will display "L1," indicating that the user may proceed with Level 1 QC testing. Following acceptable Level 1 QC, the monitor will display "L2," and the user may continue with Level 2 QC testing.
3 Test strips. Each new box of test strips contains a "code key" that is inserted into the back of the monitor to match the lot number of the test strips.
4 QC samples.
5 Dermal puncture materials.

Summary of Procedure

1 Turn on monitor.
2 Perform electronic check. Do not proceed if the electronic check does not perform to manufacturer's guidelines. Document result.
3 Verify that test strips are "coded" with the monitor. Document code.
4 Perform QC. At least two levels of QC should be tested. Do not proceed if any of the QC results are not within the manufacturer's guidelines. Document results.
5 Insert electronic check strip into monitor with electronic bars toward monitor.
6 Perform capillary puncture according to the procedure in Unit 9.
7 Obtain a large drop of blood and touch blood to the target area on test strip. Note that the monitor has a digital display readout. Error codes will appear if the sample is not completely covering the test area.
8 The result will be displayed in 40 seconds. Document result and initial.

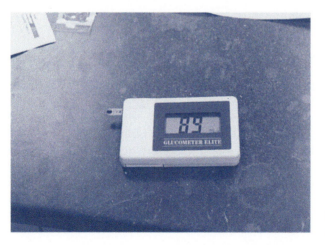

FIGURE 12–1   Glucometer Elite displaying test result.

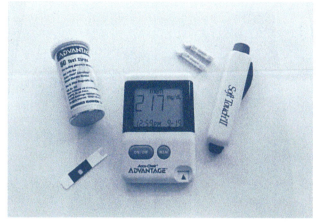

FIGURE 12–2 Accu-Chek Advantage, including dermal puncture equipment, electronic test strip, and patient testing strips.

9 Discard used materials according to Occupational Safety and Health Administration (OSHA) guidelines.
10 Make sure that testing strips are stored at room temperature in tightly closed containers.

HEMOGLOBIN

The primary function of the RBC protein hemoglobin (Hgb) is to transport oxygen to all cells in the body. A decrease in the number of RBCs or the amount of Hgb in the cells (anemia) results in a decrease in the amount of oxygen reaching the cells. Normal values for Hgb vary with age and gender, with values for adult women ranging between 12 and 15 g/dL and for adult men, between 14 and 17 g/dL. Measurement of Hgb is one of the most frequently performed screening tests in all healthcare settings and also provides a means to monitor patients known to have anemia.

Varieties of POCT analyzers that measure Hgb include instruments that provide Hgb concentration as part of a larger test menu that may analyze glucose and electrolytes or as dedicated **hemoglobinometers**. The HemoCue (Hemocue, Inc., Mission Viejo, CA) discussed in this section is designed to measure Hgb specifically.

The general principle of the HemoCue procedure is based on an optical measuring **cuvette** of small volume and short light path. The cuvette contains reagents that react with the blood sample to release the Hgb and produce a colored reaction. A **photometer** reads the absorbance of the final reaction, a modified azidomethemoglobin, at two wavelengths of light (570 mm and 880 mm) to compensate for turbidity, which may be caused by lipemic serum, elevated bilirubin, or increased white blood cells (WBCs).

Test Procedure (HemoCue)

Materials Required

1 Instrument and power source
2 Photometer check cuvette (included with the instrument)
3 Cuvettes
4 QC materials
5 Dermal puncture supplies

Summary of Procedure

1 Turn on the instrument and pull out the cuvette holder into insertion position.
2 The digital display shows "Hb" and after 6 seconds "Ready" with three blinking dashes (Fig. 12–3).

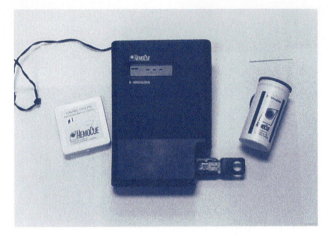

FIGURE 12–3 HemoCue containing reaction cuvette.

3 Perform photometer check. Do not proceed if the results are not within the manufacturer's guidelines. Document result.

4 Perform QC. At least two levels of QC should be tested. Do not proceed if QC does not fall within specified guidelines. Document results.

5 Take a cuvette from the container and reseal the container.

6 Perform capillary puncture according to procedure in Unit 9.

7 Make sure the blood drop is sufficient to fill the cuvette.

8 Hold the cuvette with two fingers at its square winged end and move the tip of the cuvette to the center of the blood drop. The cuvette should be filled in one step.

9 Immediately place the filled cuvette into the insertion position of the cuvette holder.

10 Push the holder to its inner position. The display area will show fixed dashes and the word "Measuring" will appear.

11 After 30 to 50 seconds the result will be displayed. Document result and initial.

12 Discard used materials according to OSHA guidelines.

URINALYSIS

Routine physical and chemical examination of urine has been performed in patient care areas for a much longer time than the term POCT has been in existence. The microscopic portion of the urinalysis is not a part of POCT and should not be performed by PCTs.

Urine is a readily available and usually easy-to-collect specimen that contains information about many of the body's major functions. It is important to obtain a patient history prior to testing urine, because ingestion of highly pigmented foods, medications, and vitamins can interfere with results. Information regarding collection and specimen types can be found in Unit 11. Urine should be tested within 1 hour of collection.

Physical Examination

Routine physical examination of urine describes the color and clarity of the specimen. Abnormal colors and increased turbidity can be indications of pathological conditions.

Normal urine color is yellow, and the intensity of the color is related to the concentration. A dilute urine is pale yellow or straw colored, and a concentrated (first-morning) urine is dark yellow. Common color descriptions of normal urine include pale yellow, straw, light yellow, yellow, dark yellow, and amber and may vary among institutions. If there are no interfering substances, a red or brown-black urine is abnormal and could indicate a disease process. An amber urine that produces yellow foam when shaken is also abnormal, if there are no interfering substances, and could indicate a disease process associated with liver function.

Normal urine is usually clear; however, normal substances such as epithelial cells may increase the turbidity. Describing clarity also varies from one facility to another. Common terms related to appearance include clear, hazy, cloudy, and turbid. A cloudy or turbid appearance from a fresh specimen may be cause for concern.

Test Procedure

Materials Required

1 Clear collection container with lid
2 Light source
3 Area with white background

Summary of Procedure

1 Obtain specimen in clear container with a lid.
2 Visually examine color under a good light, looking down through the container against a white background.
3 Report color according to facility guidelines.
4 Place lid on container and mix specimen by swirling the container.
5 Visually examine clarity while holding specimen in front of a light source.
6 Report clarity according to facility guidelines.

Chemical Examination

Routine chemical examination of urine is performed using plastic strips containing reagent-impregnated test pads. A color-producing chemical reaction occurs when the pads come in contact with urine. The color reaction can be read visually or by an automated reader. Most POCT settings use visual reading.

The two major types of urine testing reagent strips are the Bayer Diagnostics Multistix and the Boehringer Mannheim Chemstrip. They are available with single or multiple testing areas, depending on the POCT needs.

Proper handling and storage of reagent strips are critical for obtaining accurate results. Strips are stored at room temperature in opaque bottles containing a **desiccant** to protect them from exposure to excess light and moisture. Containers should be uncapped only long enough for a strip to be removed. When performing the test, strips should not be left sitting in the specimen because reagents will wash out of the pads and false-negative results will be obtained. Failure to read the reactions within the time frame specified by the manufacturer also will produce inaccurate results.

Test Procedure

Materials Required

1 Test strips with an acceptable expiration date
2 Positive and negative QC materials
3 Tissue
4 Light source
5 Timer

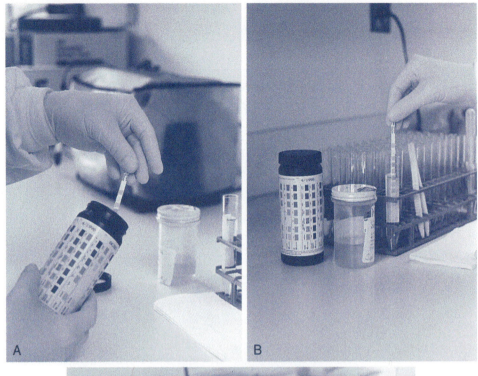

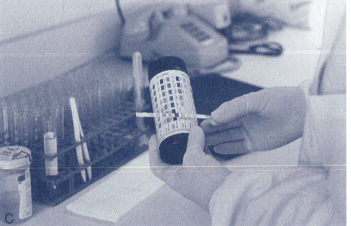

FIGURE 12–4   Chemical examination of urine. *A*, Removing reagent strip from container. *B*, Dipping reagent strip into specimen. *C*, Comparing reagent strip color reactions.

Summary of Procedure

1 Remove one strip at a time from container and recap (Fig. 12–4*A*).
2 Run positive and negative QC. Document results. If QC results are not within manufacturer's guidelines, do not proceed.
3 Mix specimen well.
4 Dip briefly, but completely, into specimen (Fig. 12–4*B*).
5 Remove excess urine when withdrawing strip from collection container and blot by touching the edge of the strip against a tissue.
6 Compare reaction colors with manufacturer's chart under a good light source at the specified time (Fig. 12–4*C*).
7 Be alert for interfering substances (Table 12–1). Obtain patient history, if necessary.
8 Document results and initial.

TABLE 12–1 **Summary of Chemical Testing by Reagent Strip**

| Test | Principle | Possible Reaction Interference | | Correlations with Other Tests |
		False-Positive	False-Negative	
pH	Double-indicator system	None	Runover from the protein pad may lower	Nitrite Leukocytes Microscopic
Protein	Protein error of indicators	Highly alkaline urine, quaternary ammonium compounds (antiseptics), detergents	High salt concentration	Blood Nitrite Leukocytes Microscopic
Glucose	Glucose oxidase, double sequential enzyme reaction	Peroxide, oxidizing detergents	Ascorbic acid, 5-HIAA, homogentisic acid, aspirin, levodopa, ketones, high specific gravity with low pH	Ketones
Ketones	Sodium nitroprusside reaction	Levodopa, phthalein dyes, phenylketones		Glucose
Blood	Pseudoperoxidase activity of hemoglobin	Oxidizing agents, vegetable and bacterial peroxidases	Ascorbic acid, nitrite, protein, pH below 5.0, high specific gravity, Captopril	Protein Microscopic
Bilirubin	Diazo reaction	Lodine Pigmented urine Indican	Ascorbic acid, nitrite	Urobilinogen
Urobilinogen	Ehrlich's reaction	Ehrlich-reactive compounds (Multistix), medication color	Nitrite, formalin	Bilirubin
Nitrite	Greiss's reaction	Pigmented urine on automated readers	Ascorbic acid High specific gravity	Protein Leukocytes Microscopic
Leukocytes	Granulocytic esterase reactions	Oxidizing detergents	Glucose, protein, high specific gravity, oxalic acid, gentamycin, tetracycline, cephalexin, cephalothin	Protein Nitrite Microscopic
Specific gravity	pK change of polyelectrolyte	Protein	Alkaline urine	None

FECAL OCCULT BLOOD

The purpose of the fecal **occult** blood test is to detect gastrointestinal bleeding that is not visible to the naked eye. Detection of occult blood is a valuable aid in the early diagnosis of colorectal cancer.

Test kits for fecal occult blood must be sensitive enough to detect a very small amount of blood; therefore, they are highly subject to interference by foodstuffs and medications. Patients should be instructed to avoid the following items 72 hours prior to testing: red meat, turnips, radishes, melons, horseradish, high doses of vitamin C, and excessive amounts of vitamin C–enriched foods. Aspirin and other nonsteroidal anti-inflammatory drugs that may cause gastrointestinal irritation should be avoided 7 days prior to testing. Test kits are available from several manufacturers, and it is important not to combine materials from different kits. Specimens should be collected following instructions provided by the test kit manufacturer. Contamination of the specimen with urine or toilet water should be avoided.

The SmithKline Hemoccult kit (SmithKline Diagnostics, Inc., San Jose, CA) consists of a packet containing filter paper areas impregnated with guaiac reagent, positive and negative control areas, and a bottle of color-developing reagent (Fig. 12–5). Note that samples can be mailed by the patient, if necessary. Hgb present in the stool sample reacts with hydrogen peroxide in the color-developing reagent to release oxygen, which then reacts with the guaiac reagent to produce a blue color.

Test Procedure (Hemoccult)

Materials Required

1 Slide test card
2 Developer specifically for use with slide card
3 Fecal sample

Summary of Procedure

1 Open the front of the card by pulling the tab.
2 Examine test areas for discoloration.
3 Apply a thin smear of stool sample inside the designated areas according to manufacturer's instructions (Fig. 12–6*A*).
4 Close the flap.
5 Allow closed card to sit for 3 to 5 minutes.
6 Open the back of the card slide.
7 Apply two drops of the developer directly over each test area (Fig. 12–6*B*).
8 Wait 60 seconds and read patient test area. Any trace of blue on or at the edge of the test area is a positive result.
9 After reading patient result, apply one drop of developer between the positive and the negative performance monitor (control) areas.
10 Visually read the performance monitor area within 10 seconds. A blue area should appear only in the positive area (Fig. 12–6*C*). Do not report a patient result if the performance monitor area does not read as expected.
11 Document patient and performance monitor results and initial.

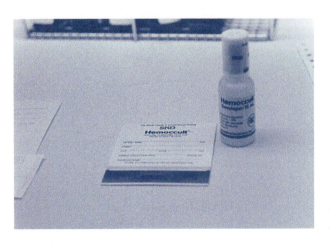

FIGURE 12–5　Hemoccult slide and developer.

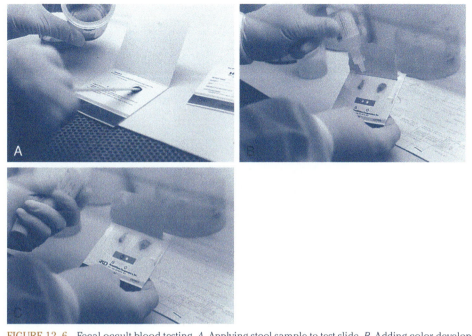

FIGURE 12–6   Fecal occult blood testing. *A*, Applying stool sample to test slide. *B*, Adding color developer to sample on test card. *C*, Reading test and controls.

PREGNANCY

Pregnancy testing is based on the detection of **human chorionic gonadotropin (HCG)** hormone in urine or serum. HCG is produced by cells of the placenta and, depending on the sensitivity of the test kit, can be detected approximately 10 days after conception. False-negative results will be obtained if not enough HCG has been produced to be detected at the time of testing. It is also important to perform urine pregnancy testing on a first-morning specimen to achieve maximum concentration. Cloudy urine specimens should be centrifuged prior to testing to avoid interference with the test reaction.

No special instrumentation is required for pregnancy testing, and a variety of commercial test kits are available. Most kits use the principle of ***enzyme immunoassay***, in which antibodies attached to a membrane in the testing receptacle bind with HCG when urine or serum is poured through the membrane. Additional antibody **conjugated** with enzyme then binds to the HCG on the membrane, and the addition of enzyme substrate produces a color reaction. The placement of the original antibody on the membrane determines the shape of the color reaction, such as a plus or minus sign, line, or circle. Areas to be used as positive and negative controls are also included on the test kit membranes.

Test Procedure (Hybritech ICON II)

Materials Required

1 HCG kit (Fig. 12–7) (remains stable at room temperature for 3 months)
   - Testing cylinder with membrane filter
   - Transfer pipets
   - Specimen diluent
   - Antibody conjugate
   - Substrate reagent (Light sensitive. Store in dark. The color should be clear; if it has turned blue, it must be replaced.)
   - Wash solution

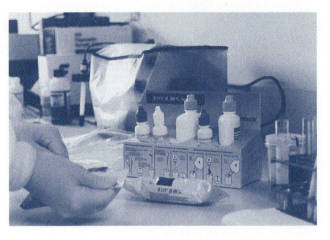

FIGURE 12–7   ICON II HCG test kit.

2 HCG-positive control

3 HCG-negative control

Note: Never mix components from different kits. Thoroughly mix components by swirling prior to testing. Complete washing and correct timing are critical to obtaining accurate results.

Summary of Procedure

1 Position the cylinder with the "P" facing toward you.

2 Dispense five drops of urine specimen with a transfer pipet or a pipet marked to 250 µL onto the center of the cylinder membrane, allowing each drop to absorb into the membrane filter (Fig. 12–8 [1]).

3 Dispense three drops of antibody conjugate in rapid succession onto the cylinder membrane filter so that the reagent covers the entire surface (Fig. 12–8 [2]). Wait 1 minute.

4 Dispense wash solution to the fill line, directing the flow toward the inner wall of the cylinder (Fig. 12–8 [3]). Wait for the wash solution to be absorbed into the membrane (less than 1 minute) before adding the next reagent.

5 Dispense three drops of substrate reagent in rapid succession onto the cylinder membrane. Wait 2 minutes. Do not allow reagent bottle tip to touch membrane surface (Fig. 12–8 [4]).

6 Stop the color development by filling the cylinder with wash solution (Fig. 12–8 [5]).

7 With the indicator "P" facing you, observe the test zone and the positive reference zone for the appearance of a blue dot, indicating a positive result (Fig. 12–8 [6]). Report as positive or negative.

8 Document patient and QC results and initial.

Note: If serum is used, it must first be diluted with two drops of specimen diluent using a sample cup included in the kit and a transfer pipet or a pipet marked to 500 µL. Let stand for 30 seconds and then transfer all of the treated serum onto the center of the cylinder membrane one drop at a time, allowing each drop to absorb into the membrane. Follow Procedure steps 4 through 7. Not all pregnancy test kits can be used for serum pregnancy tests. The capabilities of the kit are listed in the package insert.

GROUP A STREPTOCOCCUS

Symptoms of a sore throat are an indication to test for group A streptococcus (strep throat). Although only a small percentage of children and adults with sore throat symp-

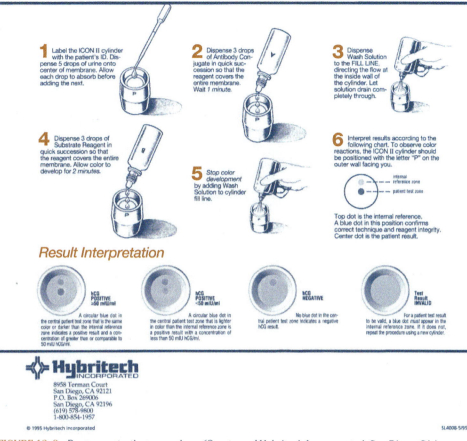

Result Interpretation

1 Label the ICON II cylinder with the patient's ID. Dispense 5 drops of urine onto center of membrane. Allow each drop to absorb before adding the next.

2 Dispense 3 drops of Antibody Conjugate in quick succession so that the reagent covers the entire membrane. Wait *1 minute.*

3 Dispense Wash Solution to the FILL LINE, directing the flow at the inside wall of the cylinder. Let solution drain completely through.

4 Dispense 3 drops of Substrate Reagent in quick succession so that the reagent covers the entire membrane. Allow color to develop for *2 minutes.*

5 *Stop color development* by adding Wash Solution to cylinder fill line.

6 Interpret results according to the following chart. To observe color reactions, the ICON II cylinder should be positioned with the letter "P" on the outer wall facing you.

— internal reference zone
— patient test zone

Top dot is the internal reference. A blue dot in this position confirms correct technique and reagent integrity. Center dot is the patient result.

hCG POSITIVE >50 mIU/ml
A circular blue dot in the central patient test zone that is the same color or darker than the internal reference zone indicates a positive result and a concentration of greater than or comparable to 50 mIU hCG/ml.

hCG POSITIVE <50 mIU/ml
A circular blue dot in the central patient test zone that is lighter in color than the internal reference zone is a positive result with a concentration of less than 50 mIU hCG/ml.

hCG NEGATIVE
No blue dot in the central patient test zone indicates a negative hCG result.

Test Result INVALID
For a patient test result to be valid, a blue dot *must* appear in the internal reference zone. If it does not, repeat the procedure using a new cylinder.

Hybritech
INCORPORATED
8958 Terman Court
San Diego, CA 92121
P.O. Box 269006
San Diego, CA 92196
(619) 578-9800
1-800-854-1957

© 1995 Hybritech Incorporated

SLA008-5/95

FIGURE 12–8   Pregnancy testing procedure. (Courtesy of Hybritech Incorporated, San Diego, CA.)

toms test positive for group A streptococcus, complications of untreated positive infections are serious; therefore, all symptomatic patients are usually tested.

Detection of group A streptococcus using a rapid test kit can be accomplished in a matter of minutes as opposed to the 1 or 2 days required when using conventional culture methods. Rapid tests work well when a high number of bacteria are collected on the throat swab. Fewer numbers of bacteria reduce the accuracy of the rapid tests and it is common policy to perform a throat culture on negative rapid test results. With this in mind, it may be necessary to collect two throat swabs, one for the rapid test and one to hold for possible culture. Specimens should be collected from the throat using a swab that does not have a cotton or calcium alginate tip and does not have a wooden shaft. When swabbing the throat, the procedures discussed in Unit 11 should be followed.

Rapid tests for group A streptococcus use the principles of enzyme immunoassay to detect group A streptococcus–specific antigens in material collected by standard swabbing of the throat. Bacterial antigens are removed from the swab using a mild acid solution. Antigens in the solution bind with antibody conjugated with enzyme. When the solution is poured through the membrane of the test cup, the antigen-antibody complexes bind with additional antibody impregnated in the test membrane. Addition of enzyme substrate to the membrane results in color production, indicating a positive result.

Test Procedure (Hybritech ICON Strep A)

Materials Required

1 Test kit (Fig. 12–9).
2 Components (can be stored at room temperature until expiration date).

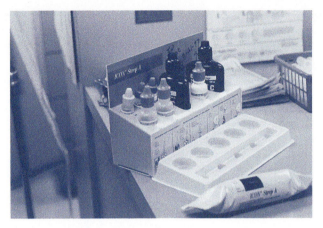

FIGURE 12–9   ICON Strep A test kit.

- Test cylinder
- Extraction reagents E1, E2, and E3 (Extraction reagents form a mild acid when mixed.)
- Antibody conjugate
- Substrate reagent (light sensitive and should be stored in the dark. It should be colorless; if it has turned blue, it must be replaced.)
- Wash solution
- Extraction cups
- Prefilter nozzles
- Reagent station
- Positive control

Note: Never mix components from different kits. Thoroughly mix components by swirling prior to testing. Complete washing and correct timing are critical to obtaining accurate results.

Summary of Procedure

1   If two swabs have been collected, rotate them together to evenly distribute specimen, and use one for the rapid test and one for the culture.
2   Add one drop of E1 and one drop of E2 to the extraction cup. The solution should change from pink to yellow (Fig. 12–10 [1]).
3   Add specimen swab to the cup within 1 minute of the color change. Rotate the swab to mix the reagents. Wait 1 minute (Fig. 12–10 [2]).
4   Add five drops of E3 and mix by rotating the swab in the cup. The solution in the cup should be pale yellow (Fig. 12–10 [3]).
5   Add one drop of antibody conjugate and mix by rotating the swab in the cup. After mixing, squeeze the sides of the cup together between thumb and index finger to remove all of the liquid from the swab (Fig. 12–10 [4]). Discard swab.
6   Place the prefilter nozzle onto the extraction cup (Fig. 12–10 [5]).
7   Position the cylinder with the "S" facing toward you.
8   Squeeze the entire sample through the prefilter onto the test cylinder (Fig. 12–10 [6]). Wait 2 minutes.
9   Add wash solution to the cylinder fill line and allow to drain completely (Fig. 12–10 [7]).
10   Add three drops of substrate reagent to the center of the cylinder (Fig. 12–10 [8]). Wait 2 minutes.
11   Add wash solution to stop the color reaction (Fig. 12–10 [9]). Allow to drain completely.
12   With the indicator mark "S" facing you, read the patient's results by looking for a purple spot of any intensity in the center of the membrane (Fig. 12–10 [10]).

PROCEDURE

EXTRACTION PROCEDURE

Bring all reagents and ICON cylinders to room temperature before running test.
Label ICON cylinder and extraction cup with patient ID.

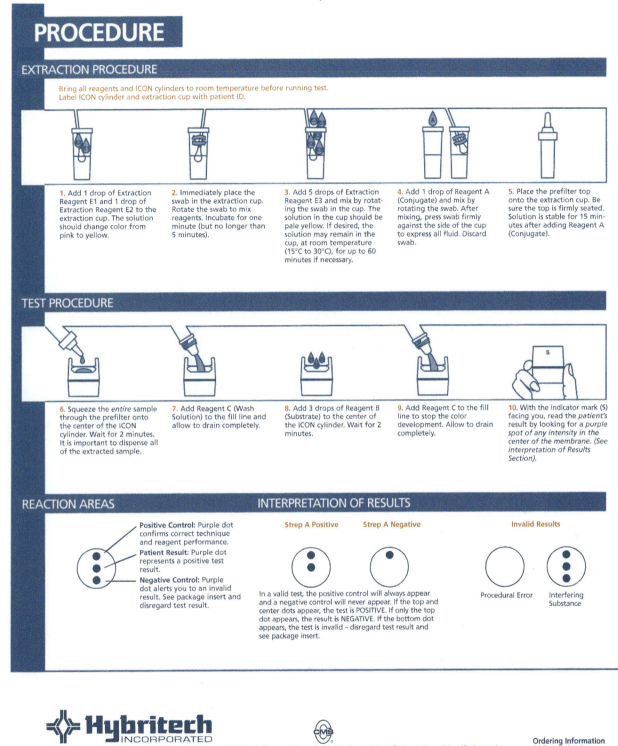

1. Add 1 drop of Extraction Reagent E1 and 1 drop of Extraction Reagent E2 to the extraction cup. The solution should change color from pink to yellow.

2. Immediately place the swab in the extraction cup. Rotate the swab to mix reagents. Incubate for one minute (but no longer than 5 minutes).

3. Add 5 drops of Extraction Reagent E3 and mix by rotating the swab in the cup. The solution in the cup should be pale yellow. If desired, the solution may remain in the cup, at room temperature (15°C to 30°C), for up to 60 minutes if necessary.

4. Add 1 drop of Reagent A (Conjugate) and mix by rotating the swab. After mixing, press swab firmly against the side of the cup to express all fluid. Discard swab.

5. Place the prefilter top onto the extraction cup. Be sure the top is firmly seated. Solution is stable for 15 minutes after adding Reagent A (Conjugate).

TEST PROCEDURE

6. Squeeze the *entire* sample through the prefilter onto the center of the ICON cylinder. Wait for 2 minutes. It is important to dispense all of the extracted sample.

7. Add Reagent C (Wash Solution) to the fill line and allow to drain completely.

8. Add 3 drops of Reagent B (Substrate) to the center of the ICON cylinder. Wait for 2 minutes.

9. Add Reagent C to the fill line to stop the color development. Allow to drain completely.

10. With the indicator mark (S) facing you, read the *patient's* result by looking for a *purple spot of any intensity in the center of the membrane. (See interpretation of Results Section).*

REACTION AREAS

Positive Control: Purple dot confirms correct technique and reagent performance.

Patient Result: Purple dot represents a positive test result.

Negative Control: Purple dot alerts you to an invalid result. See package insert and disregard test result.

INTERPRETATION OF RESULTS

Strep A Positive   **Strep A Negative**

In a valid test, the positive control will always appear and a negative control will never appear. If the top and center dots appear, the test is POSITIVE. If only the top dot appears, the result is NEGATIVE. If the bottom dot appears, the test is invalid – disregard test result and see package insert.

Invalid Results

Procedural Error   Interfering Substance

Hybritech INCORPORATED

Hybritech Incorporated
8958 Terman Court
P.O. Box 269006 (92196)
San Diego, CA 92121
(619) 578-9800
1-800-854-1957

Hybritech Canada
3650 Danforth Road
Scarborough, Ontario
Canada M1N 2E8
1-800-268-4446 (Canada)
(416) 694-3221

Hybritech Europe S.A.
B-4031 Liege (Angleur)
Belgium
32-(041)-67-70-00

Curtin Matheson Scientific, Inc.
P.O. Box 1546
Houston, Texas 77251
(713) 820-9898
We keep the best company.™
FISONS

Trace Scientific Pty, Ltd.
P.O. Box 310, Clayton, Vic. 3168
Australia
Telephone: (03) 543 1255
(07) 870 1922
(02) 899 1122
(008) 333 110

Ordering Information
24 Determinations
Hybritech Cat. No. 4509
CMS Cat. No. 304-386
50 Determinations
Hybritech Cat. No. 4504
CMS Cat. No. 262-473

© 1995 Hybritech Incorporated

SL3005-6/95

FIGURE 12–10 Group A streptococcus testing procedure. (Courtesy of Hybritech Incorporated, San Diego, CA.)

13 Check the positive control zone at the top of the cylinder and the negative control zone at the bottom of the cylinder.

14 Document results of patient and controls, and initial.

CHOLESTEROL

Cholesterol is a lipid manufactured by the body for use in cell membranes and as a precursor to steroid hormones. It is also found in high concentrations in animal fats; therefore, additional cholesterol enters the body through ingestion. When excessive amounts of cholesterol are ingested or produced by the body, the increased cholesterol circulating in the blood adheres to the walls of the blood vessels, resulting in blockage of blood flow and subsequent coronary artery disease (see Unit 13).

Normal values for cholesterol vary with age. The ideal value is less than 200 mg/dL, but it may be as high as 240 mg/dL in persons over age 50.

In the 1980s a nationwide effort was begun to educate the public on the importance of controlling blood cholesterol levels. Cholesterol testing became a routine part of health screening, necessitating the development of POCT instrumentation capable of performing a sophisticated chemical analysis while keeping sources of error to a minimum. Several instruments are currently available that meet these criteria. Operators should thoroughly understand the requirements and limitations of their particular instruments.

The Cholestech L-D-X (Cholestech Corporation, Hayward, CA) analyzer uses a cassette containing dry reagents capable of performing an enzymatic reaction when blood is added to the cassette (Fig. 12–11). Each cassette has a magnetic stripe containing calibration information; therefore, no operator calibration is required. The analyzer is designed to go into a "locking" mode if QC testing is not within acceptable limits. The operator must then contact a technical service representative at Cholestech, Inc.

Test Procedure (Cholestech L-D-X)

Materials Required

1 Instrument
2 Power source
3 Testing cassettes (room temperature)
4 Cholestech L-D-X capillary tubes containing lithium heparin
5 Cholestech L-D-X capillary plungers

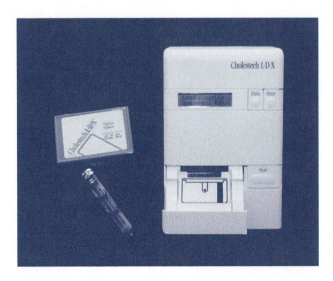

FIGURE 12–11   Cholestech L-D-X with optics cassette and capillary tubes.

6 High control
7 Low control
8 Optics check cassette

Summary of Procedure

1 Turn on analyzer and perform optics check using optics cassette. Document results.
2 Perform high and low controls. Document results.
3 Proceed with patient testing if optics and QC are within acceptable range.
4 Remove the cassette from the package. Hold the cassette by the short sides. Do not touch the black bar or magnetic stripe. Place cassette on flat surface.
5 Put a capillary plunger into the end of a Cholestech capillary tube with a red mark.
6 Press "Run." The analyzer will do a self-test. The analyzer screen will display "Selftest," "Running," then "Self-test OK." The cassette drawer will open. The analyzer screen will display "Load Cassette," followed by "Run."
7 Perform capillary puncture and fill the tube to the black mark with no air bubbles.
8 Gently push the plunger and apply the blood sample into the sample well within 5 minutes of collection.
9 Keep the cassette level and place in the analyzer drawer. The black bar must face toward the analyzer. The magnetic stripe must be on the right.
10 Press "Run." The drawer will close. During the test the screen will display "Test Name," then "Test Running."
11 When the test is complete, the analyzer will beep and the screen will display "Test Name, Result, and Date." The drawer will open. Remove and dispose of cassette.
12 Document results and initial.

ACTIVATED CLOTTING TIME

The formation of clots occurs when blood comes into contact with a foreign surface. This process is beneficial when a blood vessel is punctured and the exposed **collagen** in the vessel wall initiates the formation of a clot to stop the bleeding. This same process can be detrimental to patients if it is initiated during a surgical procedure or when the irritation to a blood vessel results in the release of clots into the circulatory system. Clinical procedures that can initiate the clotting process include cardiac catheterization, **hemodialysis**, and coronary **angioplasty**.

To prevent the formation of clots in these circumstances, patients are given the anticoagulant heparin. It is necessary to closely monitor the effects of heparin therapy because too much heparin can produce internal hemorrhaging and too little heparin may lead to clot formation (thrombosis). POCT instruments capable of measuring the time required for blood exposed to an activator to clot provide an efficient method of monitoring patients on heparin therapy.

The general principle of the Hemochron Jr. ACT-LR (International Technidyne Corporation, Edison, NJ) is based on determining the amount of time required to produce clotting in a whole blood specimen. A cuvette containing **celite** as an activator is placed into the instrument, blood is added, and the timing begins. Blood is automatically mixed with the celite and moved back and forth in the chamber between optical detectors until a clot has formed. The timing stops when the clot is detected, and the result is displayed in celite equivalent (CE) seconds. This particular instrument is intended for use in monitoring patients receiving low to moderate heparin anticoagulant therapy (up to 2.5 units [U] of heparin per cubic centimeter). Instruments using other inert clot activators, such as kaolin and glass beads, and electromagnetic timing of clot formation also are available.

Test Procedure (Hemochron Jr. ACT-LR)

Materials Required

1 Hemochron Jr. ACT-LR instrument (Fig. 12–12)
2 Power source
3 Hemochron Jr. microcoagulation ACT-LR cuvette
4 Normal and abnormal electronic controls
5 Normal and abnormal liquid controls
6 Hemochron temperature verification slide
7 Specimen collection system (capable of collecting 0.3 mL of blood [small syringe])

Note: Venous whole blood is required for testing. Capillary punctures are not acceptable for ACT Testing. Collection from an indwelling line is acceptable, providing no heparin has been administered through the line and any blood contaminated with fluid is discarded.

Summary of Procedure

1 Turn on instrument.
2 Insert cuvette (room temperature).
3 Allow instrument to proceed through prewarm/self-check mode.
4 When ready, the instrument will display "Add Sample," then "Press Start."
5 The user has 5 minutes to add the sample.
6 Dispense one drop of whole blood into the center of the sample well on the cuvette, filling from the bottom up flush to the top. Push any excess blood into the overflow well.
7 Depress "Start" key. A single "beep" marks the start of the test.
8 If too little or too much blood is added, the instrument will beep twice and display a fault code.
9 When the test is complete, a single beep will sound.
10 The result will be displayed in seconds equivalent to the celite activator (CE seconds).
11 Document results and initial.
12 QC procedures:
   • Temperature verification is performed on a daily basis using the temperature verification slide. The temperature should be $37°C \pm 1°$. Document temperature reading.
   • Normal and abnormal electronic QCs are performed on each shift in which the instrument is operated. Results should be within the range specified on the electronic control cartridge. Document control results.

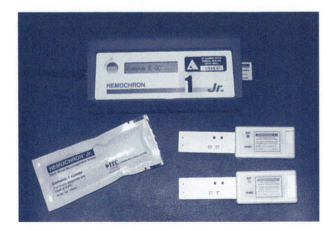

FIGURE 12–12 Hemochron Jr. ACT-LR with cuvettes and controls.

- Normal and abnormal liquid QCs are run when a new box of cuvettes is opened and when electronic QC does not yield acceptable results. Results should be within the range specified in the package insert accompanying the liquid controls. Document liquid control results.

Note: The instrument does not count in "real time" seconds, and normal values are based on CE seconds and can range between 89 and 169 CE seconds for nonheparinized patients.

BIBLIOGRAPHY

Henry, JB (ed): Clinical Diagnosis and Management by Laboratory Methods, ed. 19. WB Saunders. Philadelphia, 1996.

Manufacturer's Instructions: Accu-Chek Advantage. Boehringer Mannheim Corporation, Indianapolis, IN.

Manufacturer's Instructions: Cholestech L-D-X. Cholestech Corporation, Hayward, CA.

Manufacturer's Instructions: Hemochron Jr. International Technidyne Corporation, Edison, NJ.

Manufacturer's Instructions: HemoCue. HemoCue, Inc., Mission Viejo, CA.

Manufacturer's Package Insert: Hemoccult. SmithKline Diagnostics, Inc., San Jose, CA.

Manufacturer's Package Insert: ICON II HCG. Hybritech Inc., San Diego, CA.

Manufacturer's Package Insert: ICON Strep A. Hybritech Inc., San Diego, CA.

Strasinger, SK: Urinalysis and Body Fluids, ed. 3. FA Davis, Philadelphia, 1994.

STUDY QUESTIONS

1. State the two categories of laboratory testing that may be performed by a PCT/medical assistant according to CLIA '88 guidelines.

   a. _____

   b. _____

2. Define point-of-care testing (POCT) and name three different settings in which POCT is performed.

   a. The definition of POCT is _____ .

   b. Setting 1: _____

   c. Setting 2: _____

   d. Setting 3: _____

3. Define quality control (QC) and explain why it is required prior to any patient testing.

   _____

   _____

4. The Accu-Chek Advantage is used to test for _____ .

5. A fasting blood sugar (FBS) of 40 mg/dL is considered (a) normal (b) abnormal. (Circle one.) What would you do if you obtained the above result on a patient specimen?

   _____

   _____

6. Describe the primary function of Hgb.

   _____

   _____

7. Why does the HemoCue read the absorbance of the reaction at two different wavelengths?

   _____

   _____

8. The physical examination of urine includes visually examining the specimen for

   a. _____

   b. _____

9. A PCT has been assigned to test 10 urine specimens chemically. He or she removes 10 strips from the container and proceeds with testing. What is wrong with this scenario?

   _____

   _____

10. The Hemoccult is a slide card test for _____. List three things patients should avoid prior to having this test performed.

    a. _____

    b. _____

    c. _____

11. Pregnancy test kits are based on the presence of _____.

12. What is the purpose of the final wash solution step in the Hybritech ICON II pregnancy test kit?

    _____

    _____

13. True or false. The Hybritech ICON II kit test for pregnancy can use either urine or serum following the same procedural instructions. _____ If false, correct the statement to make it true.

    _____

    _____

14. Strep throat is caused by the presence of _____.

15. Why would two throat swabs be collected from a patient who is symptomatic for strep throat?

    _____

    _____

16. Swabs from the throat for rapid strep tests should not be made of materials that contain

    _____

17. Total timing to perform the Hybritech ICON II Strep A test is _____ minute(s).

18. The most desirable blood cholesterol level is _____ mg/dL.

19. High blood cholesterol levels have been shown to increase the risk of _____

    _____

20. What is the purpose of the magnetic stripe found on each testing cassette used with the Cholestech L-D-X?

    _____

    _____

21. The Cholestech L-D-X procedure states that the blood sample must be applied to the testing cassette within _____ minute(s) of collection.

22. Explain what has happened if the Cholestech L-D-X instrument goes into a "locking" mode and does not allow the user to continue with the procedure.

    _____

    _____

23. What is the purpose of heparin therapy?

_____

_____

24. Name three clinical procedures that may require a patient to be placed on heparin therapy.

a. _____

b. _____

c. _____

25. Heparin therapy may be monitored at the bedside by testing the _____ .

26. True or false. The Hemochron Jr. ACT-LR instrument accepts venous and capillary samples. _____ If false, correct the statement to make it true.

_____

EVALUATION OF BLOOD GLUCOSE DETERMINATION

RATING SYSTEM   2 = Satisfactory   1 = Needs improvement   0 = Incorrect/did not perform

_____ **1.** Turns on instrument

_____ **2.** Verifies that "Code Key" inserted in monitor matches lot number of test strips and documents results

_____ **3.** Performs check strip test

_____ **4.** Verifies that check strip test is acceptable and documents results

_____ **5.** Understands and follows monitor display throughout procedure

_____ **6.** Correctly removes one test strip from container

_____ **7.** Recaps container

_____ **8.** Correctly inserts test strip into monitor

_____ **9.** Performs QC and documents results

_____ **10.** Collects capillary specimen from patient according to procedure in Unit 9

_____ **11.** Correctly touches one drop of blood to the center of yellow target area

_____ **12.** Visually reads result from monitor and documents results

_____ **13.** Disposes of biohazardous materials according to OSHA guidelines

_____ **14.** Follows monitor directions for additional testing and/or appropriate instructions for turning off monitor

Total points _____

Maximum points = 28

COMMENTS

EVALUATION OF HEMOGLOBIN DETERMINATION

RATING SYSTEM   2 = Satisfactory   1 = Needs improvement   0 = Incorrect/did not perform

_____ **1.** Turns on instrument

_____ **2.** Correctly pulls out cuvette holder into insertion position

_____ **3.** Performs photometer check with photometer cuvette and documents results

_____ **4.** Removes cuvettes needed for testing from container

_____ **5.** Recaps container

_____ **6.** Performs QC and documents results

_____ **7.** Performs capillary puncture according to procedure in Unit 9.

_____ **8.** Correctly touches blood to tip of cuvette in one step, allowing blood to fill test area completely without creating air bubbles

_____ **9.** Correctly removes any excess blood without touching cuvette opening

_____ **10.** Positions filled cuvette correctly into cuvette holder

_____ **11.** Pushes cuvette holder into its inner position

_____ **12.** Understands and follows monitor display throughout procedure

_____ **13.** Correctly reads and documents patient results

_____ **14.** Disposes of biohazardous materials according to OSHA guidelines

_____ **15.** Follows directions for additional testing and/or appropriate instructions for turning off monitor

Total points _____

Maximum points = 30

COMMENTS

EVALUATION OF URINALYSIS (PHYSICAL DETERMINATION)

RATING SYSTEM   2 = Satisfactory   1 = Needs improvement   0 = Incorrect/did not perform

_____ **1.** Prepares to observe urine by ensuring specimen is in clear container with lid

_____ **2.** Positions container in a good light source

_____ **3.** Examines color visually by looking down through container against a white background

_____ **4.** Documents color of urine specimen according to facility guidelines

_____ **5.** Places lid on container

_____ **6.** Swirls container to completely mix specimen

_____ **7.** Examines clarity visually by holding specimen container in front of a light source

_____ **8.** Documents clarity of urine specimen according to facility guidelines

Total points _____

Maximum points = 16

COMMENTS

EVALUATION OF URINALYSIS (CHEMICAL DETERMINATION)

RATING SYSTEM   2 = Satisfactory   1 = Needs improvement   0 = Incorrect/did not perform

_____ **1.** Verifies and documents lot number and expiration date of test strips

_____ **2.** Removes one test strip from the container at a time

_____ **3.** Recaps container

_____ **4.** Visually checks test strip for discoloration

_____ **5.** Performs QC and documents QC positive and negative chemical reactions

_____ **6.** Mixes patient urine specimen

_____ **7.** Dips test strip completely, but briefly, into patient specimen

_____ **8.** Correctly removes excess urine from strip without causing carryover onto adjacent test pads

_____ **9.** Visually compares any color changes to test pads under a good light source at specified timing intervals

_____ **10.** Documents results

_____ **11.** Disposes of biohazardous materials according to OSHA guidelines

Total points _____

Maximum points = 22

COMMENTS

EVALUATION OF FECAL OCCULT BLOOD DETERMINATION

RATING SYSTEM   2 = Satisfactory   1 = Needs improvement   0 = Incorrect/did not perform

_____ **1.** Opens front of slide card

_____ **2.** Visually examines test areas for discoloration

_____ **3.** Correctly applies thin smear of stool to cover test areas

_____ **4.** Closes slide card by inserting cover into flap

_____ **5.** Allows card to sit for 3 to 5 minutes

_____ **6.** Opens back of slide card

_____ **7.** Correctly applies two drops of developer onto each test area

_____ **8.** Waits 1 minute and visually examines slide card for color reaction

_____ **9.** Correctly applies one drop of developer onto performance monitor area of slide card

_____ **10.** Waits 10 seconds and visually examines performance monitor area for color reaction

_____ **11.** Documents results of patient and performance monitor

_____ **12.** Disposes of biohazardous materials according to OSHA guidelines

Total points _____

Maximum points = 24

COMMENTS

EVALUATION OF PREGNANCY DETERMINATION

RATING SYSTEM   2 = Satisfactory   1 = Needs improvement   0 = Incorrect/did not perform

_____ **1.** Correctly dispenses five drops of urine specimen onto center of testing cylinder

_____ **2.** Allows each drop to absorb into filter

_____ **3.** Correctly dispenses three drops of antibody conjugate

_____ **4.** Waits 1 minute before proceeding

_____ **5.** Dispenses wash solution to fill line, directing flow toward inner wall of cylinder

_____ **6.** Allows solution to completely absorb into filter before proceeding

_____ **7.** Correctly dispenses three drops of substrate reagent

_____ **8.** Waits 3 minutes before proceeding

_____ **9.** Stops color reaction process by adding wash solution to fill line

_____ **10.** Correctly positions "P" indicator

_____ **11.** Examines visually for color reaction at test zone and reference zone

_____ **12.** Documents results from test and positive reference zone

Total points _____

Maximum points = 24

COMMENTS

EVALUATION OF GROUP A STREPTOCOCCUS DETERMINATION

RATING SYSTEM   2 = Satisfactory   1 = Needs improvement   0 = Incorrect/did not perform

_____ **1.** Correctly adds one drop of E1 and one drop of E2 to extraction cup

_____ **2.** Examines extraction cup visually for color change from pink to yellow

_____ **3.** Adds specimen swab to extraction cup within 1 minute of color change

_____ **4.** Rotates the swab in the extraction cup to mix the reagents

_____ **5.** Waits 1 minute before proceeding

_____ **6.** Correctly adds five drops of E3 and mixes by rotating swab in extraction cup

_____ **7.** Verifies visually the pale yellow color of the solution in the extraction cup

_____ **8.** Adds one drop of antibody conjugate and mixes by rotating the swab in the extraction cup

_____ **9.** Squeezes the sides of the extraction cup together, removing excess liquid from swab

_____ **10.** Discards swab

_____ **11.** Correctly places prefilter nozzle onto extraction cup

_____ **12.** Dispenses entire contents of extraction cup onto test cylinder

_____ **13.** Waits 2 minutes before proceeding

_____ **14.** Adds wash solution to cylinder fill line and allows to drain completely

_____ **15.** Adds three drops of substrate reagent to center of test cylinder

_____ **16.** Waits 2 minutes before proceeding

_____ **17.** Adds wash solution to stop color reaction and allows to drain completely

_____ **18.** Positions "S" indicator

_____ **19.** Examines visually for color change in center of test cylinder

_____ **20.** Examines visually upper and lower control zones for positive and negative reactions

_____ **21.** Documents results from test area and control zones

Total points _____

Maximum points = 42

COMMENTS

EVALUATION OF CHOLESTEROL DETERMINATION

RATING SYSTEM   2 = Satisfactory   1 = Needs improvement   0 = Incorrect/did not perform

_____ **1.** Turns on instrument

_____ **2.** Correctly performs optics check using optics cassette and documents acceptability

_____ **3.** Correctly removes cassette from package and does not touch the black bar or the magnetic stripe

_____ **4.** Places cassette on flat surface

_____ **5.** Prepares Cholestech L-D-X capillary tube by inserting plunger into end with red mark

_____ **6.** Correctly performs self-test on instrument

_____ **7.** Understands and follows instrument display throughout procedure

_____ **8.** Performs capillary puncture according to procedure in Unit 9

_____ **9.** Correctly fills capillary tube to black mark in one step without creating air bubbles

_____ **10.** Gently pushes plunger of capillary tube and applies blood sample to test well of cassette within 5 minutes of collection

_____ **11.** Keeps cassette level

_____ **12.** Correctly places cassette into analyzer "drawer"

_____ **13.** Performs test "Run" according to procedure

_____ **14.** Documents results

_____ **15.** Disposes of biohazardous material according to OSHA guidelines

_____ **16.** Follows instrument directions for additional testing and/or turning off instrument

Total points _____

Maximum points = 32

COMMENTS

EVALUATION OF ACTIVATED CLOTTING TIME DETERMINATION

RATING SYSTEM   2 = Satisfactory   1 = Needs improvement   0 = Incorrect/did not perform

_____ **1.** Turns on instrument

_____ **2.** Correctly inserts cuvette

_____ **3.** Monitors and documents acceptable prewarm/self-check mode

_____ **4.** Performs and documents electronic and liquid QC

_____ **5.** Understands and follows instrument display throughout procedure

_____ **6.** Recognizes time factor for adding sample

_____ **7.** Selects appropriate collection equipment

_____ **8.** Performs venous collection according to procedure in Unit 6

_____ **9.** Correctly dispenses one drop of venous blood into center of sample well on the cuvette

_____ **10.** Presses "Start" key

_____ **11.** Documents results when test is complete

_____ **12.** Disposes of biohazardous material according to OSHA regulations

_____ **13.** Follows instrument guidelines for additional testing and/or turning off monitor

Total points _____

Maximum points = 26

COMMENTS

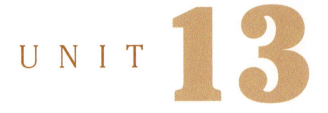
ELECTROCARDIOGRAPHY

KEY TERMS

- **Automaticity**   Ability of cardiac electrical cells to generate an impulse from within the heart

- **Bradycardia**   Slow heartbeat

- **Cardiac cycle**   One complete contraction and relaxation sequence of the heart

- **Conductivity**   Ability of cardiac electrical cells to transfer impulses

- **Depolarization**   Transmission of an electrical impulse from the SA node to the Purkinje system

- **Electrode**   Device capable of sensing electrical activity

- **Excitability**   Ability of cardiac electrical cells to transfer an impulse from one cell to another

- **Fibrillation**   Rapid, irregular movement of muscle fibrils

- **Holter monitor**   Portable system to measure cardiac activity over a prescribed time period

- **Isoelectric line**   Flat line on an electrocardiogram (ECG) indicating no electrical impulse

- ***QRS complex***   Deflection on an ECG tracing caused by the depolarization of the ventricles
- ***Repolarization***   Recovery phase following transmission of a cardiac electrical impulse
- ***Tachycardia***   Rapid heartbeat

The purpose of this unit is to prepare the PCT to perform a 12-lead electrocardiogram (ECG). This unit reviews the anatomy and physiology of the heart (Unit 4), emphasizing the electrical conduction system, the portion of the heart monitored by the ECG. It also discusses briefly the **pathophysiology** of cardiac disease, which is the main reason for electrocardiographic monitoring. Finally, it discusses the preparation of a patient for, and the conductance of, a diagnostic ECG.

Several disease processes, or pathophysiologies, can affect the functioning of the heart. **Cardiologists** use different diagnostic tests to determine the condition of the heart when a disease process is suspected or is being monitored over time. Some of these tests are very sophisticated, such as cardiac catheterization, in which dyes are injected directly into the coronary arteries, and electrode wires are inserted directly into the heart; such tests may require an operating room procedure. However, the most frequently used and one of the simplest tests is the ECG. An ECG provides the physician with a graphic representation of the heart's electrical system, the system responsible for initiating the muscular contraction that ejects blood from the heart to the lungs or the systemic circulation. An ECG can easily be performed in a physician's office, outpatient clinic, or emergency department. It can also be used to monitor the heart when stress is applied, as in controlled exercise (bicycle or treadmill), or to monitor the heart during daily activity (***Holter monitor***). The test consists of the placement of electrodes on the outside of the body in specific areas that, in turn, transmit electrical impulses to an electrocardiograph (ECG) machine. The machine then prints out the impulses on heat-sensitive paper. The task of the PCT is not to read or interpret the ECG tracing but to perform the test accurately so that the physician has the best possible tracing of the heart's activity with which to evaluate the patient. The PCT should recognize dangerous rhythms and alert a supervisor.

Structure of the Heart

The heart is a hollow, cone-shaped organ, located in the middle of the chest cavity, that rests on the **diaphragm**. It is composed of special muscle tissue and with each contraction propels blood to all parts of the body.

The heart varies in size but is generally about the size of a closed fist, about 14 cm long and 9 cm wide. The lungs are on either side of the heart, and the heart sits between the vertebrae in the back and the sternum in the front. The heart is angled slightly to the left of the midline, with its base at the level of the second rib, where the major blood vessels (aorta, pulmonary arteries, and veins) are located. The **apex** of the heart is a rounded tip located at the fifth intercostal space. A heartbeat taken at the apex is known as the **apical pulse**.

The heart is contained in a tough, fibrous membrane sac known as the **pericardium**. The heart consists of special tissue divided into three layers: the **epicardium**, a thin outer layer; the **myocardium**, a thick muscle layer; and the **endocardium**, a very smooth inner layer.

Internally the heart is divided into four chambers. The upper two chambers, the right atrium and the left atrium (the **atria**), are receiving chambers, and the lower two chambers, the right **ventricle** and the left ventricle, are pumping chambers. The right and left sides of the heart are separated by the septum. The upper and lower chambers are separated by **valves**, the **tricuspid** on the right and the **bicuspid** (mitral) on the left.

Function of the Heart

The heart functions as a four-chambered muscular pump that propels blood to all cells in the body. In reality, it is two separate pumps. One pump, the right side, propels deoxygenated blood to the lungs for reoxygenation, and the other pump, the left side, propels oxygenated blood to all of the body's millions of cells (see Fig. 4–5).

Deoxygenated blood is received into the right atrium from the superior vena cava, which collects blood from the upper portion of the body, and from the inferior vena cava, which collects blood from the lower portion of the body. As the right atrial wall contracts, blood is propelled through the tricuspid valve into the right ventricle. As the right ventricle contracts, blood is propelled into the right and left pulmonary arteries. Once the blood reaches the capillaries in the lungs, the blood is reoxygenated via the **alveoli**. Freshly oxygenated blood returns to the heart via the right and left pulmonary veins, entering the heart via the left atrium. As the left atrial wall contracts, blood is propelled into the left ventricle through the bicuspid valve. When the left ventricular wall contracts, blood is then propelled with an average force of 120 mm Hg through the aorta to begin its journey throughout the body.

Although the right and left sides of the heart function separately, they do not function independently. Instead, their action is perfectly coordinated, so that when the atrial walls contract the ventricular walls relax (**diastole**), and when the ventricular walls contract the atrial walls relax (**systole**). This series of events constitutes a complete heartbeat or *cardiac cycle*.

The heart normally continues this pumping action an average of 80 times per minute and is capable of increasing to a rate of more than 200 times per minute. Be-

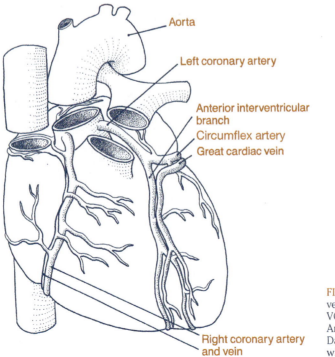

Aorta

Left coronary artery

Anterior interventricular branch

Circumflex artery

Great cardiac vein

Right coronary artery and vein

FIGURE 13–1 Coronary blood vessels. (Adapted from Scanlon, VC, and Sanders, T: Essentials of Anatomy and Physiology, ed. 2. FA Davis, Philadelphia, 1995, p. 268, with permission.)

cause of this continuous beating, the myocardium, the cardiac muscle itself, requires a significant amount of oxygen to perform the pumping task. Because the heart is a muscle, it must be fed oxygen just like any other cell in the body.

The heart receives its oxygenated blood through the right and left coronary arteries. Both coronary arteries obtain their blood from the aorta just above the aortic semilunar valve. The coronary arteries are the first branching of blood vessels off the aorta, but they receive their blood supply during the relaxation phase of the cardiac cycle rather than during the contraction phase. The coronary arteries are angled downward in a self-preservation manner. Even if the heart is capable of only a minimal ventricular contraction, the heart muscle itself benefits as blood flows downward into the coronary arteries during diastole.

The left coronary artery divides into two major branches, the **circumflex artery** and the **left anterior descending artery**. The circumflex branch curves to the posterior portion of the heart and supplies blood through various branches to the posterior wall of the left atrium and ventricle. The left anterior descending branch travels down the anterior portion of the left ventricle and supplies, through branching, the right and left walls with blood. The right coronary artery travels across the heart to the right side and branches to supply blood to the posterior and anterior walls of the right ventricle and atrium (Fig. 13–1).

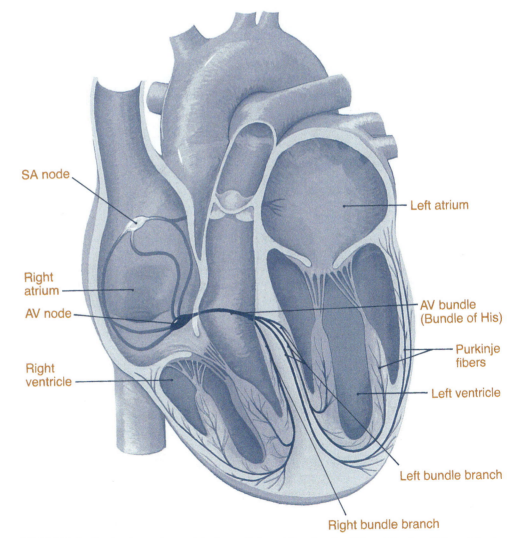

FIGURE 13–2   Conduction pathway of the heart. (Adapted from Scanlon, VC, and Sanders, T: Essentials of Anatomy and Physiology, ed. 2. FA Davis, Philadelphia, 1995, p. 271, with permission.)

The heart contains a sophisticated electrical conduction system that is controlled by the **autonomic nervous system** located within the myocardium. The purpose of the conduction system is to initiate an impulse, move it through the atria, and transmit it quickly to the apex, where it stimulates the ventricles to contract.

The cells of the conduction system have several important properties: *excitability*, *conductivity*, and *automaticity*. Excitability refers to the ability of the conduction cells to respond to an electrical impulse. Conductivity refers to the cells' ability to transfer the electrical impulse from one cell to another, and automaticity refers to the ability of electrical system cells to initiate an electrical impulse from within, rather than receiving it from an outside source.

The electrical system cells capable of generating an impulse the fastest are known as **pacemaker** (pacer) **cells**. The **sinoatrial (SA) node**, located high in the right atrium, is a small mass of pacer cells capable of generating 60 to 100 impulses per minute and is considered the dominant pacemaker of the heart. Two other pacer cell areas are also capable of generating impulses. The **atrioventricular (AV) node**, located at the junction of the right atrium and the right ventricle, generates impulses at a rate of 40 to 60 per minute, and the **Purkinje system**, located in the apex of the myocardium, generates impulses at a rate of 20 to 40 per minute. Should the SA node fail to initiate an impulse, the AV node will do so, and if the AV node fails, the Purkinje system will initiate the impulse.

Once the electrical impulse is generated by the dominant pacemaker (SA node), it is conducted down the atria via the **internodal pathways** to the AV node. The impulse is slowed slightly in the AV node and is conducted down the **bundle of His**, which transmits the impulse through the interventricular septum, subsequently dividing into the **right and left bundle branches**, where it ends at the Purkinje system at the apex. From here, the impulse is spread throughout the ventricles, producing a coordinated contraction of the myocardium (Fig. 13–2).

Pathophysiology of Cardiac Disease

Cardiovascular disease is the number one cause of death in the United States. Although the actual number of cardiac deaths is steadily decreasing, cardiac disease remains one of the primary reasons that thousands of people annually visit hospital emergency departments and physicians' offices.

The major underlying factor in most cardiac disease is atherosclerosis, hardening or narrowing of major arteries. Atherosclerosis is a progressive, degenerative disease that can affect any artery in the body, but it is most dangerous when it affects the arteries of the heart and brain. The hardening or narrowing is a result of deposits of fats (lipids) in the middle layer of the artery wall. Over time, calcium is also deposited, causing the formation of plaque. Small hemorrhages can occur in the plaque that may lead to the narrowing of the blood flow area within the artery and, in time, may entirely block (occlude) the blood flow within the artery.

Researchers have learned much over the past 30 years about the development of atherosclerosis, and the American Heart Association has mounted an aggressive campaign to make the public aware of the risk factors leading to atherosclerotic artery disease and steps to take to reduce these risks. Prominent in a long list of risk factors for the development of atherosclerosis are hypertension, smoking, elevated blood lipids (cholesterol and triglycerides), sedentary lifestyle, obesity, family history of heart disease, diabetes, male gender, and advanced age. The more risk factors an individual has, the more likely it is that he or she will develop atherosclerosis, especially at a young age, even as young as 30. Following a good program of healthy living, exercise, and stress reduction, however, has proven to help reduce the risk of developing atherosclerosis.

In addition to the healthy habits listed previously, regular cardiac evaluation by a physician can help to determine whether atherosclerosis of the coronary arteries (coronary artery disease [**CAD**]) is developing. Along with routine blood tests to determine cholesterol levels, routine ECGs and exercise stress testing are used by the physician to evaluate patients. When discovered early, CAD can be treated successfully.

Regardless of how watchful an individual may be, CAD can still develop. The PCT will be asked to perform a diagnostic 12-lead ECG for the individual who comes to the physician for routine cardiac evaluation or has experienced chest pain, the heart's primary warning symptom.

The PCT should be familiar with some of the cardiac complications that can develop as a result of atherosclerosis. Among these complications are hypertension, angina pectoris, myocardial infarction (MI), and congestive heart failure (CHF).

Hypertension, or high blood pressure, is characterized by persistent elevation of the blood pressure above 140/90 mm Hg. Of major concern is the elevation of the diastolic pressure (the second number), which in severe conditions may rise to more than 130 mm Hg. Hypertension is generally caused by an increase in peripheral vascular resistance or by the narrowing of the blood flow lumen in the arteries. Hypertension can lead to left ventricular failure, cerebrovascular accidents (CVA), dissecting aortic aneurysm, and renal failure.

Angina pectoris is a chronic cardiac condition that occurs when the oxygen demands of cardiac muscle are greater than the supply available because of constricted coronary arteries. When the blood flow to the myocardium is diminished (**ischemia**), chest pain develops. Ischemia may be a result of either coronary artery vasoconstriction or spasm. Anginal pain is diminished by decreasing the myocardium's demand for oxygen through rest or administration of oxygen, nitroglycerin, or nifedipine. The 12-lead ECG is used as both a diagnostic and a monitoring tool in angina pectoris. Changes in the electrical pattern of the patient's ECG may be indicative of increasing ischemia.

MI or acute MI (AMI) produces death (necrosis) of a portion of the heart muscle because of prolonged reduction of blood flow. An MI usually occurs when a coronary artery or one of its many branches is totally occluded by a blood clot associated with atherosclerotic plaque. The actual location and size of the infarcted area depends on the site of the obstruction. The obstruction may be in a small branch, producing acute chest pain, or it may occlude a major branch, such as one feeding the left ventricle, which results in immediate cardiac arrest. When myocardial muscle dies, scar tissue eventually develops and is often a precursor to the development of cardiac complications such as CHF, especially if a large portion of the myocardium is involved or if there are multiple infarcted areas. The major symptom of an MI, severe chest pain, is the result of the occlusion produced by a blood clot. Currently, this clot can often be successfully treated with **thrombolytic** (clot breaking) agents such as streptokinase, urokinase, or tissue plasminogen activator (**t-PA**). They are most successful when administered shortly after the onset of the chest pain. If thrombolytic treatment is successful and blood flow is restored, damage to the myocardium may be minimal. The 12-lead ECG is one of the diagnostic tools used by the physician to confirm a diagnosis of MI. Infarcted tissue will alter the normal electrical pattern of the heart's electrical conduction system, and the 12-lead ECG tracing can indicate the location of the suspected infarct.

CHF usually occurs when the left ventricle fails as an effective pump, causing blood to back up in the pulmonary system, resulting in pulmonary edema. Left ventricular failure is most often a result of one major or multiple small myocardial infarctions, but it may also be caused by valvular disease and chronic hypertension. The resultant pulmonary edema decreases the alveoli's ability to oxygenate blood, which can produce severe respiratory distress in patients. CHF is generally considered a chronic disorder and also results in retention of salt and water by the kidneys. The 12-lead ECG is used as a monitoring tool in CHF. A patient with CHF may show changes in the 12-lead ECG tracing, reflecting progressive cardiac strain, heart enlargement, or ischemia.

A number of other conditions affect the cardiac system. They include congenital anomalies, such as septal defects (inflammatory diseases), including myocarditis, endocarditis, and pericarditis; and valvular diseases (valvular stenosis or insufficiency). The 12-lead ECG is one of several diagnostic tools used by the physician to determine the status of the heart. Any condition affecting the heart can produce changes to its electrical pattern and be reflected on the 12-lead ECG tracing.

Principles of Electrocardiography

As discussed previously, the heart contains a sophisticated electrical conduction system, the purpose of which is to initiate an impulse and move it through the atria into the ventricles, where it stimulates the myocardium to contract.

Transmission of the electrical impulse initiated in the SA node through to the Purkinje system is known as **depolarization**. Once depolarization occurs, the electrical cells require a period of recovery known as **repolarization**, after which another electrical impulse may be generated by the SA node. Depolarization and repolarization can be visualized as a wavelike action spreading downward from the upper right atrium to the ventricles.

In summary, a complete cardiac cycle refers to the initiation of an impulse, depolarization leading to muscular contraction, followed by repolarization. Transmission of the impulse does not guarantee contraction. The only way to determine whether an actual muscle contraction occurs is to feel the pulse.

The electrical impulses generated by the cardiac electrical conduction system can be recorded outside the body. This is the physiological basis of the ECG. After placing **electrodes** on an individual's skin in designated positions and connecting them via cables to an ECG machine, the impulses can be recorded by a pen on moving heat-sensitive paper to create a printed ECG. The impulses form a pattern, a series of waves (positive or negative deflections). Each wave or deflection corresponds to a specific action within the cardiac cycle.

The waves or deflections are known as the P, Q, R, S, and T waves, with the QRS being known collectively as the **QRS complex** (Fig. 13–3). When the SA node initiates an impulse, the atrial fibers are stimulated to depolarize, and a deflection known as the P wave is recorded just prior to the contraction of the atria. When the impulse reaches

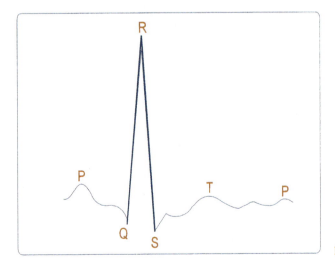

FIGURE 13–3   Normal ECG waves.

the ventricles, they are stimulated to depolarize, and, just prior to contracting, the deflection known as the QRS complex is recorded. The QRS is a greater deflection than that of the P wave because the electrical change is greater. The last deflection, the T wave, occurs as the ventricular walls repolarize. The atria also repolarize, but the deflection is lost within the QRS complex because atrial repolarization occurs at the same time ventricular depolarization occurs. Following the T wave, the system has a short rest period known as polarization, and this is seen on the ECG as a flat line because no deflections are produced while the heart is resting. Another wave, the U wave, may be seen following the T wave in patients who have low serum potassium levels or other metabolic imbalances.

Performing the Electrocardiogram

The ECG is a graphic recording of the electrical activity of the heart. As stated earlier, the electrical activity within the heart can be sensed outside the heart by placing electrodes on the skin and connecting them to an ECG machine via wires. The ECG machine records the positive and negative electrical impulses produced by the heart. The positive impulses are recorded as upward deflections, and the negative impulses are recorded as downward deflections. If no impulses are being generated, the line remains flat. This flat line is known as the baseline, or *isoelectric line*.

One of the most important aspects of the ECG machine is the heat-sensitive graph paper with internationally accepted standard measuring increments that record the heart's electrical activity. Each small square measures 1 millimeter (**mm**) by 1 mm, with every fifth line (both horizontal and vertical) appearing darker in color, indicating a larger square, 5 mm by 5 mm. The graph paper is standardized so that the horizontal axis measures time while the vertical axis measures voltage. Paper moves through the ECG machine at a standard rate of 25 mm per second (mm/sec), recorded on the horizontal axis. Thus, each time the paper moves one small box, 0.04 seconds of time have passed, and with each large box, 0.20 seconds pass ($0.04 \times 5 = 0.20$ seconds) (Fig. 13–4). The horizontal passage of time is used to measure the duration of the cardiac cycles. Time, in larger increments, is marked on the top of the ECG paper. Marks are placed at 3-second intervals (15 large boxes) and are helpful when calculating heart rate.

The voltage or amplitude of the ECG machine is also standardized, and, when properly calibrated, 1 millivolt (**mV**) deflection measures two large boxes (10 mm) on the ECG paper. Sometimes it is necessary to adjust the calibration of older ECG machines using the sensitivity knob. The newer computerized machines adjust themselves at the beginning of each recording.

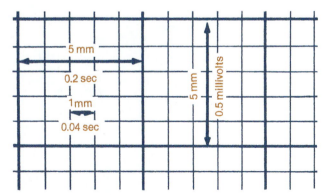

FIGURE 13–4   ECG paper grid. (From Frew, MA, Lane, K, and Frew, DR: Comprehensive Medical Assisting, ed. 3. FA Davis, Philadelphia, 1995, p. 841, with permission.)

ELECTRODES

Electrodes are patches attached to the skin that sense the heart's electrical activity. Patient cables containing wires are attached to the electrodes and connect directly to the ECG machine. Electrodes come in various forms. Early limb patches were made of metal and attached to the body with rubber straps. Suction cups with a conducting gel under the metal cup were used for the chest leads. This process was often messy and gave way to disposable round or oval foam adhesive pads with conduction gel centers. The newest electrodes are small, silver chloride vinyl tapes on which lead wires clip very easily (Fig. 13–5).

LEADS

The first ECG recording was reported by William Einthoven in the early 1900s. Einthoven placed electrodes attached to lead wires on the arms and legs of patients and connected them to a simple galvanometer to measure the heart's electrical activity.

An ECG lead is not a single wire but a combination of two wires attached to an electrode that makes a complete electrical circuit with the ECG machine. There are three types of ECG leads: bipolar limb leads, unipolar (augmented) limb leads, and precordial (chest) leads. In all ECG leads, electrical activity is measured from a negative electrode to a positive electrode. The amount of deflection associated with the electrical activity of the heart produces the positive or negative wave form seen on the ECG tracing.

There are three bipolar limb leads: lead I, lead II, and lead III. They are termed bipolar because two electrodes of opposite polarity (positive and negative) are used. In lead I, the negative electrode is on the right arm, and the positive electrode is on the left arm. In lead II, the negative electrode is on the right arm, and the positive electrode is on the left leg. In lead III, the negative electrode is on the left arm, and the positive electrode is on the left leg (Fig. 13–6). The bipolar leads actually form a triangle around the heart known as Einthoven's triangle (Fig. 13–7).

The unipolar (augmented) limb leads use the same electrode placement that the bipolar leads use, but they take a different view of the heart by combining two of the electrodes into a single electrode. The ECG machine does the combining of the electrical current. The machine also automatically records both the bipolar and the unipolar readings. Lead aVR has the positive electrode placed on the right arm, with the left arm and left leg negative electrodes combined. In lead aVL, the positive electrode is placed on the left arm, with the right arm and left leg electrodes combining to form the negative electrode. Finally, in lead aVF, the positive electrode is placed on the left leg,

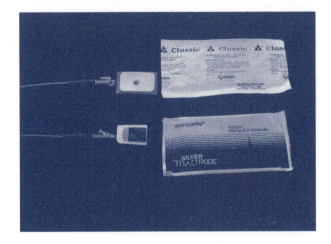

FIGURE 13–5   Examples of silver chloride electrodes and lead wires.

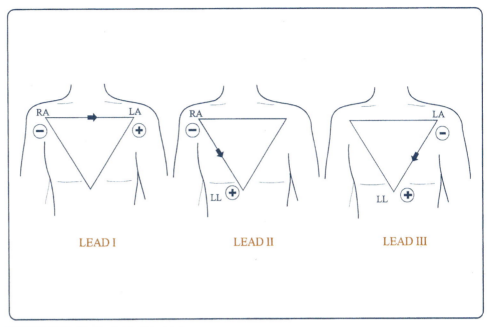

FIGURE 13–6   Bipolar lead placement.

with the right arm and left arm combining as the negative electrode. Combined into a single diagram, the augmented leads form a 360-degree circle around the heart (Fig. 13–8).

The precordial (chest) leads view the horizontal plane (front to back or sternum to spine) of the heart. The negative electrode for these leads is a common ground arranged electronically within the ECG machine, whereas the positive leads are placed on the anterior surface of the chest in positions known as V_1 through V_6. The positive electrode for the V_1 position is placed on the chest to the right of the sternum at the fourth **intercostal** space. V_2 is placed on the left side of the sternum at the fourth intercostal space, directly across from V_1. V_3 is placed on the chest in a line midway between leads V_2 and V_4. V_4 is placed midclavicularly at the fifth intercostal space and V_5 is placed on the anterior axillary line at the fifth intercostal space. V_6 is placed on the midaxillary line, fifth intercostal space. Leads V_4, V_5, and V_6 are all along the fifth inter-

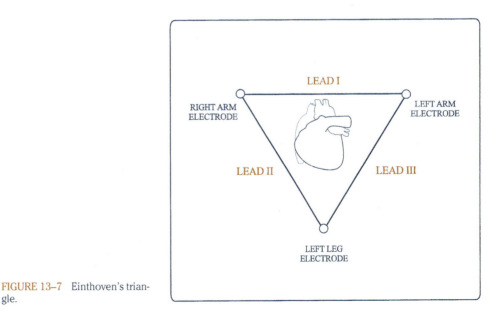

FIGURE 13–7   Einthoven's triangle.

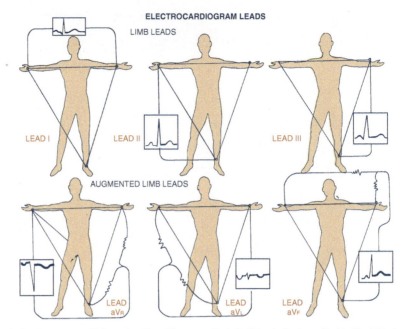

FIGURE 13–8   Augmented ECG leads. (From Thomas, CL (ed): Taber's Cyclopedic Medical Dictionary, ed. 18. FA Davis, Philadelphia, 1997, p. 612, with permission.)

costal space, moving progressively from the midclavicular line to the midaxillary line (Fig. 13–9). It is important to actually count the ribs by palpation when placing electrodes.

Although the fact that an ECG machine takes 12 different views of the heart makes it seem quite complex, it is important to realize that all 12 leads record the exact same electrical event occurring within the heart.

INTERPRETATION

Today's computerized ECG machines also provide an interpretation of the tracing. Although extremely accurate because of computer technology, the cardiologist still

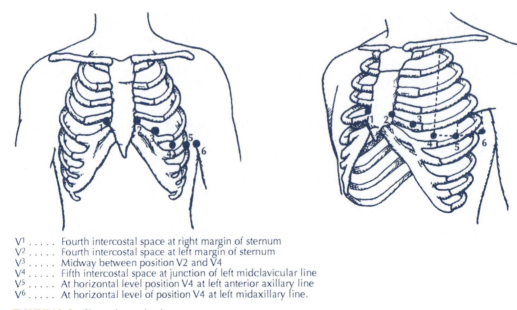

V^1 . . . . . Fourth intercostal space at right margin of sternum
V^2 . . . . . Fourth intercostal space at left margin of sternum
V^3 . . . . . Midway between position V2 and V4
V^4 . . . . . Fifth intercostal space at junction of left midclavicular line
V^5 . . . . . At horizontal level position V4 at left anterior axillary line
V^6 . . . . . At horizontal level of position V4 at left midaxillary line.

FIGURE 13–9   Chest electrode placement.

makes the final interpretation of the patient's tracing. PCTs should be able to recognize a normal tracing, along with some aberrations, such as ***tachycardia***, ***bradycardia***, ST segment elevation and depression, premature beats, atrial ***fibrillation***, ventricular tachycardia, and the lethal rhythm known as ventricular fibrillation.

To interpret a cardiac rhythm in the simplest manner PCTs must evaluate the presence of P waves and the rate and rhythm of the ECG tracing. To facilitate this analysis, a series of questions can be used:

P waves:

1 Are they present?
2 Are they upright?
3 Is there a single P wave for each QRS complex?

The presence of a single, upright P wave before each QRS complex is the expected or normal finding. If the P wave is inverted or absent, it is an indication that the SA node is not the origin of the electrical impulse, and if more than one P wave is present before the QRS complex, it is an indication that the generated impulse is not getting through the AV node. Absent or inverted P waves or the presence of multiple P waves is an indication of an abnormal ECG tracing (Fig. 13–10). It is not within the responsibilities of the PCT to determine the reason for the abnormality.

Ventricular rate:

1 Is the rate between 60 and 100 beats per minute?
2 Is the rate above 100 beats per minute?
3 Is the rate below 60 beats per minute?

Ventricular rate is measured automatically by the computerized ECG machines, but the PCT should be able to determine the ventricular rate of the ECG tracing. There are several methods for calculating the ventricular rate, but the simplest method is to follow the 6-second rhythm strip rule. Most ECG graph paper is marked with small lines on the top or bottom margin in 1-second intervals. To measure the ventricular rate, simply count the number of R waves within a 6-second span and multiply by 10. If the 1-second marks are not present, count the number of R waves in 30 large squares (30 × 0.20 seconds = 6 seconds) and multiply by 10. In Figure 13–11, there are nine R waves in the 6-second span; thus, nine R waves multiplied by 10 equals a heart rate of 90 beats per minute.

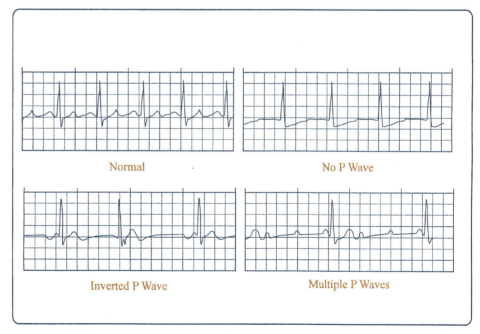

Normal

No P Wave

Inverted P Wave

Multiple P Waves

FIGURE 13–10   P-wave patterns.

6 sec interval

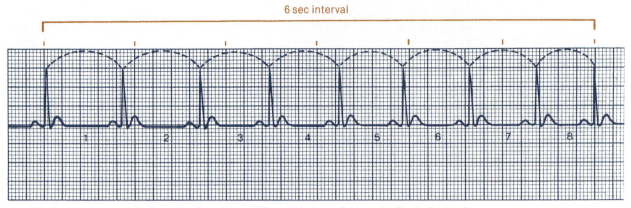

FIGURE 13–11   A 6-second rhythm strip. (From Brown, KR, and Jacobson, S: Mastering Dysrhythmias: A Problem-Solving Guide. FA Davis, Philadelphia, 1988, p. 9, with permission.)

Once the rate is calculated, it can then be determined whether the rate is normal (between 60 and 100 beats per minute) or abnormally fast or slow. Rates over 100 are termed tachycardia, and rates below 60 are termed bradycardia.

Rhythm or regularity:

Are the R to R wave intervals the same?

It is also important to determine whether the electrical stimulus occurs in a regular manner. The simplest method for determining regularity is to measure the distance between R to R intervals. This can be done by using calipers. One leg of the caliper is placed on an R wave and the second leg is placed on the next R wave. The calipers are then moved (without changing the distance of the caliper legs) to the next R to R interval. If the legs match up with the R waves, the tracing is said to be regular. If the legs do not match, the strip is considered to be irregular. If calipers are not available, a piece of paper can be marked and used to measure the intervals.

ELECTROCARDIOGRAM RHYTHMS

The PCT should be able to distinguish the following rhythms: normal (regular) sinus rhythm, sinus tachycardia, sinus bradycardia, premature ventricular contractions, **ventricular fibrillation**, **atrial fibrillation**, and **ventricular tachycardia**.

A normal ECG tracing, as shown in Figure 13–12, is known as normal sinus rhythm (**NSR**) and has the following characteristics:

P wave: Single, upright P wave before each QRS complex
Ventricular rate: 60 to 100 beats per minute
Rhythm: Regular

Sinus tachycardia (**ST**) is exactly like NSR, with the exception that the rate is above 100 beats per minute. Figure 13–13 shows the following:

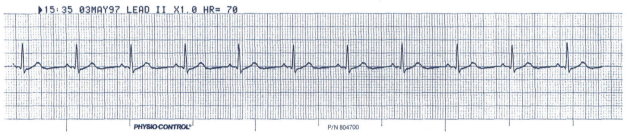

15:35 03MAY97 LEAD II X1.0 HR= 70

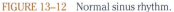

FIGURE 13–12   Normal sinus rhythm.

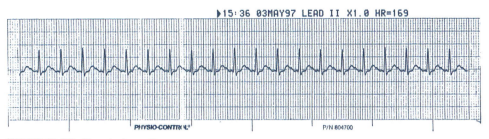

FIGURE 13–13   Sinus tachycardia.

P wave: Single, upright P wave before each QRS complex
Ventricular rate: Above 100 beats per minute
Rhythm: Regular

Sinus bradycardia (**SB**) also has an NSR, with the exception of the rate, that is below 60 beats per minute. Figure 13–14 shows the following:

P wave: Single, upright P wave before each QRS complex
Ventricular rate: Below 60 beats per minute
Rhythm: Regular

Premature ventricular contractions (**PVCs**) occur when an area of the ventricles initiates an electrical impulse out of the normal SA-AV-Purkinje sequence. PVCs are wide, bizarre, and early and look different from normal, narrow QRS complexes. The QRS complexes may exhibit positive or negative deflections. PVCs generally interrupt the normal underlying cardiac rhythm and do not produce a pulse. Patients often state that they feel their heart skipping a beat when a PVC occurs (Fig. 13–15).

Ventricular fibrillation occurs when the normal electrical system is totally disrupted. Ventricular cells fire independently, causing the heart to quiver instead of producing a coordinated contraction to pump blood. Ventricular fibrillation is considered a lethal rhythm and is the leading cause of death in cardiac arrest situations. An outside electrical shock (defibrillation or countershock) must be delivered quickly to the chaotic heart if the patient is to survive. Defibrillation causes simultaneous depolarization of all cardiac cells, thus allowing the electrical system to realign itself (Fig. 13–16).

Atrial fibrillation, caused by disorganized quivering of the atria, produces an irregular, rapid ventricular heart rate, as shown in Figure 13–17.

An extremely rapid (more than 150 beats per minute) rhythm is seen in ventricular tachycardia (Fig. 13–18). The heart is beating so fast that there is not enough time for the ventricles to adequately fill with blood between beats.

Two additional changes can occur on the ECG tracing that will also alter NSR or the normal appearance of the ECG tracing. They are ST segment elevation and depression. The ST segment occurs between the end of the QRS complex and the beginning of the T wave. The ST segment is normally an isoelectric line. Both ST elevation and ST depression are indications of ischemia, oxygen-deprived cardiac tissue, or abnormal serum potassium (K). To be considered ST elevation, the positive deflection must be at

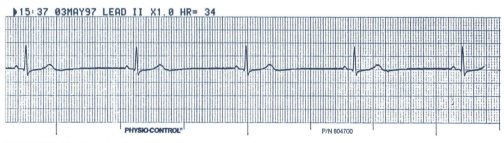
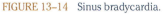

FIGURE 13–14   Sinus bradycardia.

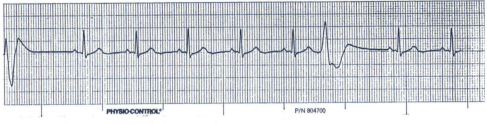

FIGURE 13–15   Premature ventricular contractions.

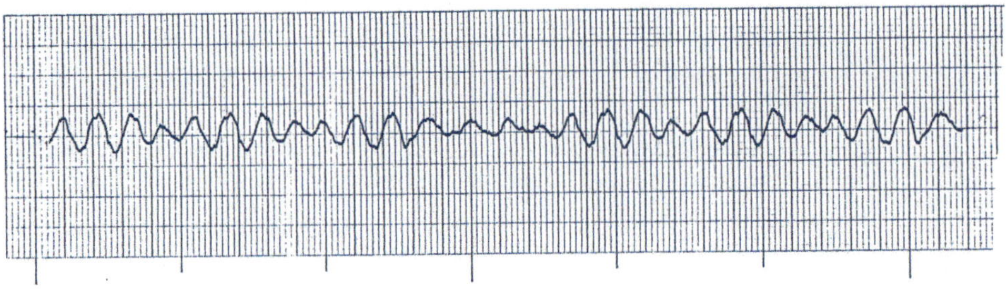

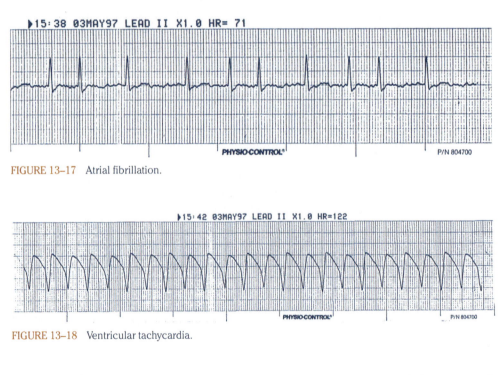

FIGURE 13–16   Ventricular fibrillation.

▶15:38 03MAY97 LEAD II X1.0 HR= 71

FIGURE 13–17   Atrial fibrillation.

▶15:42 03MAY97 LEAD II X1.0 HR=122

FIGURE 13–18   Ventricular tachycardia.

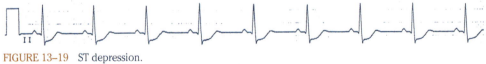

FIGURE 13–19   ST depression.

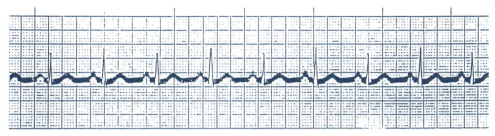

FIGURE 13–20   Electrical interference.

least 2 mm *above* the isoelectric line. To be considered ST depression, the negative deflection must be at least 2 mm *below* the isoelectric line (Fig. 13–19).

Last, there are four artifacts that can alter the appearance of the ECG tracing: 60-cycle interference, patient movement, loose leads or electrodes, and wandering baseline. Although the new computerized ECG machines often automatically correct for 60-cycle interference and wandering baselines, the PCT must be aware of these artifacts and be able to correct their cause.

Sixty-cycle interference is produced by electrical interference. It appears as a widened, spiky tracing (Fig. 13–20). The interference is from electrical sources, such as fluorescent lights or electrical appliances, or from nearby alternating current nongrounded lead wires. Correction involves eliminating the offending source. The source of interference caused by lead wires can be determined by examining a tracing of leads I, II, and III for the major areas of interference. Leads I and II indicate the right arm, leads I and III indicate the left arm, and leads II and III indicate the left leg.

Patient movement can also cause artifacts on the ECG. Natural electric voltage from muscle movement causes additional stylus movement across the ECG paper. Patient movement produces jagged peaks of irregular height and spacing and may also produce a wandering baseline (Fig. 13–21). Patient movement occurs when patients are nervous, anxious, moving, talking, suffering from body tremors, or shivering from a cold environment. Correction includes calming and relaxing the patient and asking the patient to stop unnecessary movement, such as talking and moving the arms. It is sometimes helpful to ask the patient to place his or her hands with the palms up under the buttocks. This will help keep the arms quiet while the ECG is performed. Keeping the room at an acceptable temperature is also helpful. Remember that patients are partially undressed when ECGs are performed.

Another source of artifact is loose leads or electrodes. A lead that has come loose or an electrode that is not adhering to the skin properly can give a spiky, abnormal appearance to the ECG tracing (Fig. 13–22). Causes of loose leads or electrodes include disconnected or reversed leads, poor skin contact with the electrodes, old or inadequate electrode paste, and oily or excessively hairy skin. Correction includes checking that all lead attachments are secure as well as checking the electrode placement and

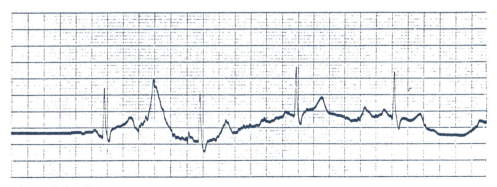

FIGURE 13–21   Patient movement.

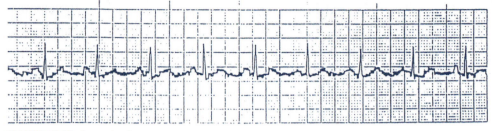

FIGURE 13–22 Loose leads.

adherence to the skin. In some patients, hair may have to be shaved and the skin scrubbed prior to placement of the electrodes.

The last artifact is the wandering baseline. A wandering baseline generally occurs with patient movement, especially with deep, rapid, or sighing breathing. It produces a baseline that is alternately up and down instead of straight (Fig. 13–23). Most computerized ECG machines correct for this artifact automatically. Should a wandering baseline occur, check the patient and have him or her lie as quietly as possible while the ECG is being taken. Removing oil or lotion from the patient's skin using an alcohol swab prior to applying the electrode may also prevent a wandering baseline.

USING A 12-LEAD ELECTROCARDIOGRAPH MACHINE

Most modern 12-lead ECG machines are menu-driven computers. They have a small display screen and standard keyboard (Fig. 13–24). PCTs should be familiar with their particular machines. Most machines require the following information to be entered:

1 Patient last name and first name
2 Patient age and gender
3 Patient ID number
4 Patient medication
5 Physician's name
6 Technician's name/ID number

Obtaining a 12-lead ECG takes very little actual time. Placement of the electrodes takes the greatest amount of time. Before the patient's arrival for an ECG, all of the equipment and supplies should be available. The ECG machine should be turned on, and the PCT should verify that it is working properly and that the cords are not frayed or broken. In addition to the ECG machine, the PCT should have 10 electrodes, the patient cable (untangled), and a patient gown and drape sheet available.

The following steps should be followed when conducting a 12-lead ECG:

1 Obtain the physician's order for an ECG.
2 Locate the patient and introduce yourself. (Indicate to the patient that you will be performing a 12-lead ECG.)

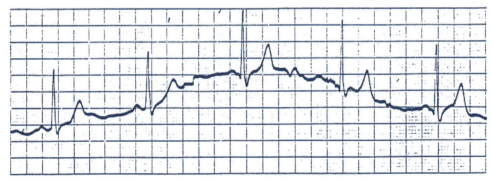

FIGURE 13–23 Wandering baseline.

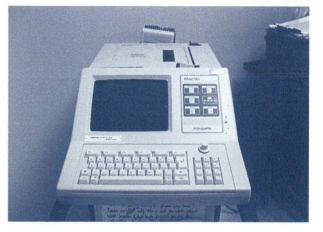

FIGURE 13–24   Electrocardiographic machine.

3 Check the patient's name using appropriate identification procedures for the area in which you are working.

4 Carefully explain to the patient the procedure you are about to conduct and the purpose of the procedure. (A careful explanation at this point will help to alleviate a great deal of the patient's apprehension, especially if this is his or her first ECG.)

5 Ask the patient to remove all of his or her clothing from the waist up and to put on the patient gown so that the opening is in the front. Also ask the patient to remove his or her shoes and socks.

6 When the patient is ready, have him or her lie on the ECG table and place the drape over the patient.

7 It is best to work from the patient's left side, because the precordial leads are placed there.

8 Place the electrodes on both upper arms and both lower legs. (On some men, it may be necessary to shave the area of electrode placement. It may also be necessary to clean the skin prior to placing the electrode. The electrodes are best placed on the fleshiest portion of the arms and legs. This helps to minimize muscle movement.)

9 Uncover the patient's chest and place the six precordial electrodes.

10 Attach the lead wires to each electrode. (Be sure that they are clipped or snapped firmly.)

11 Enter pertinent patient information into the ECG machine.

12 Ask the patient to lie perfectly still and to breathe quietly. (The patient will need to remain this way for approximately 30 seconds while the machine acquires and analyzes the heart's activity.)

13 Press "Record" on the ECG machine. "Acquiring Data" will appear on the screen. If a lead is loose or off, the screen will display a bad lead message. Check the leads and press "Record" again.

14 After 10 seconds, the screen will display "ECG Acquisition Complete," followed by "Analyzing ECG."

15 When the acquisition and analysis are complete, the screen will display "Printing Report," followed by the release of the printed 12-lead ECG. The top left of the paper (usually a white area) will display patient information, with the ECG analysis appearing in the upper right white area (Fig. 13–25).

16 Review the printed ECG tracing. If it is not acceptable, check all lead and electrode attachments and repeat steps 12 through 15.

17 Remove lead wires and electrodes from the patient, thank the patient, and instruct him or her to dress.

18 Tear off the 12-lead ECG tracing and place it in the patient's chart or give it to the ordering physician.

Name:	ID:			
25mm/s	Med:			
10mm/mV	Age:	Ht:	Wt:	
100Hz	Sex:	Race:		
Pgm 006A	Loc:	Room:		
v206				
S	Vent. rate		69 BPM	
	PR interval		136 ms	
	QRS duration		108 ms	
Cart: 1	QT/QTc		384/409 ms	
Tech.:	P-R-T axes		69 73 248	

NORMAL SINUS RHYTHM
INCOMPLETE RIGHT BUNDLE BRANCH BLOCK
ST ELEVATION CONSIDER ANTERIOR INJURY OR ACUTE INFARCT
** ** ** ** * ACUTE MI * ** ** ** **
ABNORMAL ECG

Referred by: Unconfirmed

FIGURE 13–25   ECG patient information.

ELECTROCARDIOGRAPH MONITORING

In addition to the 12-lead ECG, PCTs may be asked to assist with portable ECG monitoring, cardiac stress testing, and Holter monitoring.

Often when patients are being observed in the emergency department or cardiac care unit they are placed on continuous monitoring. The heart is monitored using one of two leads, lead II or the modified chest lead I (MCLI). The standard lead II provides a view of the electrical system by placing the negative electrode on the right arm or midclavicular area, second intercostal space, with the positive electrode placed on the left leg or just below the ribs, midaxillary area. The third electrode (ground) is placed on the left arm or midclavicular area, second intercostal space (Fig. 13–26A). The lead II electrode placement is often used by paramedics using portable ECG or defibrillator units and by emergency department personnel when patients are transferred between areas in the hospital. Cardiac care units frequently use the MCLI, where the negative electrode is placed on the left arm or midclavicular area, second intercostal space; the positive electrode is placed on the right leg or just below the ribs, midaxillary area; and the ground is placed on the left leg or just below the ribs, midaxillary area (Fig. 13–26B). The MCLI is often preferred, because this provides a better view of the depolarization of the atria.

Cardiac stress testing is frequently conducted to observe and record a patient's response to measured cardiac stress caused by exercise (Fig. 13–27). Lead placement differs according to physician preference. Some use only lead II or MCLI during the test; others use all 12 leads, with the leg leads generally placed below the ribs, midaxillary area. An ECG tracing is taken before exercise; continuously during exercise; and 5, 10, and 15 minutes post exercise. Cardiac stress testing is not without risk, and only those individuals trained in cardiopulmonary resuscitation, defibrillation, and definitive arrest procedures should conduct cardiac stress tests.

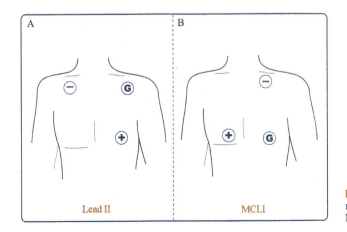

Lead II   MCLI

FIGURE 13–26   Placement of monitoring leads. *A*, Lead II. *B*, MCLI.

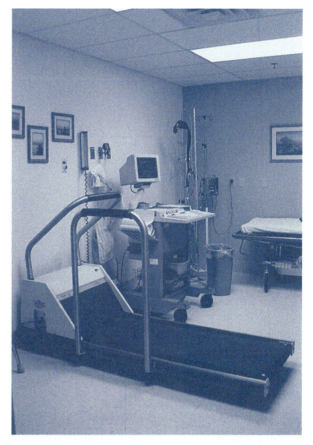

FIGURE 13–27   Cardiac stress testing equipment.

Holter monitoring is a portable monitoring system that records cardiac activity over a 24-hour period. Generally, five leads are attached to a small recording device and placed on the patient's chest. Two electrodes are placed on the right and left midclavicular areas at the second intercostal space, one electrode is placed midchest just below the sternum, and two electrodes are placed on the right and left midaxillary line at the fifth intercostal space. The electrodes and leads must be securely attached because they will remain in place for 24 hours or even longer. It may be necessary to shave the placement area to obtain good contact. Generally, the round adhesive/gel electrodes are used along with snap-on leads because they adhere more securely. Patients may be asked to keep a diary of their activities for the physician to compare with the ECG tracing. A button is also available on the monitor that patients can push when they notice any cardiac symptoms. The monitor is returned to the physician after 24 hours for interpretation.

BIBLIOGRAPHY   Atwood, S, Stanton, C, and Storey, J: Introduction to Basic Cardiac Dysrhythmics, ed. 2. Mosby-Lifeline, St. Louis, 1996.

Bledsoe, BE, Porter, RS, and Shade, BR: Brady Paramedic Emergency Care, ed. 3. Brady Prentice-Hall, Upper Saddle River, NJ, 1996.

STUDY QUESTIONS

1. Describe the size and shape of the heart.

   _____

   _____

2. Define systole and diastole.

   _____

   _____

   _____

3. What is the function of the coronary arteries?

   _____

   _____

   _____

4. Define excitability, conductivity, and automaticity.
   a. Excitability _____
   b. Conductivity _____
   c. Automaticity _____

5. List the pathway of the electrical conductance system of the heart.

   _____

   _____

   _____

6. Where is the SA node located, and how often does it initiate an impulse?

   _____

7. If the SA node does not initiate an impulse, are alternate mechanisms available? Explain your answer.

   _____

   _____

8. List the risk factors associated with the development of atherosclerotic heart disease.

   _____

   _____

9. What is a myocardial infarction?

   _____

   _____

10. Label the areas of the ECG wave shown below.

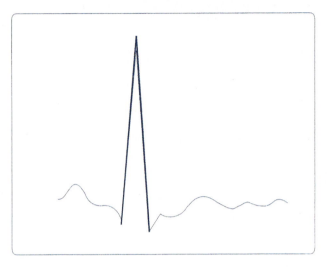

11. Determine the rate of the ECG shown below.

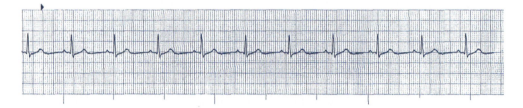

12. Identify the chest leads in the first column with the anatomic placement in the second column.

a. _____ V_1 1. Midway between V_2 and V_4

b. _____ V_2 2. Fifth intercostal space, midclavicular line

c. _____ V_3 3. Fourth intercostal space, right sternal margin

d. _____ V_4 4. Fourth intercostal space, left sternal margin

e. _____ V_5 5. Fifth intercostal space, midaxillary line

f. _____ V_6 6. Midway between V_4 and V_5

13. Match the following ECG tracings:

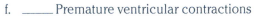

a. _____ Atrial fibrillation

b. _____ Sinus tachycardia

c. _____ Ventricular tachycardia

d. _____ Sinus bradycardia

e. _____ Ventricular fibrillation

f. _____ Premature ventricular contractions

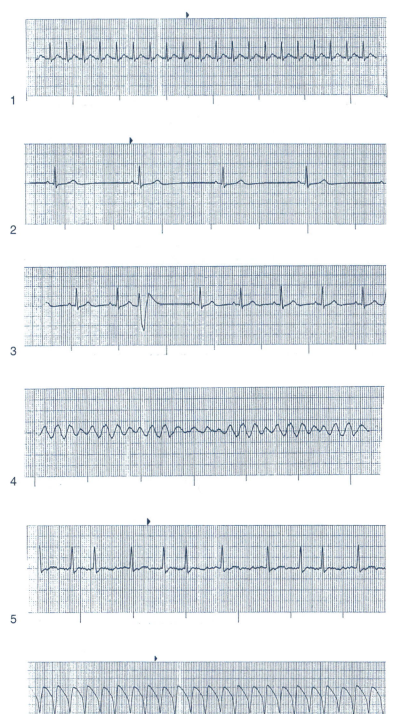

1

2

3

4

5

6

14. Describe the lead placement for the following:

a. Lead II _____

b. MCLI _____

c. Stress testing _____

d. Holter monitoring _____

15. Match the following artifacts:

a. _____ Loose leads

b. _____ Patient movement

c. _____ Electrical interference

d. _____ Wandering baseline

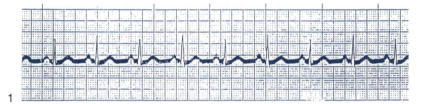

1

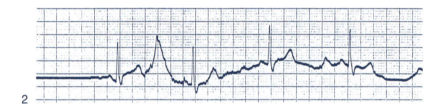

2

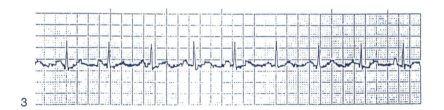

3

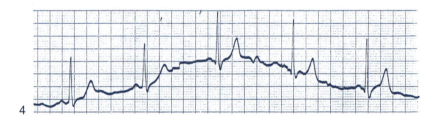

4

16. Describe how the artifacts in Study Question 15 can be corrected.

a. Loose leads _____

b. Patient movement _____

c. Electrical interference _____

d. Wandering baseline _____

EVALUATION OF 12-LEAD ELECTROCARDIOGRAM TECHNIQUE

RATING SYSTEM　　　2 = Satisfactory　　　1 = Needs improvement　　　0 = Incorrect/did not perform

_____　**1.** Obtains physician's order

_____　**2.** Prepares room and checks equipment

_____　**3.** Checks that equipment is safe and functioning properly

_____　**4.** Washes hands

_____　**5.** Identifies patient and introduces self

_____　**6.** Explains procedure to patient

_____　**7.** Provides patient with gown and disrobing instructions

_____　**8.** Positions patient on ECG table

_____　**9.** Correctly places electrodes on limbs

_____　**10.** Correctly places electrodes on chest

_____　**11.** Attaches lead wires

_____　**12.** Enters patient data into ECG machine

_____　**13.** Instructs patient to lie very quietly

_____　**14.** Presses "Record" on ECG machine

_____　**15.** Reviews printed ECG for acceptability

_____　**16.** Troubleshoots for artifacts, if necessary

_____　**17.** Removes lead wires and electrodes

_____　**18.** Thanks patient and instructs him or her to dress

_____　**19.** Returns equipment and prepares room for next patient

Total points _____

Maximum points = 38

COMMENTS

UNIT 14

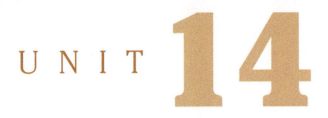

PATIENT CARE

Marsha Cornell, MSN

KEY TERMS

- **Ambulatory**   Able to walk
- **Emesis**   Vomit
- **Incontinence**   Inability to control passage of urine or feces

---

- **Infiltration** Leakage of IV fluid into the surrounding tissue
- **Medication** Administration of remedies
- **Nasogastric tube** Tube passing through the nose to the stomach
- **Pressure sores** Decubitus ulcers or bed sores
- **Sphygmomanometer** Instrument that measures blood pressure
- **Stethoscope** Instrument used to listen for body sounds
- **Vital signs** Measurement of body processes that support life—temperature, pulse, respiration, and blood pressure

Patient care is provided by a group of healthcare professionals with varied levels of skill and knowledge all directed toward the total care of the patient. The nursing service in most healthcare facilities is one of the major departments. The director of nursing service is a registered nurse (RN) who may have varied titles depending on the organizational structure of the facility. The director, together with nursing supervisors, manages the day-to-day responsibilities of the nursing department. Traditionally, each nursing unit was staffed with RNs, licensed practical nurses (LPNs), and certified nursing assistants (CNAs), and the RN assigned and supervised the work of the LPN and the CNA. Today, the PCT is a part of the nursing service and is an integral member of the healthcare team trained to perform multiple tasks. This unit addresses the PCT's duties directly related to patient care.

Observing and Recording Patient Conditions

Assessing patient conditions is an essential function of the RN. These functions may include neurology assessments to determine a patient's alertness and orientation to place and time, ability to hand grasp, and pupil status; respiratory assessment by listening to lung sounds; and general observation of the patient's overall condition. PCTs assisting the nursing staff are able to provide support in this process by reporting changes in patient status when they are observed.

As a member of the patient care team, one of the major responsibilities of the PCT is the accurate observation and documentation of patient data. Always carry a pad and pen in your pocket and make notes. Do not rely on memory. Accuracy is most important when reporting to the nurse. Information is gathered from the patient, family members and friends, and other members of the healthcare team. General observation most often means what is seen, heard, touched, or smelled. Information can be divided into two categories: subjective and objective.

Subjective signs are those reported by a patient. A patient's nausea or headache cannot be seen or felt. Information a patient relays may prompt further questions about the patient's illness or physical condition. When appropriate, ask questions that lead the patient into conversation.

Objective signs can be seen, heard, felt, or smelled. For example, sight and hearing are used when taking a blood pressure or measuring a patient's temperature. PCTs may often give or assist the patient with a bath. This is an excellent opportunity for observation. Be alert for the abnormal. Listen and watch for the normal sounds of ordinary life, for instance, the sound of normal breathing. The odor of a patient's breath may be significant. Notice how the patient sits, walks, or lies in bed. In conversation listen to how the patient talks. Notice whether the skin is flushed or pale. These observations give a great deal of information about the patient. Observation skills generally improve with experience.

Report your observations to your nurse or team leader before leaving your shift or at the end-of-shift report. Concentrate on being as accurate as possible about the conditions observed. Use your notes when making the report. Your report may have significance for the patient during the next 24 hours.

If there is a major change in the patient's condition, always report it immediately. For example, if a blood pressure reading is much higher than the reading 4 hours earlier, this observation may require immediate action and should therefore be brought to a nurse or team leader's attention.

Be careful to report as fact only those things that have been personally observed. When reporting something that a family member has stated concerning the patient, qualify the statement as unobserved.

Standard/Universal Precautions

As a member of the healthcare team, standard precautions must be practiced at all times when providing direct patient care. Proper handwashing is the number one deterrent in infection control. Handwashing is required at the beginning of each shift, after giving patient care, between caring for different patients, before administering and preparing medications, before invasive procedures, and after removing gloves. A detailed explanation of Standard/Universal Precautions, isolation procedures, and the use of personal protective equipment can be found in Unit 2.

The Patient Unit (Room Furniture and Equipment)

The hospital environment can be a potentially dangerous place for the patients it is meant to serve. PCTs must be thoroughly familiar with equipment used in patient care. Hospital patients spend long periods of time in their rooms. Recovery from illness requires rest and a comfortable environment. A patient's bed is a very important item in the patient unit or room. Hospital beds come in two types, manually operated or electrically operated. The head, foot, and height of the bed can be changed using the various controls.

Manually operated beds have the controls located at the foot of the bed, as shown in Figure 14–1. The hand crank located on the footboard is used to raise or lower the horizontal position of the bed. Located just under the footboard are two additional hand cranks. The left crank raises or lowers the head of the bed. The right crank adjusts the knee position. The hand cranks pivot up for use and down out of the way when not in use. Hand cranks can be a safety hazard if left in the up position.

Electrically operated beds have become a common item in a patient unit. Positions for these types of beds are easily changed by hand controls. The controls are located on a side panel attached to the bed, on a panel located in the side rail of the bed, or on a handheld key pad attached to a cable. Patients are instructed in using the bed controls when they are admitted to the unit.

The legs of the bed have casters or wheels. Each wheel has a lock to prevent the bed from moving. The wheels must always be locked when the bed is occupied by the patient, when giving bedside care, or when transferring a patient in or out of the bed.

All hospital beds are equipped with side rails. They come in half-, three-quarter-, or full-length sizes and are located on both sides of the bed (Fig. 14–2). Side rails move up and down and are locked in place by latches or levers. They protect the patient from falling out of bed. They also can be used by the patient to move or turn in bed.

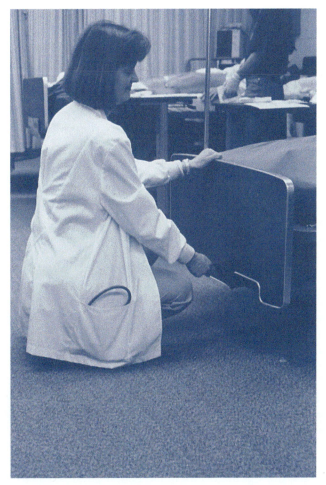

FIGURE 14–1   PCT adjusting manual hospital bed.

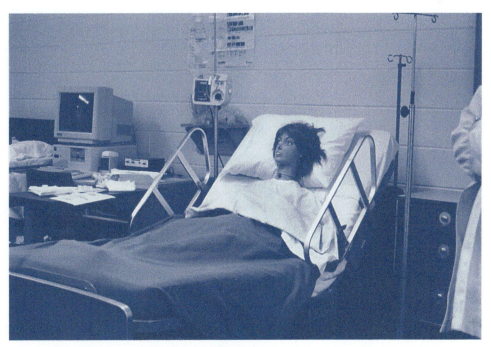

FIGURE 14–2   Hospital bed with half-length side rails.

Each bed has a mattress. Mattresses are made for a variety of uses depending on the patient's condition and treatment requirements. The mattress is covered with plastic or other waterproof material and must be fire-retardant. Many types of eggcrate and air inflation mattresses are available.

If necessary, a bed board may be placed under the mattress for additional support. Bed boards should be in two sections to allow for raising or lowering the head or foot of the bed. A footboard is an "L"-shaped device that is the width of the mattress and projects approximately 14 to 16 inches above the surface of the mattress. Footboards may be placed at the foot of the mattress to prevent footdrop (plantar flexion) or to keep bed linens off feet and legs.

A patient's bed can be a detriment to recovery or may even cause injury if not operated correctly and safely. The patient has a right to a safe environment during hospitalization. It is imperative that all personnel providing patient care protect those entrusted to their care.

All occupied beds should be in the lowest horizontal position unless bed height is needed for care procedures. Side rails should be left up to ensure that the patient does not roll or fall from the bed. Bed wheels or casters should be locked.

A very important nursing function is the positioning of the patient's bed. Figure 14–3 illustrates the four standard bed positions: **(1) Fowler's position, (2) semi-Fowler's** or contour position, **(3) Trendelenburg's position**, and **(4) reverse Trendelenburg's position.**

In the high Fowler's position, the head of the bed is elevated 90 degrees. In semi-Fowler's or contour, the head is raised to a 45-degree angle and the knee portion is raised approximately 15 degrees. This position may prove comfortable for the patient, but raising the knee portion can interfere with proper circulation. Institutions may differ on the definition of semi-Fowler's position. For patient safety always check with your supervisor before making this bed adjustment.

In Trendelenburg's position, the head of the bed is lowered and the foot is elevated. Some manually operated beds cannot make this adjustment and blocks may be used under the legs at the foot of the bed. A physician's order is required for this position. Reverse Trendelenburg's position is the opposite of Trendelenburg's. The head of the bed is elevated and the foot is lowered. Blocks may be used for this position or the

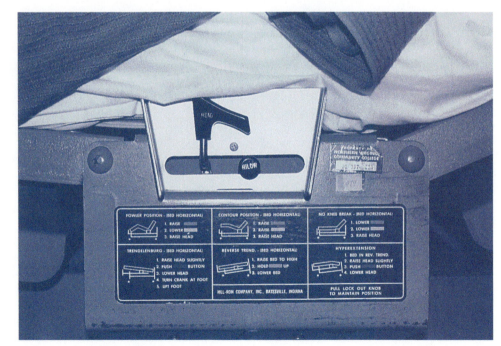

FIGURE 14–3   Examples of hospital bed positions.

entire bed frame can be tilted using the bed adjustment. This position also requires a physician's order.

Vital Signs

The measurement of temperature, pulse, and respirations (**TPR**), and blood pressure are duties of the PCT. These measurements are called *vital signs* because they indicate the function of body processes that support life. Accurate measurement, reporting, and recording of vital signs are absolutely essential. Vital signs are taken and recorded to detect changes in body function and also to determine how a patient is responding to treatment. On the patient's admission to a nursing unit, it is important to record the patient's vital signs to establish a "baseline." This baseline is used to determine changes in the patient's condition. Even minor changes in vital signs may be significant.

TEMPERATURE

Body temperature represents the balance between heat produced by **metabolism** and physical activity and heat lost through respiration, skin, and body wastes. A stable body temperature within a very narrow range is essential for healthy function of cells, tissues, and organs. A change in body temperature may signal the onset of illness or a change in an already ill patient's condition.

Sites for Taking Temperature

There are several sites for taking a patient's temperature. These sites include the mouth (**oral**), the rectum (**rectal**), the underarm (**axillary**), and the ear membrane (**tympanic**). The best site for taking a patient's temperature in the clinical setting is the oral site. The thermometer bulb is placed on the right or left under the base of the tongue or at the back of the oral cavity. The area under the tongue, the **sublingual** area, has an abundant blood supply from nearby arteries and produces a very accurate measurement. The rectal site may be used when the oral site cannot be used, when rectal temperatures are ordered by the physician, or when an infant's temperature is taken. The axillary site (underarm) is generally considered the least desirable site for taking the temperature of an adult. However, it is sometimes recommended for infants and small children. Temperatures taken at the tympanic membrane are quick and easy. A small probe is gently inserted in the ear canal.

Thermometer Types

Temperature can be measured with mercury or with electronic thermometers. Fahrenheit or Celsius thermometers are acceptable. Oral thermometers have a longer bulb, providing a greater surface area for faster reading. Rectal thermometers have a shorter, rounder bulb to facilitate entry into the rectum. Lubricants such as water-soluble K-Y jelly can make the insertion of rectal thermometers easier. Electronic thermometers are battery-operated and must remain in chargers when not in use. There are also disposable chemical thermometers that react to body heat and produce an accurate reading. An additional electronic device measures temperature at the tympanic membrane. The tympanic membrane is commonly referred to as the "eardrum." The covered probe is inserted into the ear canal and the temperature is measured in 1 to 3 seconds. Similar to other electronic devices, tympanic membrane thermometers are battery-operated and must remain in chargers when not in use. The oral/rectal electronic and mercury thermometers are the most common.

Normal Ranges of Oral and Rectal Body Temperatures

Oral temperature in adults normally ranges from 97° to 99.5°F (36° to 37.5°C). Rectal temperature, which is considered the most accurate, is generally 0.5° to 1°F higher than oral temperature. Axillary temperatures, considered the least accurate, are usually 1° to 2°F lower. Body temperature fluctuates with rest and activity. Readings in the early morning hours are the lowest, and the highest readings are usually in the late afternoon and early evening. Women generally have higher temperatures then men, especially during **ovulation**. Several other factors that affect temperature are age, emotional state, and external environment. All of the factors should be considered when taking a patient's temperature. Oral temperatures are not taken when patients are unconscious, disoriented, or seizure-prone; when patients are young children and infants; or when oral or nasal impairment makes mouth breathing necessary. Oral temperatures can be affected by hot or cold foods, routine breathing, and smoking.

Procedure for Taking an Oral or Rectal Temperature

1 Assemble the following equipment:
   Thermometer (mercury or electronic)
   Water-soluble lubricant (for rectal temperature)
   Disposable probe covers for electronic thermometer
   Tissue
   Gloves
2 Wash hands.
3 Put on the gloves.
4 Explain procedure to the patient.
5 With your thumb and forefinger, hold the mercury thermometer by the end opposite the bulb and shake down the thermometer with a snapping motion.
6 Hold the thermometer at eye level and rotate it to see the mercury line. The line should not be above the 95° mark. For an electronic thermometer, insert the temperature probe into a probe cover.
7 Position the bulb of the thermometer or tip of the temperature probe under the patient's tongue as far back as possible. Instruct the patient to close the lips but to not bite down with the teeth.
8 For rectal temperature, position the adult patient on the side. Expose the rectal area and drape the patient for privacy. Have the top leg flexed. Lubricate the thermometer; then gently insert it about 1 1/2 inches into the rectum. Children should be placed on their stomachs when rectal temperature is being taken. Place a hand on their buttocks to prevent them from moving. Insert the thermometer 1 inch into a child's rectum.
9 Leave the oral thermometer in place for 2 to 3 minutes. For a rectal temperature leave in place for 3 minutes. An electronic thermometer will signal when finished.
10 Remove the thermometer and wipe with a tissue for easier reading.
11 Read the mercury thermometer at eye level, record the temperature, and then shake down the thermometer. Disinfect and store appropriately.

PULSE

The arterial pulse is a rhythmic recurring wave that occurs through the arteries during normal pumping action of the heart. The pulse is most easily detected by **palpation** of the area where an artery crosses over a bone or firm tissue. Common pulse sites are shown in Figure 14–4. In adults and children over age 3 years, the **radial artery** is usually the easiest to locate by pressing two fingers against the **radius** just above the wrist on the thumb side (Fig. 14–5).

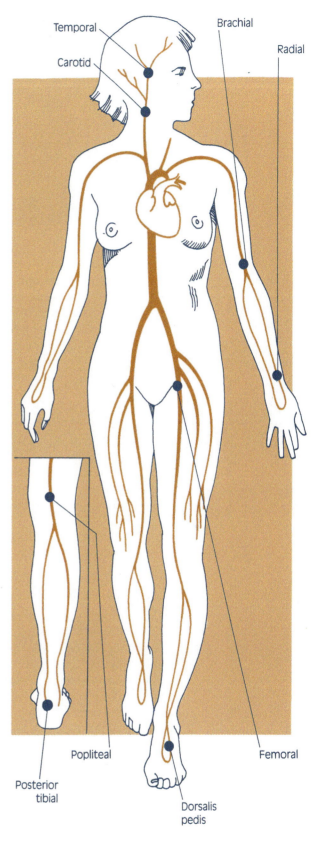

FIGURE 14–4   Pulse points. (From Taylor, C, Lillis, C, and Lemone, P: Fundamentals of Nursing: The Art and Science of Nursing Care, ed 2. JB Lippincott, Philadelphia, 1993, p. 407, with permission.)

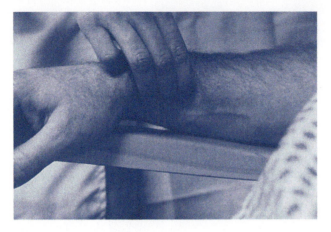

FIGURE 14–5   Proper placement of the fingers along the radial artery. (From Taylor, C, Lillis, C, and Lemone, P: Fundamentals of Nursing: The Art and Science of Nursing Care, ed 2. JB Lippincott, Philadelphia, 1993, p. 404, with permission.)

The pulse reveals heart function and is therefore considered a vital sign and is taken routinely. When taking the pulse, the rate (number of beats per minute), the rhythm (pattern of beats or regularity), and the volume (strength) are determined. If the patient's pulse is irregular, it should always be counted for a full 60 seconds. Counting for an even longer period provides more information about irregularities. If in doubt, recount the pulse. Pulse irregularities are important signs. Experience will aid an individual in more accurately identifying pulse patterns.

Normal pulse rates are shown in Table 14–1.

Procedure for Taking the Pulse

1 Prepare equipment.
2 Wash hands.
3 Have the patient sitting or lying down with the arm at the side or across the chest.
4 Gently press the fingers on the radial artery inside the patient's wrist on the thumb side.
5 When the pulse is located, count the beats for a full 60 seconds.
6 Record the pulse rate, rhythm, and volume and the time the pulse was taken.

Apical Pulse

The heartbeat is strongest over the apical area of the heart, which is located on the left side of the chest, specifically at the fifth intercostal space, midclavicular line, or just below the left nipple (Fig. 14–6). The apical pulse is taken by listening with a stethoscope (**auscultation**) over this location and counting the beats per minute. Each heartbeat sounds like two quick sounds, "lubb-dupp." These two sounds count as one heartbeat. The apical pulse is used for children who are under the age of 2 years, anyone who has heart disease or is taking heart medications, anyone who has chest pain, anyone who has an irregular peripheral pulse, or anytime you cannot get an accurate peripheral pulse.

TABLE 14–1   **Normal Pulse Rates**

Age	Rate/Minute
4 weeks to 1 year	80–160
1 year to 6 years	80–120
6 years to 12 years	70–110
12 years and older	60–100

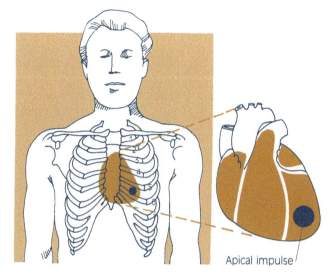

FIGURE 14–6 Schematic depiction of the thorax showing location of apical pulse. (From Taylor, C, Lillis, C, and Lemone, P: Fundamentals of Nursing: The Art and Science of Nursing Care, ed 2. JB Lippincott, Philadelphia, 1993, p. 406, with permission.)

Apical impulse

Procedure for Apical Pulse Recording

1 Identify patient.
2 Prepare equipment by cleaning eartips and diaphragm of stethoscope with alcohol.
3 Wash hands.
4 Position patient in sitting position in bed or chair, if possible.
5 Locate apical area and expose chest area.
6 Position stethoscope and count for 60 seconds.
7 Assess for presence of any irregularity.
8 Replace patient gown and assist patient to a comfortable position.
9 Record rate and report any abnormal findings.
10 Wash hands.

RESPIRATION

The process of supplying the cells of the body with oxygen and removing carbon dioxide from the cells is called respiration. Respiration involves inhalation (breathing in) and exhalation (breathing out). Each respiration consists of one inhalation and one exhalation. Respirations are normally regular, even, quiet, and effortless. The act of breathing is involuntary but can be affected by some voluntary control. In a healthy adult a rate of 14 to 20 respirations per minute is considered within normal limits. In the process of taking vital signs, count the pulse first; then, while continuing to hold the wrist, count the respirations. Some people have a tendency to change their breathing patterns when they are aware that they are being observed. If this recommended sequence is followed and fingers are kept on the pulse, the patient is unaware that respirations are being observed and counted. The depth and character of respirations should be described as well as the number of respirations. Respirations can be affected by all of the same factors that cause the pulse rate to vary from normal. Respirations are counted by observing the rise and fall of the chest. They are counted for a full 30 seconds. The number is then multiplied by two to get the total respirations for 1 minute. If any abnormal pattern in breathing is observed, the count should be for 1 full minute.

BLOOD PRESSURE

Blood pressure is the force exerted by the blood on the arterial walls. A number of physiological factors can determine or have an effect on blood pressure. Among these factors are the force of ventricular contractions of the heart, peripheral vascular resistance, blood volume, anxiety, recent activity, and medications. The systolic, or maximum, pressure occurs when the left ventricle contracts. This pressure reflects the integrity of the heart, arteries, and arterioles. The diastolic, or minimum, pressure occurs when the left ventricle relaxes and indicates blood vessel resistance. Blood pressure is measured in millimeters of mercury (**mm Hg**) and is taken using a ***sphygmomanometer*** and a ***stethoscope*** at the **brachial artery** of the right or left arm. The systolic pressure is recorded over the diastolic pressure. Blood pressure in combination with other vital signs and observations serves as an indicator of the circulatory status of the patient. Blood pressure varies considerably with the individual. A "normal" reading is usually identified as being within a certain range. Generally, blood pressure increases with age, being lowest in the newborn and gradually increasing from childhood through adult life. For example, the normal range for adults is 110 to 140 over 60 to 90. A persistent systolic pressure over 160 or a diastolic pressure over 100 is known as hypertension. Any pressure over 140 mm Hg should be reported to the supervisor immediately.

Sphygmomanometers come in three types: aneroid, mercury, and electronic. The aneroid **manometer** is an air pressure gauge that registers the blood pressure by a pointer on a dial. The mercury manometer, which is more accurate than the aneroid, comes in a variety of models: a portable one in a small box, a wall model, and a floor model often on wheels for easy movement. The mercury rises in a calibrated glass tube as the cuff is inflated and then falls as the air is released.

There are many types of electronic manometers that provide a digital readout of the systolic and diastolic pressures. Some also display the pulse rate, and other models have automatic inflation and deflation of the cuff.

The sphygmomanometer (Fig. 14–7), or what is commonly referred to as the blood pressure cuff, consists of a rectangular rubber bladder covered with a nonexpandable fabric. A hand bulb is attached to the rubber bladder by a small tube through

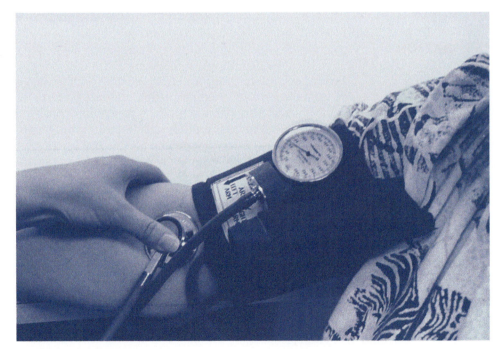

FIGURE 14–7   Sphygmomanometer.

which air is pumped. The hand bulb has a thumbscrew valve that allows the air to escape from the bladder at the desired rate. Hook, bandage, snap, or Velcro cuffs come in six standard sizes ranging from newborn to extra-large adult. Disposable cuffs are also available.

A stethoscope is used with all types of manometers to listen for the sounds that determine the blood pressure reading. Most stethoscopes have two sides, one bell-shaped and one with a flat diaphragm. Low-pitched sounds heard when determining the diastolic pressure are heard more readily with the bell side of the stethoscope.

Procedure for Measuring Blood Pressure

1 Collect the following equipment:
   Sphygmomanometer (blood pressure cuff)
   Stethoscope
   Alcohol wipes
2 Wash hands.
3 Identify the patient.
4 Explain the procedure to the patient.
5 Clean stethoscope diaphragm and earpieces with alcohol wipes.
6 The patient may lie supine or sit erect with the arm extended and supported at the level of the heart.
7 The mercury measuring device should be at eye level, and the aneroid gauge should be directly in front of you.
8 Expose the upper arm and place the arrow on the cuff over the brachial artery, wrapping the cuff around the arm at least an inch above the elbow.
9 With thumb and index finger, close the valve on the rubber inflation bulb.
10 Place the stethoscope in the ears and place the diaphragm of the stethoscope over the brachial artery.
11 With the tips of your fingers, locate the radial artery and inflate the cuff until you no longer feel the pulse, usually between 160 and 170 mm Hg.
12 Using thumb and index finger carefully, open the bulb valve and slowly deflate the cuff—no faster than 5 mm Hg/second.
13 When you hear the first beat, note the pressure on the column or on the gauge. This is the systolic pressure reading.
14 Continue to deflate slowly. Listen carefully for the sound. Note the point at which the sound disappears. This is the diastolic pressure reading.
15 Completely deflate the cuff. Remove it from the patient's arm.
16 Record the patient's blood pressure.
17 Return the equipment to its proper place.

Height and Weight Measurements

Determining and recording height and weight measurements are routine admission procedures in most healthcare facilities. Knowing exact height and weight is essential for calculating dosages of medications, determining an individual patient's fluid status, and assessing nutritional status. This information, along with temperature, pulse, respiration, and blood pressure, is added to the baseline status of the patient. The patient's clothing adds weight and shoes add to height; therefore, unnecessary clothing items should be removed prior to determining height and weight. The patient usually wears only a gown or pajamas. A full bladder may add to weight so the patient should be asked to empty the bladder before being weighed. If this is an admission weight and a urine sample is also needed, it is a good time to obtain the sample.

Weight can be measured with a standing scale, a chair scale, or a lift scale. In most instances a standing scale with a measuring bar is used for **ambulatory** patients. However, if the patient is very **debilitated**, a chair scale or lift scale may be necessary. Standing scales often become unbalanced if they are the type that can be transported from room to room. Prior to weighing the patient, make certain that the weights are placed at the "0" position and that the balance pointer is in the center. Most standing scales have two riders with sliding weights. The upper rider is divided in 1/4-lb marks with the printed numbers in 2-lb increments (10, 12, 14, 16, and so on). The lower rider is divided in 50-lb increments (0, 50, 100, 150, and so on) and is adjusted first to the number closest to the patient's estimated weight. With the patient standing on the scale platform, the weight is determined by sliding the weights on the upper and lower riders until the balance pointer is in the center (Fig. 14–8). The figure indicated on the lower rider is added to the figure indicated on the upper rider to determine the weight.

Ideally the patient's weight should be taken at the same time each day (preferably before breakfast), in similar clothes, and with the same scale. If a patient must use crutches to walk or stand, weigh the patient with the crutches. Then, weigh the crutches and subtract the figure from the patient's weight. If a patient is very obese, check the scale capacity. Most scales have a 350-lb capacity. It may be necessary to have the patient weighed on a large commercial scale, which is typically located near the facility's loading dock or kitchen.

The height-measuring bar is located on the front of the standing scale and has a folding end. Have the patient stand as erect as possible facing forward. Raise the measuring bar above the head and extend the folding end to the horizontal position. Next, lower the bar until it touches the top of the patient's head (Fig. 14–9). Then, read the height from the figures located on the front of the measuring bar.

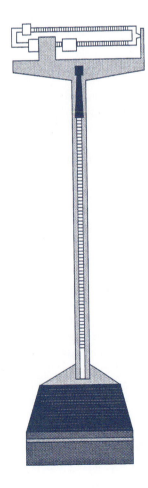

FIGURE 14–8   Standing scale.

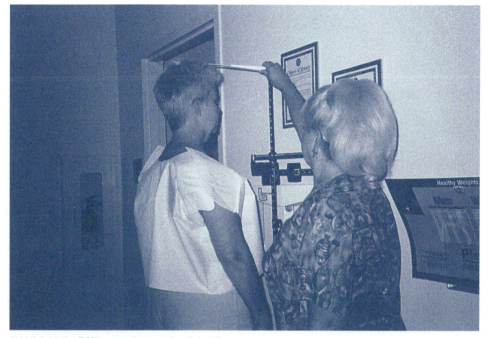

FIGURE 14–9   PCT measuring a patient's height.

PROCEDURE FOR MEASURING HEIGHT AND WEIGHT

1 Gather the following equipment:
   Scale, standing, with measuring bar
   Paper towels
2 Identify the patient.
3 Ask the patient to empty the bladder.
4 Wash hands.
5 Provide for privacy.
6 If the scale has wheels, lock them or otherwise secure the scale.
7 Ask the patient to remove robe and slippers or shoes.
8 Place a paper towel on the scale platform.
9 Ask the patient to stand on the scale, looking straight ahead; assist, if necessary.
10 Raise the height-measuring bar and determine the patient's height.
11 Record the height on a notepad.
12 Fold the end and lower the measuring bar.
13 Slide the weight on the lower rider to a groove estimated as the patient's weight.
14 Slide the weight on the upper rider until the balance beam is level.
15 Add the upper and lower rider figures to determine the patient's weight.
16 Record the weight on a notepad.
17 Assist the patient off the scale and assist while putting on robe and slippers.
18 Return the scale to its designated storage area.
19 Record the measurements on the patient's chart.

Principles of Body Mechanics in Daily Activities

PCTs engaged in clinical care of patients perform a variety of physical tasks, including reaching, pushing, stooping, lifting, and carrying. Any one of these activities performed incorrectly has the potential to cause excess fatigue, strain, or injury and threatens the safety of the patient. Proper body mechanics means using the body in an

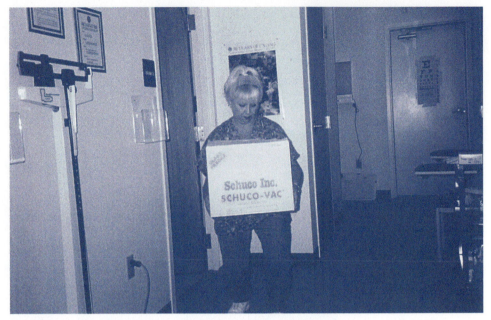

FIGURE 14–10   Person lifting a box, using her hips and knees for support, rather than her back.

efficient and careful way by using the largest and strongest muscle groups to perform work. Cleaning, washing laundry, mowing the yard, and picking up a baby are examples of routine activities that require good body mechanics. With daily practice, using the principles of body mechanics will minimize personal strain and promote safety, comfort, and confidence of patients.

The basic principles of body mechanics include:

Maintain good posture. Stand correctly with feet apart, placing equal weight on both legs, making sure to have a wide base of support.

Face in the direction of the task to be performed. Turn the whole body when changing direction. Avoid twisting.

Use the larger and stronger muscle groups. These are the shoulders, upper arms, thighs, and hips.

Push, pull, or slide heavy objects on a smooth surface when possible rather than lifting them.

Bend hips and knees, rather than the back, when lifting (Fig. 14–10). Use leg and thigh muscles to lift.

Carry objects close to the body and stand close to objects to be moved.

Use smooth motions when working. Avoid quick and jerky movements.

When moving patients, use a pulling motion whenever possible.

During patient care, adjust the bed height to avoid unnecessary bending and reaching.

PCTs are often required to help move patients. A patient may be moved or turned in bed or moved from bed to wheelchair or stretcher. These and other activities require efficient use of body strength. Use of correct body mechanics prevents injury to self and patients. Besides using correct body mechanics, individual physical limitations must be considered. Examine the task at hand. Determine whether coworker assistance is necessary to avoid strain or injury. Ask for help when it is needed.

Mobility and Body Position

Mobility is very often the first activity the patient loses when illness occurs. Loss of mobility as a result of bed rest affects all body systems and can be as serious as the primary illness. The combined psychological and physical effects of immobility can hinder the patient's recovery; therefore, the goal is to motivate the patient toward independence and to restore mobility as soon as possible.

Ambulation means the physical act of walking. It can be very helpful in restoring health in an ill patient. Ambulation maintains and restores muscle tone and joint flexibility and stimulates circulation and respiration. Physical activity improves mental health as well as physical health.

There is a general approach that can be used to assist ambulation that can be modified as needed for each individual patient. First determine the patient's capabilities. Identify the ordered activity, and check the previous level of activity. Find out whether any special equipment such as a cane or walker is needed. Plan where you will walk the patient and how far and how long it will take. Explain to the patient the activity and ask if there are any questions before beginning. If the patient has been in bed for an extended period, have him or her sit on the side of the bed for 3 to 5 minutes before standing. It is often a good idea to check the vital signs before beginning ambulation.

In simple assisted ambulation, walk on the patient's weaker or affected side. The weaker or affected side is defined as that side that is impaired because of surgery, bone or joint injury, paralysis, or degenerative illness. Transfer belts are often used to transfer patients from the bed to a wheelchair, commode, or shower chair, as shown in Figure 14–11. Many transfers require two care providers. Transfers must be undertaken with the correct body mechanics or patient care providers may be injured.

You should also extend an arm bent at the elbow. The patient can then determine how much support is needed. Walk slowly, synchronizing your steps with the patient's.

PROCEDURE FOR ASSISTED AMBULATION

1 Explain the activity to the patient.
2 Wash hands.
3 Lower the bed to the lowest position. Lock the bed wheels.

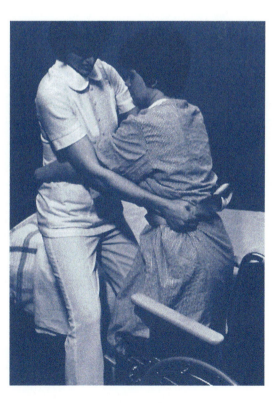

FIGURE 14–11.   PCT transferring a patient to a wheelchair using a safety transfer belt. (From Swearingen, PL, and Howard, CA: Photo Atlas of Nursing Procedures, ed 3. Addison-Wesley Publishing, Redwood, CA, 1996, with permission.)

4 Assist the patient with robe and shoes.
5 Put the transfer belt on the patient.
6 Assist the patient into a sitting position, with feet and legs off the side of the bed, resting on the floor.
7 Help the patient stand, grasping the transfer belt at the side and back.
8 Assist the patient to walk, providing support using the transfer belt if necessary.
9 Encourage normal walking, and discourage shuffling or sliding.
10 Walk the planned distance. Do not rush.
11 Observe the patient for any difficulties caused by the activity.
12 Assist the patient back into bed.
13 Place the call bell within reach.
14 Raise the side rails of the bed.
15 Wash hands.
16 Report how well the patient tolerated the activity and the distance walked.

PCTs may also assist patients to move from the bed to a chair. This transfer is frequently to a wheelchair, which can be positioned close to the bed for patients with limited mobility. Persons who have been lying in bed sometimes experience a drop in blood pressure (**orthostatic hypotension**) and should be watched carefully and moved slowly to a standing position.

PROCEDURE FOR TRANSFERRING PATIENT TO A CHAIR

1 Wash hands.
2 Identify the patient.
3 Explain the procedure.
4 Position the wheelchair on the patient's stronger side.
5 Lock the brakes on the wheelchair.
6 Assist the patient to sit on the side of the bed.
7 Assess the patient for orthostatic hypotension before moving the patient from the bed.
8 Place the transfer belt snugly around the patient's waist.
9 Use proper body mechanics as the patient is assisted into the chair.
10 Assist the patient to a position of comfort. Check body alignment.
11 Adjust gown for privacy.
12 Provide access to the call bell before leaving the patient.
13 Wash hands.

POSITIONING

Proper positioning and alignment are necessary for all patients but especially for those with impaired mobility. When combined with scheduled position changes, proper positioning can promote comfort, maintain and help circulation, and prevent ***pressure sores*** (decubitus ulcers) and **contracture**. Many alert patients automatically reposition themselves and readily move about in bed. They may not need special attention, but they often need a reminder that comfort and good body alignment are sometimes not the same. Two large pillows may seem comfortable, but if they are improperly placed under the head they may cause neck problems. During sleep or rest, the majority of healthy people turn often in bed. Repositioning of patients unable to move on their own is essential. It is usually done every 2 hours. For some patients more frequent turning may be necessary. *Without a 24-hour repositioning schedule, patients who are unable to move about on their own will develop pressure sores.* Certain positions or position restrictions may be ordered by the patient's physician. Positioning aids may be necessary to maintain good alignment and position. These aids are readily available in most facilities. Pillows, towels, washcloths, sandbags, and footboards can all be used to assist in maintaining a position, as shown in Figure 14–12*A* through *D*.

Three common resting positions are (1) supine, (2) prone, and (3) lateral. The definitions and guidelines discussed next will help to safely position patients.

Supine Position

The patient lies on the back with the face upward and the spine in straight alignment. Place a low pillow under the head to prevent neck extension. The arms may be at the patient's side with palms of hands down. The forearms can also be elevated with pillows. If the patient's hands are paralyzed, handrolls should be used. Place the roll in the palm of the hand. The fingers and thumb should be flexed around it. Position the legs so that external rotation is prevented. External rotation is the turning of the hip and leg outward. A **trochanter roll** placed at the hip joint is effective in preventing external rotation of the leg and hip. Ankle rolls or sandbags may be placed at the ankles for further stabilization. Both feet should be supported so that the toes point upward. A manufactured footboard or sandbags can be used to maintain this support.

Prone Position

In this position the patient is on the abdomen with the head turned to one side. The prone position is not used frequently because respirations may be compromised. However, if it is done correctly, many patients can tolerate it. This position is used very effectively with a patient who has pressure sores. It relieves pressure on the buttocks and both hips.

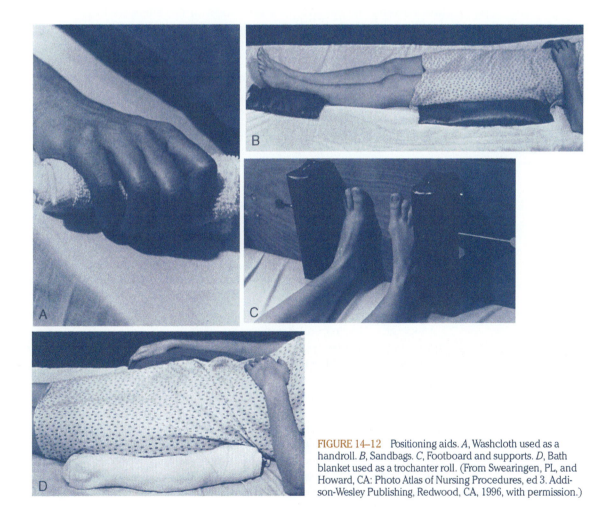

FIGURE 14–12   Positioning aids. *A*, Washcloth used as a handroll. *B*, Sandbags. *C*, Footboard and supports. *D*, Bath blanket used as a trochanter roll. (From Swearingen, PL, and Howard, CA: Photo Atlas of Nursing Procedures, ed 3. Addison-Wesley Publishing, Redwood, CA, 1996, with permission.)

With the patient on the abdomen, turn the head to one side. A standard pillow is usually not used, but a folded towel or small pillow under the head may provide added comfort. Maintain straight alignment of the spine. For comfort, female patients may require a low pillow under the abdomen to prevent added pressure on the breasts.

The arms may be flat at the patient's side or flexed at the elbow with hands near the head. Feet should be extended beyond the end of the mattress or the knees flexed using pillows at the ankles to keep the toes pointed down.

Lateral Position

In this position, the patient is on one side with the head supported on a pillow. When used correctly, the lateral or side-lying position can be very comfortable for a patient. A patient who is paralyzed on one side can be placed on that side as well as the unaffected side unless contraindicated by the physician. A pillow is tucked in at the back to provide support and hold the position. Bring the underlying arm forward and flex it onto the pillow used for the head. Flex the top arm, bring it forward, and rest it on a pillow in front of the body. The upper leg and thigh are supported with pillows. Provide support for the feet to prevent footdrop.

Position in a Chair

Patients are often neglected when sitting in a chair. Maintaining good alignment and position is as important here as in the bed. The patient must be able to hold the upper body and head erect. In a chair the patient's feet should be flat against the floor or on wheelchair footrests, with the knees and hips at right angles. The buttocks should rest firmly against the back of the chair. Backs of the knees and calves should not press against the edge of the seat. Try to avoid placing pillows at the back, as they may interfere with proper alignment. Support the elbows with armrests. Various postural supports help maintain body alignment. Cushions and stabilizers maintain correct sitting posture. Some of these supports limit movement; therefore, rules and safety measures for restraints apply.

Bathing, Skin Care, and Comfort

A hospitalized patient has the same needs for comfort and personal hygiene measures in daily life as the individual not in the hospital. In some cases the patient may have more hygiene requirements. However, the routine of the institution may prevent the completion of these measures without assistance. PCTs may provide the patient with the opportunity to perform personal care needs, assisting them as needed, taking into consideration their personal preferences and physical limitations.

ORAL CARE

Illness and subsequent medications may cause a bad taste in the mouth or a coating of the tongue and mouth. Oral care is important for patients with **nasogastric tubes** in place and those who are on nothing by mouth (**NPO**) status. Oral care prevents mouth odors and infections, increases comfort, and makes food taste better. Proper oral care is too often neglected in daily patient care. Ideally, each patient should be offered the opportunity for oral care before breakfast, after meals, and at bedtime. Every patient may not want oral care this often but it should be offered. The type of care and the amount of assistance needed varies among patients. When assistance is required for oral care, standard precautions should be followed carefully. If patients can perform their own oral care but are confined to bed, they should be provided the necessary articles: toothbrush, toothpaste, mouthwash, dental floss, water glass with water, emesis basin, and towel.

Procedure for Brushing a Patient's Teeth

1 Explain the procedure to the patient.
2 Wash hands.
3 Collect equipment and place on an over-the-bed table within easy reach.
4 Adjust the bed to a comfortable working height.
5 Raise the head of the bed so the patient sits comfortably.
6 Place a towel across the chest and under the chin.
7 Put on gloves.
8 Apply toothpaste to a moistened toothbrush.
9 Brush the teeth using a back-and-forth motion, covering all surfaces of the teeth to the gum line.
10 Allow the patient to rinse the mouth, holding the emesis basin under the chin.
11 Follow rinsing with mouthwash, if desired.
12 Wipe the patient's mouth.
13 Remove the towel.

Care of Dentures

Dentures are expensive, and losing or damaging them is negligent conduct for hospital personnel. Mouth care is given and dentures are cleaned as often as natural teeth. Patients often want to care for their dentures themselves. If so, they should be offered the necessary articles for cleaning as previously listed. If the patient must remain in bed, furnish a partially filled bath basin lined with a washcloth or towel so that if the dentures fall they will not break. Should a patient be unable to clean dentures, assist with denture removal and place the dentures in a denture cup. Take them to the bathroom sink and line it with a towel. Using a toothbrush, toothpaste, and cool water, brush all surfaces of the denture, rinse well, and return to the denture cup. Do not use hot water to clean or store dentures. Have the patient rinse the mouth with water or mouthwash before reinserting the dentures.

BATHING

A complete bath, whether in bed, tub, or shower, cleanses the skin, stimulates circulation, provides mild exercise, and promotes comfort. Bathing allows for observation of skin color and condition, joint mobility, and muscle strength. Depending on the general condition of the patient and the length of hospitalization, the patient may require a complete bath each day. Assistance is provided depending on the limitations and personal preferences of the patient. Take a few minutes to plan what will be needed for giving or assisting with the bath. Determine whether a coworker is needed for additional assistance. Check the patient's chart for any information related to this procedure. Always allow the patient to participate to the extent possible in bathing. This is a very personal activity of daily living and each patient should be approached with a respect for privacy. Whenever possible, bed linens should be changed at the time of patient bathing.

Equipment

The same equipment listed here is needed for a partial bath as well as a complete bed bath. The quantity of each item may differ, depending on the condition of the patient. Find out the patient's preference for soap and other personal toiletries such as deodorant, body lotion, or powders. Some patients are allergic to soap or their skin is very dry, and soap can cause itching and discomfort. Some bar soaps contain bath oil or creams that reduce this effect. The equipment should be assembled on an over-the-bed table or bedside stand, whichever is more convenient for the patient and PCT. Collect the following:

Wash basin and emesis basin
Equipment for oral hygiene or mouth care
Soap
Body lotion or talcum powder
Washcloths
Bath towels
Bath blanket
Clean gown or pajamas
Patient's personal toilet articles
Gloves
Paper towels/toilet tissue
Clean bed linen
Bag for soiled linen

Partial Bath

A partial bath involves bathing the following areas in the order listed:

1 Face
2 Neck
3 Hands and arms
4 Axillae
5 Back
6 Genital and rectal areas

The partial bath can replace the complete bath for the patient with very dry skin or with extreme weakness due to debilitating illness or surgery. This type of bath can supplement the complete bath for the **diaphoretic** (perspiring) patient or one who is incontinent for stools or urine. Patients who are able may do a partial bath themselves in bed or at the bathroom sink. PCTs should be available to assist as needed, especially with washing the back. If the patient is unable to do any of the bathing, follow the steps outlined in the Complete Bed Bath procedure that cover washing the required areas.

Procedure for Partial Bath

1 Explain the procedure to the patient.
2 Ask the patient whether the temperature of the room is comfortable, and close windows or doors to prevent drafts.
3 Adjust the bed height to a comfortable working level.
4 Provide for privacy.
5 Wash hands.
6 Assist with or give oral care.
7 Remove the top linens and cover the patient with a bath blanket.
8 Fill the wash basin with warm water and place on the over-the-bed table.
9 If allowed, raise the head of the bed so the patient can bathe comfortably.
10 Assist with removing of gown or pajamas.
11 Ask the patient to wash areas that he or she can reach. Explain that you will wash the back and any area that cannot be reached.
12 Place the call bell within reach and leave the patient alone to bathe.
13 When the patient has finished, change the bath water.
14 Make a mitt out of the washcloth (Fig. 14–13).
15 Wash areas the patient is unable to reach. Note the order of areas listed previously.

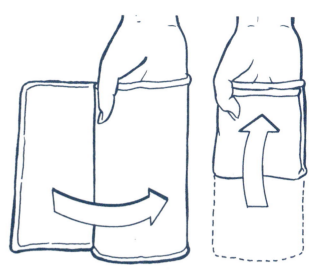

FIGURE 14–13 Folding a mitt for bathing. (From Gomez, GE, Hord, EV, and Gettrust, KV: Fundamentals of Clinical Nursing Skills. John Wiley & Sons, New York, 1988, p. 113, with permission.)

16 Wash from cleanest to dirtiest area. Rinse the washcloth often and change the water if it becomes too dirty or soapy.
17 Give the patient a back rub with body lotion.
18 Assist with dressing.
19 Change the bed linen.
20 Clean and dry the wash basin and emesis basin. Return them to storage area.
21 Make the patient comfortable.
22 Report the procedure and observations to nurse or team leader.

Complete Bed Bath

A complete bed bath consists of washing the patient's entire body while the patient remains in bed. Complete bed baths are given to patients who are paralyzed, unconscious, or otherwise physically impaired because of illness or surgery and unable to bathe themselves. When planning a complete bed bath, consult with the nurse for information about the patient's activity level and ability to assist with the bath. Many patients have never had a bed bath and the activity may be embarrassing and/or frightening. Each patient must be given a complete explanation about the procedure and how the body is covered to avoid unnecessary exposure and to protect privacy.

Procedure for Complete Bed Bath

1 Identify the patient.
2 Explain the procedure to the patient.
3 Ask whether a urinal or bedpan is needed before beginning.
4 Wash hands.
5 Collect bath equipment (see equipment listed previously). Use the over-the-bed table and bedside stand for a working surface.
6 Raise the bed to a comfortable working height.
7 Give oral care.
8 Place the patient in a supine position, if possible.
9 Remove the top bed linen and cover the patient with a bath blanket.
10 Assist with removal of gown or pajamas. Do not expose the patient.
11 Fill the bath basin approximately 2/3 full with warm water. Place the basin on the over-the-bed table within easy reach.
12 Spread a towel across the patient's chest under the chin.
13 Wash the face beginning with the eyes. Do not use soap. After the eyes, apply soap to the cloth and wash the face, ears, and neck. Use gentle, firm strokes.

14 Rinse the skin well and dry.

15 The male patient may want to shave at this point. This task is also your responsibility. If you are unfamiliar with this task, ask for assistance.

16 Place a towel under the far arm. Wash the far hand, arm, and axilla, in that order. Rinse and dry thoroughly.

17 Wash the hand, arm, and axilla near you in the same manner.

18 Turn down the bath blanket and drape the chest with a towel. Wash and rinse the chest. Be certain to rinse and dry thoroughly under the breasts of the female patient. Leave the towel over the chest.

19 Turn the bath blanket down to the groin area. Wash and rinse the lower abdomen. Remove the towel from the chest and replace with the bath blanket.

20 Change the bath water.

21 Remove the blanket from the far leg only, placing a towel lengthwise underneath the leg. When possible, place a basin of warm water on the bed, flex the leg at the knee, and place the foot in the basin. Allow the foot to soak. Wash, rinse, and dry the leg. Wash the foot and toes and rinse and dry carefully, especially between the toes.

22 Wash the near leg and foot in the same manner.

23 Change the bath water.

24 Next, wash the back and buttocks. Turn the patient on the side facing away from you. Drape the patient with the blanket to avoid exposure and chill. Begin at the neck and wash toward the buttocks. Rinse and dry thoroughly.

25 The perianal area may need careful washing if soiled with stool. Wear gloves when washing this area.

26 Change the bath water.

27 Wash the genital area, rinse, and dry well.

28 A back massage may be given at this point, or the patient may prefer it after the bath is finished.

29 Comb or brush and arrange the patient's hair.

30 Inspect the patient's fingernails and toenails. Report your observations to the nurse. Some facilities do not permit nail cutting. Be sure to know the policy and comply with it.

31 Change the patient's bed linen.

32 Wash and replace the bath equipment in the patient's storage unit. Put away the patient's personal articles.

33 Lower the bed and raise the side rails.

34 Follow facility policy for soiled linen.

35 Wash hands.

36 Report the procedure and observations to the team leader or nurse.

Many times the hair and scalp are neglected on patients who are hospitalized for 2 weeks or more. A shampoo helps a person on bed rest to feel better and should be provided to all patients when possible. Put the patient in a supine position. Place towels under the back, shoulders, and head and over the chest. Use a large plastic bag, unopened, and place it under the shoulders and head to make a trough to drain to a basin placed on the floor or a low table.

BED LINEN CHANGES

It is sometimes necessary to perform a complete bed linen change while the patient is in bed. This requires the patient to be on a side in the lateral position. Remove bottom linens from head to toe behind the patient and roll them neatly up to the patient's back logroll style. Place new linens on the bed from head to toe behind the patient and roll neatly up to the patient (Fig. 14–14). Assist the patient to roll over the lump of dirty and

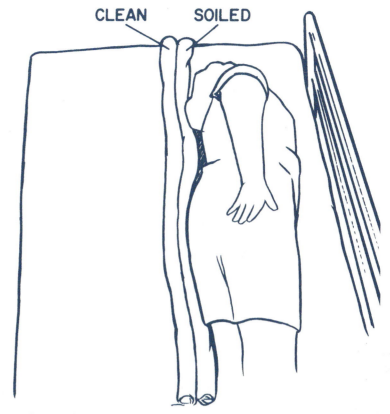

CLEAN   SOILED

FIGURE 14–14 Position of sheets when changing an occupied bed. (From Gomez, GE, Hord, EV, and Gettrust, KV: Fundamentals of Clinical Nursing Skills. John Wiley & Sons, New York, 1988, p. 140, with permission.)

clean linens and position the patient on the other side in the lateral position. Remove dirty linens, unroll clean linens, and finish making the bed with clean linens following the procedure described next for making an unoccupied bed.

Making an Unoccupied Bed

1 Wash hands.
2 Gather clean linens. (Do not place on another patient's bed.)
3 Check the dirty linens for the patient's belongings, call bell, and so on before removing from the bed.
4 Loosen linens starting at the head of the bed, moving down the bed and around the other side.
5 Place the pillow on the bedside chair after removing the pillowcase.
6 Roll all soiled linen inside the bottom sheet and, holding the linens away from the uniform, place directly in a hamper.
7 Apply the bottom sheet and draw sheet, being sure to tuck in well at the top of the mattress and to miter the upper corners of the bottom sheet. Tuck in the sides of the bottom sheet and draw sheet.
8 Apply top sheet and bedspreads. Tuck in securely at the bottom of the mattress. Miter the bottom corners. Fold the top edge of the top sheet over the spread, making a cuff of about 6 inches.
9 Make a toe pleat and leave the bed linens in the open position.
10 Put on a clean pillowcase, using the correct method of turning the case wrong-side out and grasping the pillowcase and pillow at the center of one short side. Pull the pillowcase over the pillow and place at the head of the bed.

11 Do not shake linens throughout the process.
12 Attach the call bell to the bed in a convenient place for patient use.
13 Lower the bed to its lowest position.
14 Wash hands.

Toileting and Continence

Assisting patients with elimination is a basic responsibility of PCTs. Solid waste is called *feces* or *stool.* The process of eliminating stool is called a *bowel movement* (**BM**) or *defecation.* Liquid waste is called *urine,* and the process of eliminating urine is called *urination* or *voiding.* The patient's ability to eliminate waste can be affected by age, disease, diet, activity, and medications.

The following terms refer to elimination problems:

- ***Incontinence***—involuntary, uncontrollable passage of urine or feces
- **Constipation**—decreased frequency or difficulty in passing feces
- **Ostomies**—surgical openings for the elimination of wastes
- Urinary Catheter—a tube used to drain urine from the bladder
- Catheterization—A sterile procedure for inserting a catheter
- **Enema**—an irrigation of the rectum to promote defecation

When assisting patients with elimination procedures it is important to be sensitive to the patient's feelings and emotions and to respond to the patient quickly. The urge to eliminate may happen suddenly and be uncomfortable or difficult to control, which may cause the patient to be embarrassed, irritable, or incontinent. Be sure to provide the patient with as much privacy as possible by closing doors, pulling curtains, and covering him or her during elimination. If the patient experiences incontinence, wash the affected areas and change the bed linens promptly, taking care not to blame or belittle the patient. Remember to wear gloves when performing these procedures. Keep equipment used for elimination clean and in proper storage areas. Equipment that may be needed includes bedpans, fracture pans, and urinals (Fig. 14–15*A* through *D*). Specimen hats are placed in the commode for specimen collection. A calibrated measuring device should also be available. The PCT is responsible for observing elimination, recognizing problems, and reporting results. When the patient is on intake and output (**I & O**) it is necessary to measure all liquid elimination such as urine, stool, and *emesis* and to report the amounts and observations. Normal urine is clear, pale yellow, with a faint odor. Normal feces are brown and soft-formed. Any discoloration, unusual odor, or appearance of urine or feces should be reported to the nurse.

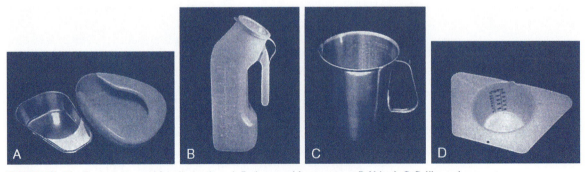

FIGURE 14–15   Equipment used for elimination. *A,* Bedpan and fracture pan. *B,* Urinal. *C,* Calibrated measuring device. *D,* Specimen hat. (From Taylor, C, Lillis, C, and LeMone, P: Fundamentals of Nursing: The Art and Science of Nursing Care, ed 2. JB Lippincott, Philadelphia, 1993, p. 856, with permission.

Other sources of output may include wound drainage and mechanical suction devices such as nasogastric tubes, chest tubes, Hemovac, and Jackson-Pratt wound drains. Follow the institution's procedure and your job description for proper emptying procedures. You will need to observe, measure, and report all types of drainage.

CATHETER CARE

Patients with a **retention urinary catheter (Foley)** require special care. The insertion of the catheter is a sterile procedure. Improper handling can contaminate the catheter or drainage system and cause infection. Catheter care must be provided daily and the drainage bag should be emptied every shift and/or as indicated. Catheter care is a clean procedure and involves cleansing around the urinary opening using soap, water, and a clean cloth. Some institutions may use povidone-iodine (Betadine) applicators or a catheter care kit. Clean around the urinary opening and several inches down the catheter by wiping gently away from the tube's entrance at the urinary opening. The catheter should be secured to the inside of the patient's thigh and the drainage bag should always be kept below the level of the bladder. Coil extra drainage tubing on the bed, making sure there are no kinks, and secure with a clip or rubber band and safety pin to provide a short, straight section of tubing from the bed to the drainage bag to maintain gravity drainage as shown in Figure 14–16.

When emptying the drainage bag, wear gloves. Do not allow the spout to touch the inside of the measuring container, and always close and replace the spout in the protective holder when the bag is empty. Observe, measure, dispose of, and record the urine volume. An external catheter, sometimes called a condom catheter, may be used

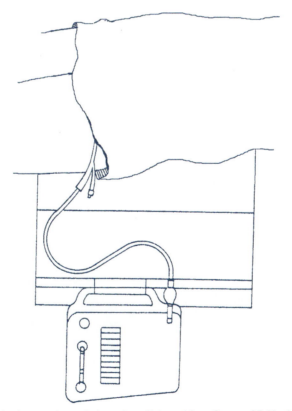

FIGURE 14–16 Positioning a catheter drainage bag. (Adapted from Gomez, GE, Hord, EV, and Gettrust, KV: Fundamentals of Clinical Nursing Skills. John Wiley & Sons, New York, 1988, p. 142, with permission.)

on male patients to contain leakage. It fits over the penis and attaches to a drainage bag. Application of a condom catheter is a clean procedure and the catheter is replaced daily. A condom catheter should not be applied over broken or irritated skin.

OBTAINING A SPECIMEN FROM A CATHETER

A catheterized specimen should be a fresh, sterile urine specimen. Never obtain a urine specimen from the drainage bag because this is old urine. Urine goes through chemical changes when standing at room temperature, which will invalidate diagnostic tests. Follow these steps in obtaining a urine specimen from a patient with a retention catheter (Fig. 14–17A and B):

1. Obtain necessary equipment:
   Sterile specimen container
   10-cc syringe
   Gloves
   Alcohol
2. Clamp the catheter tubing for 15 minutes, if there is no urine in the tube.
3. Wearing gloves, cleanse the aspiration port of the drainage tube with an antimicrobial or alcohol swab.
4. Insert the needle into the port and aspirate the urine sample and remove the needle.
5. Wipe the aspiration port again and remove the clamp.
6. Empty the urine sample into a sterile container, taking care not to touch the inside of the container or lid.
7. Safely dispose of the needle and syringe.
8. Label the container and take to the lab within 15 minutes or refrigerate.

DISCONTINUING A CATHETER

A catheter should never be discontinued without verifying the physician's order with the nurse. Remember that a Foley catheter is held in place by a balloon inflated with water and must be deflated prior to removal of the catheter.

To discontinue or remove a catheter, use the following procedure:

1. Wash hands and don gloves.
2. Place a towel or disposable pad between the patient's legs and over the legs for privacy.

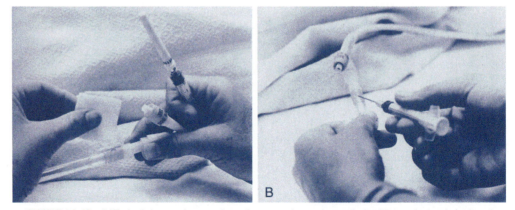

FIGURE 14–17   PCT obtaining a urine specimen from a patient using an indwelling catheter. *A,* Antiseptic cleaning of the area where a sterile needle will be inserted. *B,* Inserting the needle and withdrawing the specimen. (From Taylor, C, Lillis, C, and LeMone, P: Fundamentals of Nursing: The Art and Science of Nursing Care, ed 2. JB Lippincott, Philadelphia, 1993, p. 859, with permission.)

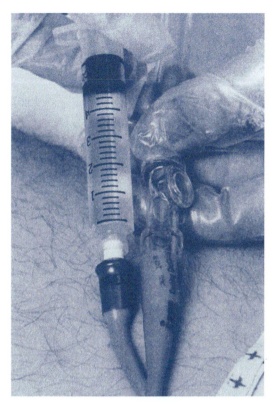

FIGURE 14–18   Deflating the balloon prior to removing a Foley catheter. (From Swearingen, PL, and Howard, CA: Photo Atlas of Nursing Procedures, ed 3. Addison-Wesley Publishing, Redwood, CA, 1996, with permission.)

3 Use a 10-cc syringe (without needle) to deflate the balloon (Fig. 14–18).

4 Slowly and steadily withdraw the catheter, observing for intactness.

5 Cleanse and dry the **perineum**.

6 Empty and measure the urine in the drainage bag.

7 Explain to the patient that you should be notified the first time the need to void occurs so that you can measure the output and assess for any problems.

8 Explain to the patient that it is normal to feel some irritation after the catheter is removed and to have slight burning with the first voiding. These sensations should subside quickly. The patient also needs to increase fluid intake unless otherwise ordered.

9 Report findings to the supervisor.

Intravenous (IV) Care

Monitoring patients who are receiving IV fluids may be a PCT responsibility. Patients receiving IV fluids will be on I & O measurements; IV fluids are a source of intake. The rate of flow of IV fluids is ordered by the doctor and is specifically calculated and regulated by the nurse. A mechanical device (IV pump or controller) may also be used to regulate the IV flow. The PCT may assist the nurse in monitoring the IV flow and in preventing and reporting signs of complications. Three main IV complications to monitor for are **thrombophlebitis**, *infiltration*, and obstruction of flow. **Phlebitis** is inflammation of the vein and may be present with or without a clot. When a clot is also present, the condition is known as thrombophlebitis. Signs of phlebitis are warmth, redness, pain, and swelling of the IV site. Infiltration is leaking of the IV fluid into the surrounding tissue. Signs of infiltration are paleness, coolness, swelling, and pain at the site. Obstruction is a decreased or stopped flow of the IV fluids, which may be caused by many things. If not corrected, obstruction may cause the IV to clot at the insertion point, resulting in the need to restart the IV in another site. One of the first things to check when obstruction occurs is for kinks in or pressure on the IV tubing, caused by the patient's lying on the tubing. Signs of these complications or any other problem with the IV should be reported to the nurse immediately.

CHANGING A GOWN OVER AN IV

When changing a gown for a patient with an IV, the IV tubing should never be broken or opened because this will cause contamination of the sterile system and may cause the patient to develop a serious infection.

To safely change the gown of a patient with an IV, follow these steps (Fig. 14–19):

1 Remove the gown from the free arm.
2 Gather the sleeve on the IV arm for better control, and move it down the arm and over the hand, being especially careful not to pull on the tubing when passing over the IV site.
3 Remove the IV from the pole and slip it through the gathered sleeve.
4 To put on a clean gown, reverse these steps by gathering the sleeve, slipping the IV through first and rehanging, carefully moving the clean gown over the IV arm and tubing, then placing the other arm in the gown, and fastening the gown.

DISCONTINUING THE IV

Before discontinuing an IV, always check with the nurse to make sure the doctor has ordered the procedure for this patient. It is painful and expensive for patients to have an IV removed by mistake. Always follow universal precautions when performing this procedure. Turn off the IV and carefully remove the tape and dressing (remove tape in the direction of the dressing on both sides to decrease the pulling sensation). Hold a cotton ball or 2- by 2-inch dressing over the IV site, and quickly remove the needle or catheter by pulling it straight out. Immediately exert pressure on the site with the dressing, and elevate the site for at least 1 minute to control bleeding. Check the needle or catheter to be sure no part has broken off or remains in the patient. Check to make sure the bleeding from the site is controlled, and apply a bandage. Check the site again in 10 to 15 minutes. Report and/or record the procedure and the patient's response.

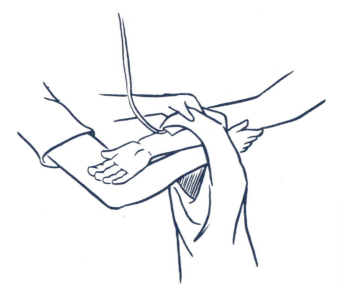

FIGURE 14–19 Changing a gown with an IV in place. (From Gomez, GE, Hord, EV, and Gettrust, KV: Fundamentals of Clinical Nursing Skills. John Wiley & Sons, New York, 1988, p. 143, with permission.)

Oral Medications

Occasionally the PCT's duties may include giving oral ***medications***. Medications are one form of treatment ordered by the physician to relieve symptoms or to control a condition or disease. The PCT must follow procedure carefully and take every precaution to prevent errors in giving medications (Fig. 14–20*A* through *E*). Check the drug literature and consult with the nurse to prevent drug errors. Occasionally, the dose supplied will not be the same as the dose ordered, and the PCT must consult with the nurse to determine the proper amount to give. Preparation of the patient is also necessary for safe and accurate administration of medication. The patient should know what medication is being given and why, as well as any special instructions, such as to take before meals or to not take with milk. The patient must always be identified before giving a medication even when you know the patient well or have worked with the same patient for a long time. Always check the patient's chart as well as ask about drug allergies. The PCT must always stay with the patient and witness that the medicine is taken. Oral medication includes drugs that are swallowed (tablets, capsules, caplets, liquids) as well as tablets that are dissolved when placed under the tongue (sublingual) or inside the pocket of the cheek (**buccal**). It is important that the patient understand not to swallow buccal or sublingual medications. To ensure accuracy when preparing

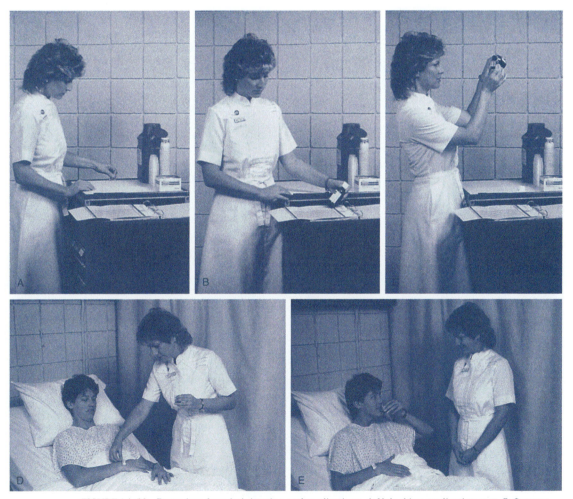

FIGURE 14–20   Procedure for administering oral medications. *A*, Unlocking medication cart. *B*, Comparing medication with order. *C*, Measuring at eye level. *D*, Checking patient's identification. *E*, Observing patient swallowing medication. (Photos © Ken Kasper.)

medications, the medication label should be checked with the medication order three times: when selecting the proper medication, before pouring, and when returning the medication to its proper location. When preparing medications it is important not to handle the drug; therefore, shake the tablets or capsules into the lid and then into a medicine cup. Liquids should be poured at eye level into a measured cup. Always pour liquids away from the labeled side and wipe the lip before re-capping. Some liquids may require mixing or shaking, so check the label carefully. Some patients, especially children and the elderly, may have difficulty swallowing and need to have solid medication crushed and/or mixed with food or liquids. Always check with your nurse first, because some medications cannot be crushed or mixed. After the patient has taken the medication, document on the patient's record according to institutional policy. If you have any questions, always consult with the nurse before you give any medication. Medications are an important part of a patient's treatment, but medication errors can cause patient injury or even death. Careful attention to detail and concentration on the procedure is necessary to avoid harmful errors.

BIBLIOGRAPHY

Ignatavicius, D, Workman, L, and Mishler, M: Medical-Surgical Nursing, ed 2. WB Saunders, Philadelphia, 1995.

Smith, S, and Duell, D: Clinical Nursing Skills, ed 4. Appleton & Lange, Norwalk, CT, 1996.

Taylor, C, Lillis, C, and Lemone, P: Fundamentals of Nursing, ed 2. JB Lippincott, Philadelphia, 1993.

STUDY QUESTIONS

1. List three categories of personnel working on a nursing unit who report to the RN.

   a. _____

   b. _____

   c. _____

2. Give an example of:

   a subjective observation _____

   an objective observation _____

3. State the purpose of the three major controls on a hospital bed.

   a. _____

   b. _____

   c. _____

4. State two purposes of a footboard.

   a. _____

   b. _____

5. Describe the routine position of an occupied hospital bed.

   _____

6. Describe the following hospital bed positions and indicate which require a physician's order:

   Fowler's _____

   Semi-Fowler's _____

   Trendelenburg's _____

   Reverse Trendelenburg's _____

7. List six baseline measurements that the PCT may perform and record when a patient is admitted to a nursing unit.

   a. _____

   b. _____

   c. _____

   d. _____

   e. _____

   f. _____

8. List four body sites used to take a patient's temperature.

a. _____

b. _____

c. _____

d. _____

9. Select the temperature site that most closely matches the following statements:

a. _____ Readings are lower and less accurate

b. _____ Measurements are always taken electronically

c. _____ Common site for infant temperatures

d. _____ Affected by breathing and smoking

10. The most common site used to take a pulse is the _____ .

11. State the three parameters that are assessed when taking a pulse.

a. _____

b. _____

c. _____

12. What vital sign measurement is taken at the same time as a pulse reading? Why?

_____

_____

13. Where should the PCT place the stethoscope when taking an apical pulse?

_____

14. Differentiate between systolic and diastolic blood pressure. Which reading is made when the first beat is heard? Which reading when the beats end?

_____

_____

_____

15. What should a PCT do if an adult patient's baseline blood pressure is 135/85?

_____

16. List three reasons for recording baseline height and weight measurements on a patient.

a. _____

b. _____

c. _____

17. Label the following body movements as either safe ("S") or unsafe ("U"):

_____ Moving patients by pushing them

_____ Using the back muscles for lifting

_____ Carrying objects close to the body

_____ Bending the knees when picking up objects

_____ Lifting objects rather than pulling or pushing them

18. When assisting a patient with ambulation, on which side of the patient should the PCT be positioned?_____

_____

19. When assisting patients out of bed, why should the PCT observe them closely and move them slowly to a standing position? _____

20. When a patient develops a decubitus ulcer, what aspect of patient care has been neglected?

_____

21. Describe the following resting positions:

Lateral _____

Supine _____

Prone _____

Which position may require a trochanter roll? _____

Which position may compromise respiration? _____

With what patient condition are hand rolls used? _____

22. When cleaning dentures, what precaution should be taken to prevent them from breaking?

_____

23. Place the following areas of the body in the correct order of bathing by putting the numbers 1 through 8 in the blanks:

_____ back

_____ eyes

_____ axillae

_____ genitals

_____ face

_____ rectum

_____ arms

_____ hands

24. When performing a linen change in an occupied bed, in what position is the patient placed?

_____

25. Describe a PCT's responsibilities when caring for a patient on intake and output orders.

_____

_____

26. Where should a catheter drainage bag be located? Why?

_____

27. What should a PCT do when noting a pink coloration to the urine in a patient's catheter drainage bag?

_____

28. What are two requirements of a catheterized urine specimen collected for laboratory testing?

a. _____

b. _____

29. Why is a 10-cc syringe needed when removing a Foley catheter?

_____

30. List the three main complications of IV therapy and the observations associated with each.

Complication	*Observations*
a.	
b.	
c.	

31. When preparing oral medications, when should the label be checked with the order?

_____

_____

32. List three ways that oral medications may be administered.

a. _____

b. _____

c. _____

33. True or False. Oral medications are left at the bedside for patients to take at their convenience. _____ Explain your answer.

_____

_____

EVALUATION OF ORAL OR RECTAL TEMPERATURE PROCEDURE

RATING SYSTEM   2 = Satisfactory   1 = Needs improvement   0 = Incorrect/did not perform

_____ **1.** Identifies patient

_____ **2.** Properly assembles equipment

_____ **3.** Washes hands

_____ **4.** Puts on gloves

_____ **5.** Explains procedure to patient

_____ **6.** Properly handles thermometer and shakes down the reading

_____ **7.** Checks that the thermometer reading is below 95°

_____ **8.** Properly positions the bulb or tip of the thermometer for taking temperature

_____ **9.** Leaves the thermometer in place for the necessary period of time

_____ **10.** Removes the thermometer and cleans before reading

_____ **11.** Reads the thermometer at eye level

_____ **12.** Records the temperature and shakes down thermometer

_____ **13.** Washes hands

Total points _____

Maximum points = 26

COMMENTS

EVALUATION OF PULSE AND RESPIRATION RECORDING PROCEDURE

RATING SYSTEM   2 = Satisfactory   1 = Needs improvement   0 = Incorrect/did not perform

_____ **1.** Identifies patient

_____ **2.** Properly prepares equipment

_____ **3.** Washes hands

_____ **4.** Properly positions patient

_____ **5.** Locates pulse beat

_____ **6.** Counts pulse rate for 60 seconds

_____ **7.** Continues to hold wrist while counting respirations for 30 seconds

_____ **8.** Records rate, rhythm, volume of pulse, respiration rate, and time observed

_____ **9.** Washes hands

Total points _____

Maximum points = 18

COMMENTS

EVALUATION OF BLOOD PRESSURE MEASURING PROCEDURE

RATING SYSTEM   2 = Satisfactory   1 = Needs improvement   0 = Incorrect/did not perform

_____ **1.** Identifies patient

_____ **2.** Assembles necessary equipment

_____ **3.** Washes hands

_____ **4.** Explains the procedure to the patient

_____ **5.** Properly cleans stethoscope diaphragm and earpieces

_____ **6.** Properly positions patient

_____ **7.** Properly aligns equipment

_____ **8.** Properly applies cuff

_____ **9.** Closes valve

_____ **10.** Properly applies diaphragm

_____ **11.** Locates artery and inflates cuff

_____ **12.** Opens valve and slowly deflates cuff

_____ **13.** Observes systolic reading

_____ **14.** Observes diastolic reading

_____ **15.** Deflates and removes cuff

_____ **16.** Records blood pressure

_____ **17.** Returns equipment

_____ **18.** Washes hands

Total points _____

Maximum points = 36

COMMENTS

EVALUATION OF HEIGHT AND WEIGHT RECORDING TECHNIQUE

RATING SYSTEM   2 = Satisfactory   1 = Needs improvement   0 = Incorrect/did not perform

_____   **1.** Identifies patient

_____   **2.** Assembles equipment

_____   **3.** Requests patient to empty bladder

_____   **4.** Washes hands

_____   **5.** Provides for privacy

_____   **6.** Properly secures scales

_____   **7.** Requests patient to remove robe and slippers or shoes

_____   **8.** Places paper towel on scale platform

_____   **9.** Properly positions patient on scale

_____   **10.** Measures and records patient's height

_____   **11.** Folds and lowers measuring bar

_____   **12.** Positions weight on lower bar to estimated weight

_____   **13.** Positions weight on upper bar until beam is leveled

_____   **14.** Determines and records patient's weight

_____   **15.** Assists patient off scale and donning robe and slippers or shoes

_____   **16.** Returns scale to storage area

_____   **17.** Records and reports measurements

_____   **18.** Washes hands

Total points _____

Maximum points = 36

COMMENTS

EVALUATION OF ASSISTING AMBULATION

RATING SYSTEM   2 = Satisfactory   1 = Needs improvement   0 = Incorrect/did not perform

_____ **1.** Identifies patient

_____ **2.** Explains procedure to patient

_____ **3.** Washes hands

_____ **4.** Lowers bed and locks wheels

_____ **5.** Assists patient with robe and shoes

_____ **6.** Applies transfer belt and assists patient to stand

_____ **7.** Properly assists patient to walk normally for the planned distance

_____ **8.** Observes patient for any difficulty

_____ **9.** Assists patient back into bed and places call bell within reach

_____ **10.** Raises the side rails of the bed

_____ **11.** Washes hands

_____ **12.** Reports distance walked and patient's tolerance

Total points _____

Maximum points = 24

COMMENTS

EVALUATION OF BED-TO-CHAIR TRANSFER TECHNIQUE

RATING SYSTEM   2 = Satisfactory   1 = Needs improvement   0 = Incorrect/did not perform

_____ **1.** Identifies patient

_____ **2.** Washes hands

_____ **3.** Explains procedure to patient

_____ **4.** Properly positions wheelchair

_____ **5.** Locks wheelchair brakes

_____ **6.** Assists patient to sit on side of bed

_____ **7.** Assesses patient before moving from bed

_____ **8.** Secures transfer belt and assists patient into chair

_____ **9.** Properly positions patient in chair and adjusts gown for privacy

_____ **10.** Provides access to call bell before leaving patient

_____ **11.** Washes hands

Total points _____

Maximum points = 22

COMMENTS

EVALUATION OF BATH PROCEDURE

RATING SYSTEM   2 = Satisfactory   1 = Needs improvement   0 = Incorrect/did not perform

_____ **1.** Identifies patient

_____ **2.** Washes hands

_____ **3.** Explains procedure to patient

_____ **4.** Provides privacy

_____ **5.** Offers bedpan before starting

_____ **6.** Prepares water and brings supplies to bedside

_____ **7.** Raises bed to high position

_____ **8.** Covers patient with bath blanket to prevent exposure at all times

_____ **9.** Washes eyes using a different corner of washcloth for each eye

_____ **10.** Applies soap and washes face, ears, and neck; rinses and dries areas

_____ **11.** Washes arms from hand to armpit, rinses and dries areas

_____ **12.** Washes chest and abdomen, rinses and dries area

_____ **13.** Places feet in water, washes legs from ankle upward, then feet; rinses and dries areas

_____ **14.** Changes bath water

_____ **15.** Washes back and buttocks, rinses and dries areas

_____ **16.** Puts on gloves

_____ **17.** Washes perianal area, rinses and dries area

_____ **18.** Changes bath water

_____ **19.** Washes genital area, rinses and dries area

_____ **20.** Observes patient's skin condition throughout bath

_____ **21.** Cleans and replaces equipment

_____ **22.** Adjusts bed and side rails

_____ **23.** Washes hands

Total points _____

Maximum points = 46

COMMENTS

EVALUATION OF PROCEDURE FOR MAKING AN UNOCCUPIED BED

RATING SYSTEM   2 = Satisfactory   1 = Needs improvement   0 = Incorrect/did not perform

_____ **1.** Washes hands

_____ **2.** Assembles clean linens

_____ **3.** Inspects dirty linens for client's belongings, call bell, and so on

_____ **4.** Loosens linens starting at head of bed, moving down bed, and around to other side

_____ **5.** Places pillow on bedside chair after removing pillowcase

_____ **6.** Properly rolls all soiled lines inside bottom sheet and places directly in linen hamper

_____ **7.** Properly applies bottom and top sheets

_____ **8.** Properly installs clean pillowcase

_____ **9.** Does not shake linens

_____ **10.** Properly attaches call bell to bed

_____ **11.** Lowers bed to its lowest position

_____ **12.** Washes hands

Total points _____

Maximum points = 24

COMMENTS

EVALUATION OF PROCEDURE FOR OBTAINING A SPECIMEN FROM A CATHETER

RATING SYSTEM   2 = Satisfactory   1 = Needs improvement   0 = Incorrect/did not perform

_____ **1.** Verifies procedure with nurse

_____ **2.** Assembles equipment

_____ **3.** Identifies patient and explains procedure

_____ **4.** Washes hands

_____ **5.** Clamps tubing for 15 minutes

_____ **6.** Puts on gloves

_____ **7.** Cleanses aspiration port

_____ **8.** Inserts needle into aspiration port

_____ **9.** Aspirates urine sample and removes needle

_____ **10.** Wipes aspiration port and removes clamp

_____ **11.** Empties syringe into sterile specimen container

_____ **12.** Correctly disposes of syringe and needle

_____ **13.** Removes gloves and washes hands

_____ **14.** Labels container and delivers to laboratory

Total points _____

Maximum points = 28

COMMENTS

EVALUATION OF IV CARE AND DISCONTINUATION TECHNIQUE

RATING SYSTEM   2 = Satisfactory   1 = Needs improvement   0 = Incorrect/did not perform

_____ **1.** Checks IV site hourly

_____ **2.** Checks tubing for kinks/obstruction

_____ **3.** Checks site dressing for leakage

_____ **4.** Inspects site for redness, swelling, pain, heat or coolness, and paleness

_____ **5.** Appropriately changes gown, without breaking line

_____ **6.** Verifies discontinuation order with nurse

_____ **7.** Assembles equipment

_____ **8.** Identifies and explains procedure to patient

_____ **9.** Washes hands and puts on gloves

_____ **10.** Stabilizes needle/catheter while removing tape toward the dressing

_____ **11.** Removes catheter quickly and smoothly and inspects for intactness

_____ **12.** Quickly applies pressure with sterile pad until bleeding stops

_____ **13.** Applies dressing

_____ **14.** Rechecks site in 15 minutes

_____ **15.** Properly disposes of equipment/needle

_____ **16.** Removes gloves and washes hands

_____ **17.** Reports and records

Total points _____

Maximum points = 34

COMMENTS

EVALUATION OF ORAL MEDICATION ADMINISTRATION

RATING SYSTEM   2 = Satisfactory   1 = Needs improvement   0 = Incorrect/did not perform

_____ **1.** Verifies doctor's order with medication record

_____ **2.** Checks with nurse for dosage calculations and/or accuracy

_____ **3.** Washes hands

_____ **4.** Assembles equipment

_____ **5.** Obtains medication

_____ **6.** Checks label with medical record

_____ **7.** Removes drug dose and places in proper container, checks label

_____ **8.** Pours liquid at eye level, away from the label, and wipes bottle before closing

_____ **9.** Checks label with medical record

_____ **10.** Returns drug

_____ **11.** Identifies patient, explains drug use, and asks about allergies

_____ **12.** Administers medication and witnesses patient swallowing drug

_____ **13.** Washes hands

_____ **14.** Documents on medical record

Total points _____

Maximum points = 28

COMMENTS

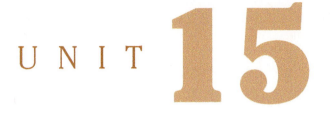
RESPIRATORY CARE

KEY TERMS

- ***Bourdon gauge*** — Gauge that displays gas pressure on a dial
- ***Bronchodilator*** — Medication that relaxes bronchial smooth muscle
- ***Fraction of inspired oxygen*** — The fractional concentration of oxygen being inhaled
- ***Metered-dose inhaler*** — Nebulizer designed to administer a small amount of aerosolized medication to the airways without an external pressurized gas source
- ***Nebulizer*** — Device that creates an aerosol
- ***Partial pressure*** — Amount of pressure exerted by an individual gas within a mixture of gases
- ***Pulse oximeter*** — Instrument that measures the oxygen saturation of blood
- ***Small-volume nebulizer*** — Instrument designed to administer a small amount of aerosolized medication to the airways using an external pressurized gas source
- ***Spacer*** — Reservoir to hold the aerosol from a metered-dose inhaler
- ***Spirometry*** — The measurement of respiratory gases

- ***Steroid***   Chemical compound that may be used to depress immune function
- ***Thorpe tube***   Type of flowmeter that uses a float to indicate flow rate

PCTs are frequently responsible for providing basic respiratory care to their patients. This unit is designed to provide PCTs with a basic understanding of the principles of oxygen therapy and the procedures to be performed.

Oxygen Delivery

Oxygen (O_2) is a colorless, odorless, tasteless gas that exists at normal atmospheric pressure and temperature. Oxygen composes 20.95%, or one fifth, of the earth's atmosphere and has the unique ability to support life. It also has the ability to support combustion. Oxygen itself is not flammable, but materials that will burn in room air will burn faster and hotter in the presence of increased amounts of oxygen. The percentage of oxygen in the atmosphere does not change, but the ***partial pressure*** of oxygen varies as barometric pressure changes. (The most common cause of a significant change in barometric pressure is a change in altitude.) Partial pressure is a term that describes the pressure exerted by a single gas present in a mixture of gases or in a mixture of gases and liquids (such as oxygen and carbon dioxide [CO_2] in the blood). For example, two different gases, nitrogen (N_2) and oxygen, make up most of the air in the atmosphere. Because 20.95% of the atmosphere is oxygen, it exerts 20.95% of the total atmospheric pressure. That pressure is called the partial pressure of oxygen in the atmosphere. The term partial pressure is often used in respiratory care.

Oxygen is given to patients with a variety of respiratory diseases. The three reasons for oxygen delivery are to treat **hypoxemia**, to reduce the work of breathing, and to reduce the work of the heart.

Hypoxemia is defined as a partial pressure of oxygen in the arterial blood (**PaO$_2$**) of less than 80 mm Hg, which indicates an inadequate amount of oxygen in the blood. Oxygen moves into the blood because of a difference in pressure between the alveolus and the pulmonary capillary. The delivery of supplemental oxygen increases this pressure difference and causes more oxygen to move into the blood, causing the PaO$_2$ to rise and effectively relieving the hypoxemia.

The first and primary response of the body to hypoxemia is an increased rate and force of contraction of the heart. This is an effort to provide more oxygen to the tissues by increasing the rate of blood flow through the tissues, but it also causes the work of the heart to increase. Hypoxemia also causes the patient to breathe faster and deeper in an effort to move more oxygen into the blood, and this causes an increase in the work of breathing. Relieving the hypoxemia by administering supplemental oxygen relieves the increased work of breathing and the increased work of the heart that accompany hypoxemia.

The administration of supplemental oxygen is not without hazards. Because PCTs will provide care to many patients receiving oxygen, they must be familiar with its hazards. Oxygen can be toxic to living tissues. In normal atmospheric amounts, living tissues have adequate defense mechanisms against this toxicity. However, at increased levels of oxygen, such as those present when administering supplemental oxygen, the defense mechanisms of the tissues can be overwhelmed. If the tissues are exposed to levels of oxygen of 40% or greater for extended periods, tissue damage may occur. Most of the damage occurs to lung tissue, because that is the tissue exposed to the increased oxygen levels.

Other hazards are associated with oxygen delivery. Some patients with chronic obstructive pulmonary disease (COPD) may slow down or stop breathing altogether when given supplemental oxygen. This response is called oxygen-induced **hypoventilation**, and it may occur with the administration of relatively small amounts of oxygen or with small increases in the amount of oxygen the patient is receiving. Patients with COPD must be observed closely when changing the delivered dose of oxygen. The PCT must be alert to changes in the condition of COPD patients receiving oxygen. If a patient with COPD becomes difficult to arouse or shows other signs of oxygen-induced hypoventilation, immediately notify the patient's nurse, respiratory therapist, or physician. Do not decrease the amount of oxygen being delivered, because it can cause severe hypoxemia. If necessary, the patient must be ventilated artificially.

DELIVERY SYSTEMS

Oxygen is delivered through a variety of systems that can be broken down into two primary components: a pressurized source of oxygen and a delivery device. The pressurized oxygen source provides oxygen at a variety of flow rates to the delivery device. The delivery device is the piece of equipment chosen to actually administer oxygen to the patient.

Common pressurized oxygen sources are high-pressure, steel gas cylinders; bulk liquid oxygen systems (used to provide oxygen to wall outlets in hospitals); and small, low-pressure, portable liquid oxygen containers.

Gas Cylinders

A variety of gases are stored in steel cylinders capable of maintaining high pressures (Fig. 15–1). The high pressure allows a relatively large amount of gas to be stored in the

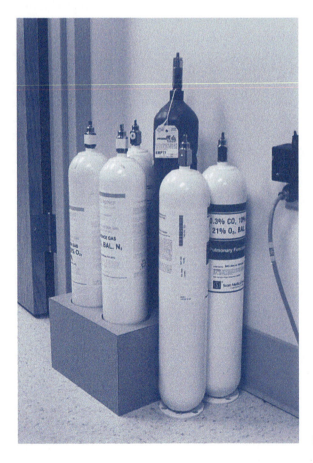

FIGURE 15–1   Gas cylinders.

cylinder. High-pressure gas cylinders come in several sizes, identified by a coding system of letters. The earlier the letter in the alphabet, the smaller the cylinder. Common cylinder sizes and capacities are shown in Table 15–1.

Gas cylinders may be color coded for easy identification of their contents; however, color coding is not internationally standardized. The United States color code for oxygen is green. Cylinders are required to have a label attached to the shoulder of the cylinder identifying the contents. This label should always be used to determine the contents of the cylinder because color coding is not a reliable means of determining the contents of a gas cylinder.

High-pressure gas inside the cylinder is reduced to a working pressure of 50 pounds per square inch (**psi**) by the use of a **reducing valve**, a device that attaches to the cylinder outlet and reduces the pressure of the gas from the cylinder. The reducing valve contains a pressure gauge that displays the amount of pressure remaining in the cylinder. The pressure gauge is read by observing the position of the needle relative to the markings on the gauge. Most reducing valves used for the administration of medical gases such as oxygen also incorporate a **flowmeter**. The combination of a reducing valve and a flowmeter is called a **regulator**.

There are two common types of flowmeters incorporated into regulators used on high-pressure gas cylinders. They are the ***Bourdon gauge*** and the ***Thorpe tube***. The Bourdon gauge is actually a pressure gauge with a dial that has been calibrated to read flow, as shown in Figure 15–2. The Thorpe tube has an upright tube containing a float that rises in the tube as the valve is opened (Fig. 15–3). Flow is read on the Bourdon gauge by observing the position of the needle relative to the markings on the gauge, whereas flow is read on the Thorpe tube by observing the position of the float relative to the markings on the tube. If the float is flat, the flow leaving the flowmeter is read according to the top of the float in relation to the markings on the tube. If the float is round (a ball float), the flow leaving the flowmeter is read at the center of the float in relation to the markings on the tube. All pressure gauges and flowmeters must be read at eye level while standing directly in front of the device or an inaccurate reading will result.

Regulators designed to fit on oxygen cylinders may be used only on those cylinders and will not fit on cylinders containing other gases. This is a safety system designed to reduce the possibility of administering the wrong gas to a patient. On cylinder sizes E and smaller, the Pin Index Safety System (PISS) is used. In the PISS, a set of two pins is used in the yoke of the regulator along with two holes in the valve of the cylinder to prevent the connection of the wrong regulator. On cylinders larger than size E, the American Standard Safety System (ASSS) uses different nut sizes, thread sizes, and thread directions to prevent the connection of the wrong type of regulator to the cylinder.

The gas cylinder should be "cracked" before attaching a regulator. "Cracking" means to rapidly open and close the valve of the cylinder while no regulator is attached. This practice allows a burst of gas to leave the cylinder to clear out any dirt or debris that may be in the valve. The cylinder valve is opened with a key (special wrench) on smaller cylinders and with a small wheel on larger cylinders. Once the cylinder has been cracked, the regulator can be attached. If a washer is present, make sure it is placed properly before attaching the regulator. Once the regulator is attached,

TABLE 15–1   **Common Gas Cylinder Sizes and Capacities**

Cylinder Size	Diameter (inches)	Height (inches)	Capacity (cu ft)
D	4.5	20.0	12.7
E	4.5	30.0	22.0
G	8.5	55.0	187.0
H or K	9.0	55.0	244.0

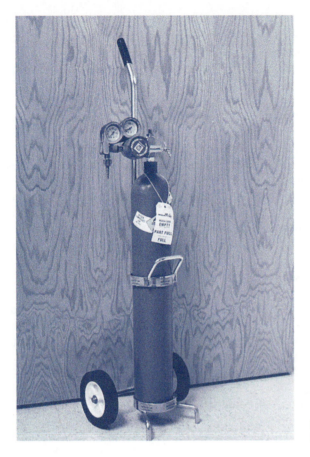

FIGURE 15–2   Bourdon gauge attached to portable oxygen tank.

slowly open the cylinder valve. The pressure reading on the pressure gauge (the one closest to the valve) will rise.

Flowmeters must also be used for the correct type of gas. The Diameter Index Safety System (DISS) is used on all connections for which pressures are less than 200 psi, which is typically when flowmeters are used (the working pressure for most respiratory therapy

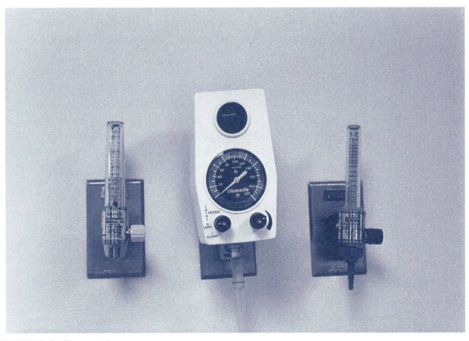

FIGURE 15–3   Thorpe tube.

equipment is 50 psi). The DISS also uses nut and thread designs to prevent the accidental connection of the wrong type of flowmeter. There are also a variety of quick-connect systems for flowmeters. These systems allow the rapid connection of flowmeters to wall outlets in hospitals. There is no standard system for quick-connect systems because these systems are developed by, and are unique to, the specific manufacturer.

When delivering oxygen from a cylinder, the PCT must know how long the cylinder will last. Oxygen is delivered through a regulator (reducing valve–flowmeter combination) at a flow calibrated in liters per minute (L/min). The only readily available information about a gas cylinder is its pressure; however, there is no gauge that tells us how many liters of gas are in the cylinder. To calculate the duration of flow from a gas cylinder, the pressure of gas in the cylinder in pounds per square inch must be converted to liters. A set of conversion factors used to accomplish this task is given in Table 15–2.

To determine the amount of gas in liters in the cylinder, multiply the pressure reading from the pressure gauge on the cylinder by the appropriate conversion factor. For example, an E cylinder with 2200 psi (a full cylinder) contains 2200 psi $\times$ 0.28 L/psi = 616 L of oxygen.

To determine how long this cylinder will last, we need to know how many liters per minute of oxygen are leaving the cylinder and going to the patient. When we know how many liters of oxygen are in the cylinder and how many liters per minute are leaving the cylinder (reading of the flowmeter), it is easy to determine how long the cylinder will last. Just divide the number of liters in the cylinder by the number of liters per minute leaving the cylinder. We know that our full E cylinder contains 616 L of oxygen; if the flow leaving that E cylinder is 2 L/min, then the cylinder will last 308 minutes (616 L ÷ 2 L/min) before becoming empty. When determining the duration of a cylinder of oxygen, it may be more convenient to convert the time from minutes to hours (divide the answer in minutes by 60). The duration of an E cylinder of oxygen with a working pressure of 2200 psi and a flow rate of 2 L/min is calculated as follows:

EXAMPLE:

$$2200 \text{ psi} \times 0.28 \text{ (L/psi)} = 616 \text{ L}$$

$$\frac{616 \text{ L}}{2 \text{(L/min)}} = 308 \text{ minutes}$$

$$\frac{308 \text{ minutes}}{60 \text{ (min/h)}} = 5.1 \text{ hours (cylinder duration)}$$

The PCT can calculate the duration of a cylinder of oxygen to determine when a cylinder needs to be replaced. For example, a patient being transported to an ancillary department, such as Radiology, for a lengthy procedure may need to have oxygen administered from an oxygen cylinder during the transport and the procedure because not all radiology departments have piped-in oxygen. The duration of the cylinder must be calculated to determine when to replace the cylinder. When making this calculation, a margin of error should always be included. In other words, give yourself extra time to go back and change the cylinder. If the cylinder will be empty in 1 hour, return to change it in 45 minutes. Another alternative is to calculate how long the cylinder will last until only 500 psi remain by subtracting 500 psi from the starting pressure and changing the tank at that time.

TABLE 15–2 **Oxygen Cylinder Conversion Factors**

Cylinder Size	Conversion Factor
D	0.16 L/psi
E	0.28 L/psi
G	2.41 L/psi
H or K	3.14 L/psi

Liquid Oxygen Containers

Large containers of liquid oxygen are used to supply oxygen to entire buildings, such as hospitals. The PCT generally will not come in contact with bulk liquid oxygen systems other than the wall outlets for flowmeter connections.

Liquid oxygen containers are also used for home delivery of oxygen. These systems usually consist of a stationary container that is used to provide oxygen to patients at home and a portable unit that weighs between 5 and 15 lb that patients can take with them outside the home. The portable unit is filled from the stationary unit. PCTs may come in contact with portable liquid oxygen systems when patients bring one with them, for example, to the doctor's office, or when patient transport takes place in the hospital. Many hospitals are using portable liquid oxygen systems instead of steel cylinders for patient transport (Fig. 15–4).

The operating pressure of a home liquid oxygen system is about 20 psi. Because of the nature of liquid oxygen systems, pressure inside the container does not decrease as a direct result of gas leaving the container. Therefore, it is not possible to determine the amount of oxygen inside the container by the pressure inside the container. To determine the amount of oxygen left in a liquid oxygen container, the container must be weighed on scales provided by the container manufacturer, and the weight must be used to calculate the amount of liquid oxygen left in the tank. The amount of liquid oxygen is not the same as the amount of gaseous oxygen, however, so the amount of liquid oxygen must be converted to a gaseous amount. Once the amount of gaseous oxygen has been determined, the flow rate from the container can be used to determine how long the cylinder will last.

EXAMPLE:

Step 1: Converting liquid weight to gaseous oxygen. (Note: This step combines the conversion of both liquid weight to liquid volume and liquid volume to

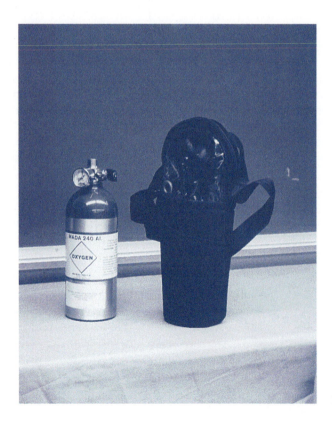

FIGURE 15–4   Portable oxygen unit.

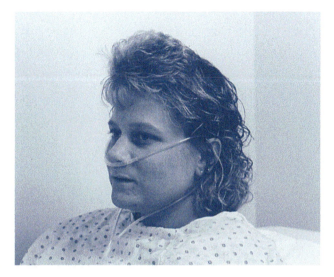

FIGURE 15–5   Nasal cannula.

gaseous volume. The conversion factors are as follows: 2.5 lb of liquid oxygen = 1 L of liquid oxygen; 1 L of liquid oxygen = 860 L of gaseous oxygen.)

$$\text{Gas Remaining (liters)} = \frac{(\text{liquid weight in pounds} \times 860)}{2.5}$$

Step 2: Calculating the duration of the contents of a liquid container.

$$\text{Duration of Contents (minutes)} = \frac{\text{gas remaining}}{\text{flow (L/min)}}$$

DELIVERY DEVICES

Nasal Cannula

The most common oxygen delivery device used by the PCT is the nasal **cannula**, shown in Figure 15–5. The nasal cannula is a continuous tube with a loop at one end containing two prongs that are partially inserted into the nose. The other end of the cannula is attached to a flowmeter. A nasal cannula is used for oxygen flow rates of up to 6 L/min.

The ***fraction of inspired oxygen* (FiO_2)** is a term similar to partial pressure and is the percentage of oxygen a patient is breathing, expressed as a decimal. To express a percentage as a decimal, divide the percentage by 100. For example, if a patient is breathing 40% oxygen, the FiO_2 the patient is breathing is 0.40 (40/100). The FiO_2 delivered by a nasal cannula can only be estimated, because the cannula provides only a portion of the gas the patient is breathing because the oxygen from the cannula mixes with room air. We do not know how much room air is being inhaled; therefore, we cannot know precisely what FiO_2 the patient is receiving. In fact, the

TABLE 15–3   **FiO_2 Delivered by Nasal Cannula**

Flow (L/min)	Estimated FiO_2
1	0.24
2	0.28
3	0.32
4	0.36
5	0.40
6	0.44

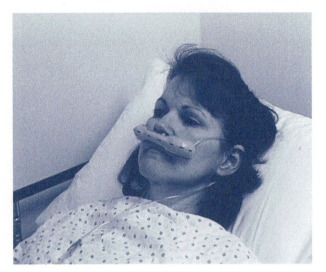

FIGURE 15–6 Nasal cannula with reservoir at the nasal prongs.

FiO_2 at any given flow rate from the cannula varies from patient to patient or even from moment to moment in any particular patient. The FiO_2 can be estimated for a patient with a normal respiratory rate and pattern of breathing using Table 15–3. An oxygen delivery system that delivers a variable FiO_2 is called a **variable** (low-flow) **performance system**.

Some nasal cannulas incorporate a reservoir called an oxygen-conserving device to conserve oxygen used in the home. The reservoir may be in a variety of places on the cannula, but two common designs put the reservoir at the nasal prongs or at the beginning of the loop in the tubing (Figs. 15–6 and 15–7). These devices are capable of providing oxygen therapy at a lower flow rate, thus conserving oxygen.

Oxygen Masks

When an FiO_2 greater than 0.40 is required, an oxygen mask can be used. The simple oxygen mask is made of plastic and rests on the bridge of the nose and the chin (Fig. 15–8). The mask increases the reservoir for oxygen, which in turn increases the FiO_2 delivered to the patient. Simple masks are variable performance devices, like the nasal cannula. Flow to a simple mask should be at least 5 L/min to ensure that exhaled car-

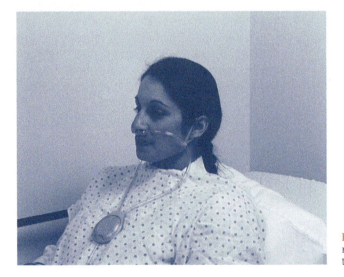

FIGURE 15–7 Nasal cannula with reservoir at the beginning of the tube.

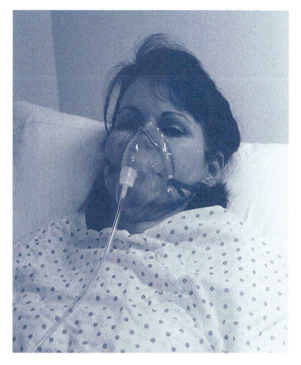

FIGURE 15–8   Simple oxygen mask.

bon dioxide is flushed from the mask before the next breath. The simple mask delivers an FiO_2 between 0.30 and 0.60.

A partial rebreathing mask can be used to deliver an FiO_2 higher than that of a simple mask by incorporating a plastic bag at the entrance to the mask to increase the reservoir for oxygen above that of a simple mask (Fig. 15–9). The opening between bag and mask allows the patient's exhaled gas to enter the bag. Only about the first third of the exhaled gas enters the bag, however, and because that gas comes primarily from

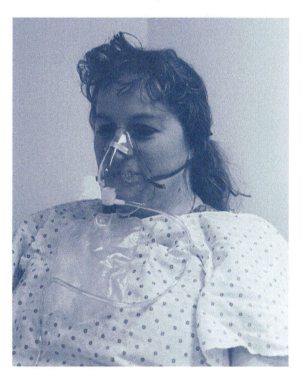

FIGURE 15–9   Partial rebreathing mask.

the trachea and upper airways, it is low in carbon dioxide. When the patient breathes in, this exhaled gas, plus the gas filling the bag from the flowmeter, is inhaled. Partial rebreathing masks should provide a flow sufficient to keep the bag from deflating more than half way when the patient breathes in. This is usually a flow rate between 8 and 15 L/min. The partial rebreathing mask is also a variable performance device and delivers an FiO_2 between 0.40 and 0.70.

A nonrebreathing mask is used to deliver the highest FiO_2 generally achievable with a variable performance device. The nonrebreathing mask is similar to the partial rebreathing mask, except that it has a one-way valve between the bag and the mask and a one-way valve on the mask itself (Fig. 15–10). The one-way valve between the mask and the bag prevents exhaled gas from entering the bag and being rebreathed on the next breath, and it reduces the **entrainment** of room air during inspiration. These two modifications effectively increase the delivered FiO_2 over that of the partial rebreathing mask, although the nonrebreathing mask is still a variable performance device. The flow delivered to the nonrebreathing mask should be enough to prevent the bag from collapsing on inspiration, usually 10 to 15 L/min or more. The FiO_2 delivered from a nonrebreathing mask is between 0.60 and 0.80.

When it is necessary to deliver a precise FiO_2, a system capable of providing all of the gas the patient inhales must be used. These devices are called **fixed** (high-flow) **performance systems**. The most common fixed performance device is the Venturi mask (Fig. 15–11), which uses a system of flow from the oxygen source and air entrainment to provide a precise FiO_2 at relatively high flow rates. At a high FiO_2 these devices may not provide enough gas flow to meet the patient's entire inspiratory demand. Under such conditions, these masks function as variable performance devices. Under most conditions, however, these masks are classified as fixed performance devices. The correct flow rate must be provided to the Venturi mask to achieve the correct FiO_2 through a specific adapter that is used for each FiO_2. The adapter has the FiO_2 and the correct flow rate inscribed on its base. Table 15–4 lists the FiO_2 available from various Venturi masks, the flow rate required to run them, and the total flow from the mask (notice that the total flow decreases as FiO_2 increases).

HUMIDIFICATION

In some cases, it is necessary to humidify the oxygen being delivered to the patient because oxygen is dry when it leaves its source, whether the source is a cylinder or a liq-

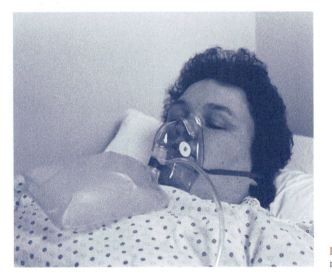

FIGURE 15–10   Nonrebreathing mask.

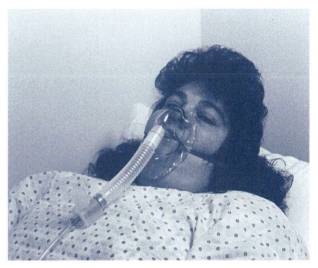

FIGURE 15–11   Venturi mask.

uid container (bulk or home system). In the case of the nasal cannula, the simple mask, and the partial rebreathing mask, this is done with a bubbletype humidifier, as shown in Figure 15–12. The bubble humidifier is simply a bottle of water that attaches to the flowmeter and allows the gas leaving the flowmeter to bubble through the water in the bottle. As the gas passes through the water, some of the water evaporates into the gas. The bubble humidifier is not commonly used with a nasal cannula at flow rates of less than 4 L/min, unless the patient is experiencing nasal dryness or discomfort. The use of the bubble humidifier with the various oxygen masks is optional, based on the patient and the particular policy of the institution. Flow rates through the nonrebreathing mask are generally too high to allow the use of a bubble humidifier. Humidification is usually not needed with Venturi masks because they entrain so much room air, which typically has a relative humidity of approximately 40%. If necessary, humidification to a Venturi mask can be provided by an external ***nebulizer***.

A nebulizer is a device that creates an aerosol, which is a collection of particles suspended in a gas. Humidity, on the other hand, refers to the existence of molecular water (water vapor) in a gas. A nebulizer can be used to add humidity (water vapor) to a dry gas. The aerosol that is produced is suspended in the gas, and the tiny particles of water evaporate, becoming water vapor and increasing the humidity of the gas. Some nebulizer systems are designed to provide both an aerosol and a specific FiO_2 to a patient and are called large-volume nebulizers. The specific FiO_2 is achieved through the same principle of air entrainment used by the Venturi mask. Nebulizers are also used to create an aerosol from a medication that the patient then inhales. These are called small-volume nebulizers and are discussed in more detail in the next section.

TABLE 15–4   **FiO$_2$ Flow Requirements and Total Flow from Venturi Masks**

FiO$_2$ Setting	Oxygen Flow (L/min)	Total Flow (L/min)
0.24	4	104
0.28	4	44
0.31	6	48
0.35	8	48
0.40	8	32
0.50	12	32
0.60	12	24
0.70	12	19

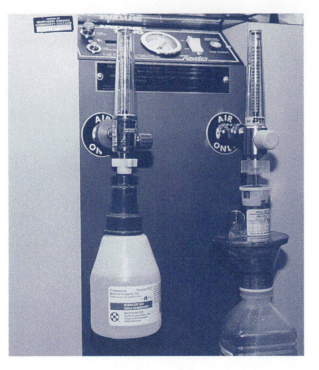

FIGURE 15–12 Bubbletype humidifier.

Aerosol Delivery of Medications

Aerosols are used to provide humidity to dry gases (as described in the previous section) and also to deliver medications to the lungs. The PCT frequently provides care to patients receiving medications inhaled by aerosol. A significant advantage to delivering medications by the inhaled route is that a much lower dose can be used, compared with the oral or intravenous routes, because the drug is going directly to the site of action, which leads to fewer side effects. Two types of nebulizers are used to deliver aerosol medications, and the PCT needs to recognize both. They are called the ***small-volume nebulizer*** (**SVN**) and the ***metered-dose inhaler*** (**MDI**).

SMALL-VOLUME NEBULIZERS

SVNs are devices used to continuously aerosolize a medication for the patient to inhale (Fig. 15–13). The SVN can nebulize almost any type of medication that can be provided in a liquid form. Because the SVN nebulizes the medication continuously, the patient does not need to coordinate breathing with the SVN; whenever the patient inhales, medication is received. The advantage is that patients who cannot follow directions or have difficulty with coordination can still receive medications. In fact, aerosol medications can be delivered with an SVN through a face mask (instead of a mouthpiece) to comatose patients. The disadvantage of aerosol medication delivery with a mask is that it wastes large amounts of medication, because when the patient is not inhaling, the medication is nebulized into the room.

SVNs are powered by a compressed gas source. In the hospital, this is often a flowmeter connected to either an oxygen or an air wall outlet. In the home or in a physician's office, this is usually a small, electrically powered air compressor. Most SVNs should be attached to a flowmeter using regular oxygen tubing and run at a flow rate of between 6 and 8 L/min. An extra piece of large-bore tubing is usually added to the end of the nebulizer opposite the mouthpiece to act as a reservoir for the aerosol to increase the amount of aerosol the patient breathes in and therefore reduce the

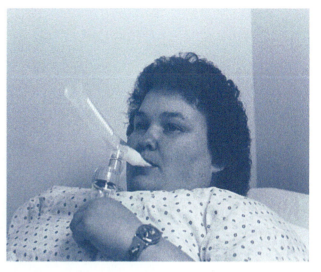

FIGURE 15–13 Small-volume nebulizer.

loss of medicine. The reservoir tubing is removed when using a mask to deliver the aerosol.

The way the patient inhales has an effect on the amount of the aerosol medication that actually enters the lungs. The PCT must coach the patient in the proper technique to help the patient receive as much benefit from the treatment as possible. The patient should be instructed to sit upright and breathe in slowly and deeply through the mouth. The patient should then hold his or her breath for up to 10 seconds, if possible, to give the aerosol time to settle into the lungs. Some patients will not be able to follow these directions, particularly if they are short of breath. They should still be encouraged to breathe in slowly and to hold their breath for as long as they can for as many breaths as possible. Comatose patients, of course, will be able to breathe normally only through a mask.

METERED-DOSE INHALERS

MDIs are small, pressurized canisters that discharge a specific amount of medication in a single dose when they are activated (Fig. 15–14). MDIs are frequently used for patients with respiratory diseases, both in and outside the hospital. Because MDIs do not continuously create an aerosol, they conserve medication. Patients must accurately coordinate the discharge of the aerosol from the MDI with their inspiration to receive the full dose of medication. This can be extremely difficult for many patients, especially the very young and very old and those who cannot follow directions.

The way the patient inhales is more important with an MDI than it is with an SVN because the dose from an MDI is much smaller. Also, the aerosol is rapidly discharged from the MDI, and if the proper technique is not used, the aerosol will simply impact in the mouth and throat. Patients should be instructed to warm the MDI canister in their hands before using it. After the canister is warmed and properly assembled, it should be shaken. The MDI should not be placed in the mouth but should be held about two finger widths away from the lips with the mouth open. The patient should then be told to sit upright, exhale normally, and then inhale slowly. Just after beginning to inhale, the patient should activate the MDI and continue to inhale as deeply as possible, followed by a breath hold of up to 10 seconds. There should be a pause of a few minutes, up to 10 minutes, between doses.

Because these directions are difficult for so many patients to follow correctly, a device called a **"*spacer*"** has been developed to make the use of an MDI easier and more effective. A spacer is a reservoir that holds the aerosol once the MDI has been activated, as shown in Figure 15–15. The patient immediately inhales slowly and as

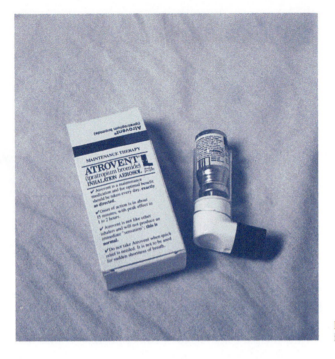

FIGURE 15–14   Metered-dose inhaler.

deeply as possible from the spacer. A 10-second breath hold is still required. The major advantage of the spacer appears to be less need for the patient to coordinate the activation of the MDI with the inhalation.

MEDICATIONS DELIVERED

There are two major types of medication delivered by aerosol to patients with respiratory disease. The PCT must be familiar with the side effects of these medications to alert the patient's other caregivers if the patient begins to experience any of the side effects.

Bronchodilators

The most common type of medication delivered by aerosol is the **bronchodilator**. The term *bronchodilator* means to dilate (widen) the airways, or bronchi, which are small airways made up primarily of muscle. In many respiratory diseases, such as

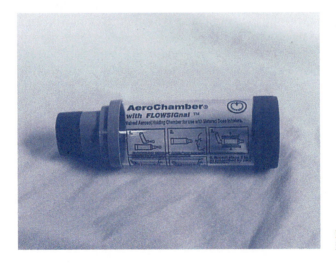

FIGURE 15–15   Metered-dose inhaler with reservoir.

TABLE 15–5   **Common Inhaled Bronchodilators**

Generic Name	Trade Name(s)	MDI	SVN	Duration (hours)
Isoetharine	Bronkosol	—	Yes	3–4
Metaproterenol	Alupent	—	Yes	3–4
	Metaprel	Yes	—	3–4
Albuterol	Ventolin	—	Yes	4–6
	Proventil	Yes	—	4–6
Pirbuterol	Maxair	Yes	—	4–6
Terbutaline	Brethine	—	Yes	3–7
	Brethaire	Yes	—	3–7
Ipratropium	Atrovent	Yes	Yes	5–7
Bitolterol	Tornalate	Yes	—	5–8
Salmeterol	Serevent	Yes	—	12

asthma, the muscle in these small airways spasms. The muscle spasm makes the airways smaller, and it becomes difficult for the patient to breathe. The patient's breathing appears labored, and air moving through the smaller-than-normal airways may make wheezing sounds that can sometimes be heard without a stethoscope. If the patient's condition changes significantly during the administration of an aerosolized medication, the PCT should notify the appropriate personnel.

The most common bronchodilators in use today are listed in Table 15–5. The usual effects of most bronchodilators delivered by aerosol are an increase in heart rate, arrhythmias, palpitation, skeletal muscle tremor, anxiety, nervousness, insomnia, and nausea. The patient should be observed closely for these side effects during treatment. The patient's pulse should be taken before, during, and after the treatment, and if the pulse rate changes by more than 20 beats per minute, the treatment should be stopped and the appropriate personnel notified.

Steroids

The PCT will encounter many patients with asthma who are receiving inhaled aerosolized corticosteroids, which are some of the primary drugs used to manage patients with asthma. **Steroids** are not classified as bronchodilators because they do not cause the smooth muscle in the airways to relax and dilate. Instead, they are classified as anti-inflammatory medications. The airways become inflamed during an asthma attack, in addition to the spasm of the airway smooth muscle, and steroids are effective at reducing this inflammation.

The most commonly inhaled steroids in use today are listed in Table 15–6. The primary immediate side effect of inhaled steroids is the development of an oral fungal infection called *candidiasis*. Having the patient use the proper inhalation technique and rinse the mouth after treatment can help reduce the incidence of candidiasis. There are few other immediate side effects from the use of inhaled steroids. There are many

TABLE 15–6   **Common Inhaled Steroids**

Generic Name	Trade Name(s)	MDI	SVN
Beclomethasone	Beclovent	Yes	Yes
	Vanceril	Yes	—
Dexamethasone	Decadron	Yes	—
Flunisolide	AeroBid	Yes	—
Triamcinolone	Azmacort	Yes	—

significant side effects of long-term steroid use, but most of these are not common when using inhaled steroids.

Pulse Oximetry

A ***pulse oximeter*** is a device that noninvasively measures oxygen-hemoglobin saturation (**SpO$_2$**) in the red blood cell (Fig. 15–16). SpO$_2$ is a measurement of the amount of hemoglobin (Hgb) that is combined with oxygen. Therefore, SpO$_2$ is a good indicator of how much oxygen is being carried in the blood.

Pulse oximeters measure SpO$_2$ using the principle of light absorption, which states that different molecules absorb light of different wavelengths. The pulse oximeter works by transmitting the specific wavelengths of light that are absorbed by both oxygenated and deoxygenated Hgb through the skin. The oximeter then measures the amount of light that is transmitted through the skin and determines how much light was absorbed; the more oxyhemoglobin present, the more light absorbed. Using this information, the oximeter calculates the percentage of Hgb combined with oxygen (Fig. 15–17).

Because the pulse oximeter transmits light through a tissue capillary bed, both oxygenated arterial blood and deoxygenated venous blood are present. Because the SpO$_2$ of arterial blood is of most interest, the oximeter must filter out the absorption of light by the deoxygenated venous blood. It is able to do this because the amount of light absorbed changes with each arterial pulsation. With each arterial pulsation, there is a rush of arterial blood into the capillary bed, which contains many Hgb molecules saturated with oxygen, and thus more light is absorbed. After one arterial pulsation and before the next pulsation, there is less Hgb present and less light is absorbed. By measuring the difference in absorption during and after each pulsation, the oximeter is able to do two things: determine the pulse rate and distinguish the absorption of light through arterial blood from the absorption of light through venous blood.

The pulse oximeter is a unique monitoring device because it does not require calibration. However, the probe that is used to transmit light through the tissue must be positioned correctly to obtain accurate data. If light passes from one side of the probe to the other without passing through the tissue, an inaccurate reading will result. The probe must not be exposed to light from the room (ambient light), which is a particular problem when a high-intensity external light is in use. Also, the probe cannot be

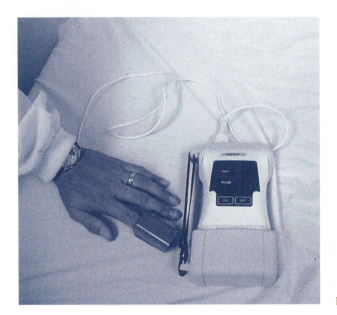

FIGURE 15–16   Pulse oximeter.

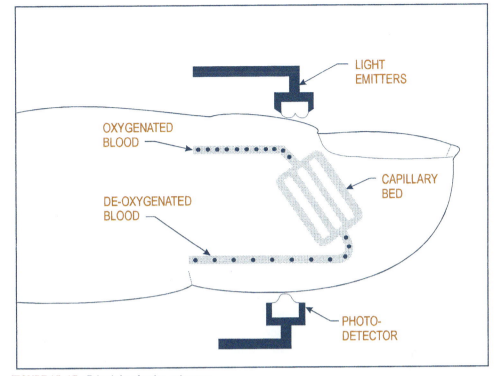

FIGURE 15–17   Principle of pulse oximetry.

placed in an area that has an opaque material, such as fingernail polish or artificial fingernails, between the two sides of the probe. Probes are available for fingers, toes, and ears. These probes may be reusable or may be for single-patient-use. Follow the manufacturer's instructions for the proper placement of the probe.

Various other factors affect the accuracy of pulse oximeter readings, including poor peripheral **perfusion**, motion artifact, abnormal varieties of Hgb, and venous pulsation.

Poor peripheral perfusion will make it difficult for the oximeter to distinguish the arterial pulse, resulting in an inaccurate reading. Motion artifact occurs when the probe is moved suddenly or often. This movement makes it difficult for the oximeter to distinguish the arterial pulsation, just as in the case of poor peripheral perfusion, and again makes the readings inaccurate. Abnormal varieties of Hgb occur in several clinical conditions, and these abnormal Hgbs absorb light differently, affecting the accuracy of pulse oximeter readings. Venous pulsations are present in some clinical conditions, and they also make it difficult for the oximeter to distinguish the arterial pulsation.

Pulse oximetry has limitations. Most pulse oximeters are accurate only to within 5%, and readings below 90% may not accurately reflect the actual SpO_2. Pulse oximeters do not give any indication of the patient's acid-base balance or cardiovascular status. Whenever the pulse rate and the pulse reading on the oximeter differ significantly, the accuracy of the oximeter should be questioned. If the patient appears to be experiencing difficulty, the cause should be assessed. Do not assume the patient is stable because of a satisfactory pulse oximeter reading when the patient appears to be in distress.

Bedside Spirometry

Spirometry is a term that means to measure lung volumes. Pulmonary function tests (PFTs) are performed to determine the type and extent of lung disease. PFTs measure lung volumes and flow rates, and these two variables are used to classify the type of pulmonary disease present. A restrictive lung disease is one in which lung volumes are reduced below normal. An obstructive lung disease is one in which the flow rates are below normal. Another way to think about this is to say that an individual with a restrictive lung disease cannot inhale or exhale as big a breath as normal, and an individual with obstructive disease cannot inhale or exhale a breath as fast as normal. Examples of restrictive lung disease include pneumonia and pulmonary edema, and examples of obstructive diseases include bronchitis, emphysema, asthma, and cystic fibrosis. It is also possible to have a combination of restrictive and obstructive lung diseases.

To learn how to measure basic PFTs at the bedside, the PCT must first understand how the lung is divided into the various volumes. There are four lung volumes (Fig. 15–18). The **tidal volume** (V_T) is the normal amount of gas that is exhaled after a normal breath. In other words, V_T is the size of a normal relaxed breath. The **inspiratory reserve volume** (**IRV**) is the maximum amount of gas that can be inhaled after a normal tidal inhalation. The **expiratory reserve volume** (**ERV**) is the maximum amount of gas that is exhaled after a normal tidal exhalation. So the ERV is the amount of gas that can be exhaled beyond that exhaled in the V_T. Finally, the **residual volume** (**RV**) is the amount of gas that remains in the lungs after a maximum exhalation. No matter how hard we try, all of the gas in the lungs cannot be exhaled, and the gas remaining after a maximum exhalation is the RV.

These four lung volumes can be combined in various ways to form lung capacities, as shown in Figure 15–18. The most important lung capacity in pulmonary function testing is the vital capacity (**VC**). VC is the maximum amount of gas that can be exhaled after a maximum inhalation. Another way of describing VC is that it is the sum of the IRV, V_T, and ERV (VC = IRV + V_T + ERV). VC is the basic spirometry test conducted at the bedside. The inspiratory capacity (**IC**) is the maximum amount of gas that can be inhaled after a normal tidal exhalation or the sum of the V_T and the IRV (IC = V_T + IRV). An important lung capacity that cannot be measured at the bedside is the **functional residual capacity** (**FRC**), which is the amount of gas left in the lungs after a normal tidal exhalation. The FRC is the sum of the RV and the ERV (FRC = RV + ERV). Finally, there is the total lung capacity (**TLC**), which is the amount of gas in the lungs after a maximum inhalation or the sum of all four lung volumes (TLC = RV + ERV + IRV + V_T). Not all lung volumes can be measured at the bedside; because the RV can never be exhaled, it can be measured only using sophisticated equipment available in pulmonary laboratories. Because FRC and TLC include RV, they cannot be measured at the bedside. Also, because the size of the ERV and the IRV are not of much value in the diagnosis of pulmonary disease, the most common procedure at the bedside is to

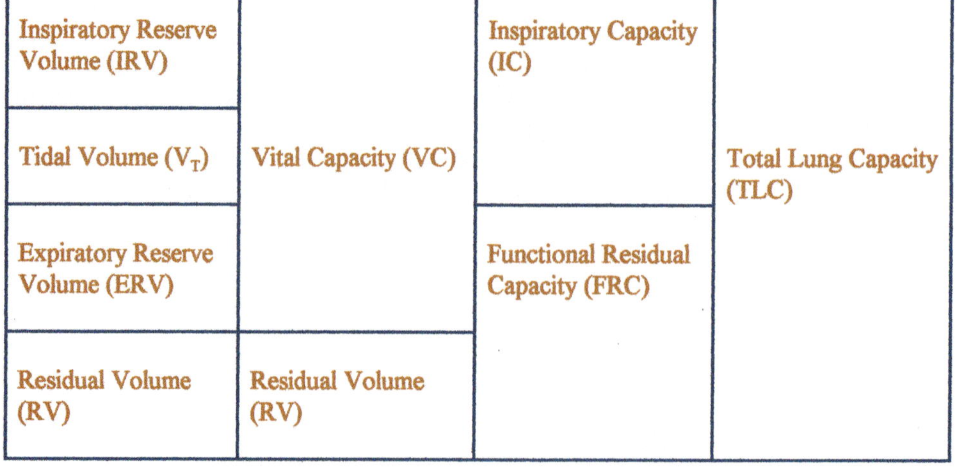

Inspiratory Reserve Volume (IRV)		Inspiratory Capacity (IC)	
Tidal Volume (V_T)	Vital Capacity (VC)		Total Lung Capacity (TLC)
Expiratory Reserve Volume (ERV)		Functional Residual Capacity (FRC)	
Residual Volume (RV)	Residual Volume (RV)		

FIGURE 15–18   Lung volumes and capacities.

measure VC and calculate the remaining values from the VC measurement. The normal lung volumes and capacities for a 165-lb, 6-ft tall, 25-year-old man are shown in Table 15–7.

VC is measured using a forced maneuver, which means that patients are instructed to exhale their VC as fast as possible. Next, patients are instructed to take in as deep a breath as possible and then to exhale as fast and as hard as they can. The reasons for doing a forced maneuver are to get an accurate measure of the maximum flow rate the patient can generate through the airways and to account for the airflow resistance caused by the constricted airways. In this one forced vital capacity (**FVC**) maneuver, we can measure both the VC and the various flow rates.

The FVC maneuver is an effort-dependent maneuver, which means that, if the patient is not giving his or her best effort, the results will not be accurate. It is extremely important for the PCT to be aware of this fact. The PCT must have the patient sit upright and must coach the patient to give the best effort possible or decisions about the diagnosis and treatment of the patient may be based on inaccurate information. To be certain that patients are giving their best effort, there should be a minimum of three FVC maneuvers, and the values for the largest and second largest FVC should not vary by more than 100 mL. Most modern bedside spirometers will determine whether the FVC maneuvers are within the acceptable range. Once three acceptable maneuvers have been performed, the results of the best maneuver are reported. Again, most modern bedside spirometers automatically provide these results. The criteria for the minimum number of tests to be undertaken and the acceptability of results may vary by institution.

Once the FVC maneuver is completed, the spirometer calculates various values based on and including the FVC. The forced expiratory volume in 1 second (FEV_1) is determined by measuring the amount of gas exhaled during the maneuver in the first second. The FEV_1% is the percentage of the FVC exhaled in the first second. The peak expiratory flow rate (**PEFR**) is the maximum flow rate generated during the maneuver, usually at the beginning of the test. There may be other calculated values, depending on the particular machine in use; these are the most common, however. The PEFR is a good measure of the effort expended by the patient and, if the patient is giving his or her best effort, the PEFR should be relatively stable between tests.

The result of PFTs are usually reported in three columns: the actual value recorded, the predicted value for that patient, and the percentage of predicted value (actual/predicted $\times$ 100). The actual values are obtained by the performance of the FVC maneuver. The predicted values are obtained by the spirometer based on information the PCT enters before the test. The patient's age, gender, and height are used to predict the individual's values. Predicted normal values may also vary based on race, ethnic background, socioeconomic factors, environmental exposures, occupation, or place of residence. Most spirometers have a correction factor for normal values of individuals of African-American descent. The PCT must be careful to enter the correct informa-

TABLE 15–7 **Normal Values of Lung Volumes and Capacities**

Volume or Capacity	Normal Value (mL)
Total lung capacity (TLC)	6000
Vital capacity (VC)	4800
Inspiratory capacity (IC)	3600
Inspiratory reserve volume (IRV)	3100
Functional residual capacity (FRC)	2400
Residual volume (RV)	1200
Expiratory reserve volume (ERV)	1200
Tidal volume (V_T)	500

tion for the patient before the test, or the interpretation of the results will be inaccurate.

The interpretation of PFTs can be quite complex and is not routinely performed by PCTs. The important thing to remember is that the interpretation is used to determine the type of treatment the patient receives, making accuracy of the values extremely important. Therefore, the PCT must be careful and accurate in performing bedside spirometry.

BIBLIOGRAPHY

Branson, RD, et al: Respiratory Care Equipment. JB Lippincott, Philadelphia, 1995.
Burton, GG, et al: Respiratory Care: A Guide to Clinical Practice, ed. 3. JB Lippincott, Philadelphia, 1991.
Karmarek, RM, Mack, CW, and Dimas, S: The Essentials of Respiratory Care. Mosby Year Book, CV Mosby, St. Louis, 1990.
Scanlon, CL, et al: Egan's Fundamentals of Respiratory Care, ed. 6. CV Mosby, St. Louis, 1995.

STUDY QUESTIONS

1. List the three indications for oxygen delivery.

   a. _____

   b. _____

   c. _____

2. Define the term *hypoxemia*.

   _____

3. List two hazards of oxygen delivery.

   a. _____

   b. _____

4. Describe the process of "cracking" a medical gas cylinder and explain why it is done.

   _____

   _____

5. Explain why it is important to know the duration of a medical gas cylinder.

   _____

6. List the estimated FiO_2 delivered by a nasal cannula for each liter per minute of flow between 1 and 6.

   a. 1 minute _____

   b. 2 minutes _____

   c. 3 minutes _____

   d. 4 minutes _____

   e. 5 minutes _____

   f. 6 minutes _____

7. Give the estimated FiO_2 delivered by a simple, a partial rebreather, and a nonrebreather oxygen mask. Also list the proper FiO_2 flow rate to be applied to these flow rate devices.

	Estimated FiO_2	*Flow Rate*
a. Simple	_____	_____
b. Partial rebreather	_____	_____
c. Nonrebreather	_____	_____

8. Differentiate between variable performance and fixed performance oxygen delivery systems.

   _____

   _____

9. Describe when it may be necessary to humidify oxygen.

_____

10. Describe the type of patient that would require an SVN instead of an MDI for aerosol medication delivery.

_____

11. Describe the proper technique for aerosol medication delivery by both the SVN and the MDI.

a. SVN _____

_____

b. MDI _____

_____

12. What are the two classifications of medications delivered by aerosol?

a. _____

b. _____

13. Describe the importance of proper pulse oximetry probe placement.

_____

_____

14. List four factors that may cause inaccurate readings by a pulse oximeter.

a. _____

b. _____

c. _____

d. _____

15. Define and give the normal values for the four lung volumes and the four lung capacities.

Volume/Capacity	_Normal Value_
a. _____	_____
b. _____	_____
c. _____	_____
d. _____	_____
e. _____	_____
f. _____	_____
g. _____	_____
h. _____	_____

16. Describe the performance of the forced vital capacity (FVC) maneuver.

_____

_____

_____

17. Discuss the importance of securing maximal patient effort during bedside spirometry.

_____

_____

EVALUATION OF CYLINDER SAFETY AND TRANSPORT

RATING SYSTEM   2 = Satisfactory   1 = Needs improvement   0 = Incorrect/did not perform

_____   **1.** Selects appropriate cylinder

_____   **2.** Properly secures cylinder in cart or stand

_____   **3.** Removes valve stem cover and "cracks" cylinder

_____   **4.** Selects appropriate regulator

_____   **5.** Attaches and tightens regulator to cylinder

_____   **6.** Slowly opens cylinder valve

_____   **7.** Checks for leaks

_____   **8.** Reads cylinder pressure

_____   **9.** Connects appropriate oxygen supplies to regulator (e.g., nasal cannula, oxygen mask)

_____   **10.** Initiates proper gas flow

_____   **11.** Estimates duration of flow

_____   **12.** Transports cylinder properly to destination

_____   **13.** Schedules cylinder to be checked or changed at appropriate time

_____   **14.** Follows oxygen safety precautions

Total points _____

Maximum points = 28

COMMENTS

EVALUATION OF OXYGEN ADMINISTRATION

RATING SYSTEM   2 = Satisfactory   1 = Needs improvement   0 = Incorrect/did not perform

_____ **1.** Verifies physician's order

_____ **2.** Washes hands

_____ **3.** Selects, gathers, and assembles appropriate equipment

_____ **4.** Identifies patient and introduces self

_____ **5.** Explains procedure to patient and confirms patient understanding

_____ **6.** Prepares and connects humidifier (if applicable)

_____ **7.** Initiates gas flow at proper rate

_____ **8.** Tests equipment for proper function

_____ **9.** Applies device to patient

_____ **10.** Modifies procedure to accommodate patient response

_____ **11.** Follows oxygen safety precautions

_____ **12.** Records pertinent data in appropriate places

Total points _____

Maximum points = 24

COMMENTS

EVALUATION OF AEROSOL DRUG ADMINISTRATION (SMALL-VOLUME NEBULIZER)

RATING SYSTEM   2 = Satisfactory   1 = Needs improvement   0 = Incorrect/did not perform

_____ **1.** Verifies physician's order

_____ **2.** Washes hands

_____ **3.** Selects, gathers, and assembles appropriate equipment

_____ **4.** Identifies patient and introduces self

_____ **5.** Explains procedure to patient and confirms patient understanding

_____ **6.** Checks patient's pulse rate

_____ **7.** Connects aerosol generator to appropriate gas source

_____ **8.** Adds prescribed drug and diluent to nebulizer

_____ **9.** Initiates gas flow at proper rate

_____ **10.** Tests equipment for proper function

_____ **11.** Properly positions patient

_____ **12.** Applies nebulizer to patient and encourages proper breathing pattern

_____ **13.** Checks patient's pulse rate during treatment

_____ **14.** Terminates therapy when complete or when patient demonstrates an adverse response

_____ **15.** Checks patient's pulse rate after treatment

_____ **16.** Records pertinent data in appropriate places

Total points _____

Maximum points = 32

COMMENTS

EVALUATION OF AEROSOL DRUG ADMINISTRATION (METERED-DOSE INHALER)

RATING SYSTEM   2 = Satisfactory   1 = Needs improvement   0 = Incorrect/did not perform

_____ **1.** Verifies physician's order

_____ **2.** Washes hands

_____ **3.** Selects, gathers, and assembles appropriate equipment

_____ **4.** Identifies patient and introduces self

_____ **5.** Explains procedure to patient and confirms patient understanding

_____ **6.** Checks patient's pulse rate

_____ **7.** Warms and shakes MDI

_____ **8.** Properly positions patient

_____ **9.** Applies MDI to patient and encourages proper breathing pattern

_____ **10.** Checks patient's pulse rate between deep inhalation maneuvers

_____ **11.** Terminates therapy when complete or when patient demonstrates an adverse response

_____ **12.** Checks patient's pulse rate after treatment

_____ **13.** Records pertinent data in appropriate places

Total points _____

Maximum points = 26

COMMENTS

EVALUATION OF PULSE OXIMETRY TECHNIQUE

RATING SYSTEM   2 = Satisfactory   1 = Needs improvement   0 = Incorrect/did not perform

_____ **1.** Verifies physician's order

_____ **2.** Washes hands

_____ **3.** Selects, gathers, and assembles appropriate equipment

_____ **4.** Identifies patient and introduces self

_____ **5.** Explains procedure to patient and confirms patient understanding

_____ **6.** Tests equipment for proper function

_____ **7.** Applies probe to appropriate site

_____ **8.** Ensures proper positioning of probe

_____ **9.** Modifies procedure to accommodate patient response

_____ **10.** Records pertinent data in appropriate places

Total points _____

Maximum points = 20

COMMENTS

EVALUATION OF BEDSIDE SPIROMETRY TECHNIQUE

RATING SYSTEM   2 = Satisfactory   1 = Needs improvement   0 = Incorrect/did not perform

_____ **1.** Verifies physician's order

_____ **2.** Washes hands

_____ **3.** Selects, gathers, and assembles appropriate equipment

_____ **4.** Identifies patient and introduces self

_____ **5.** Explains procedure to patient and confirms patient understanding

_____ **6.** Properly positions patient

_____ **7.** Provides spirometer mouthpiece to patient

_____ **8.** Has patient take full inspiration

_____ **9.** Elicits a forced expiration to residual volume

_____ **10.** Reassures patient

_____ **11.** Repeats procedure for best results and ensures reproducibility

_____ **12.** Obtains actual, predicted, and percentage of predicted values

_____ **13.** Monitors patient until stabilized

_____ **14.** Records pertinent data in appropriate places

Total points _____

Maximum points = 28

COMMENTS

UNIT 16

BASIC RADIOGRAPHY

KEY TERMS

■ *Bucky tray*	Radiographic examination table cassette holder
■ *Cassette*	Portable, lightproof container that holds radiographic film
■ *Centering light*	Directs an x-ray beam to the center of a radiographic cassette
■ *Collimator*	Lead shutters that shape and restrict x-ray beams
■ *Costophrenic angles*	Angles relating to the ribs and diaphragm
■ *Directional controls*	Controls that allow movement of an x-ray tube
■ *Film badge*	Material that records the amount of exposure to x-rays

- ***Film bin*** — Lightproof container for storage of unexposed radiographic film
- ***Gonadal shielding*** — Covering that prevents exposure of the gonads to x-rays
- ***Lateral*** — Pertaining to a side of a structure
- ***Posteroanterior*** — From back to front
- ***Radiograph*** — X-ray image
- ***Radiographic contrast*** — Visible difference in radiographic densities on film
- ***Radiographic density*** — Overall blackness of a radiographic image (the darkness of a film)
- ***Radiographic film*** — Material on which an x-ray image is produced

Medical imaging is a rapidly expanding specialty in which images (pictures) of the human body are obtained in various ways for diagnostic purposes. The methods for imaging range from computerized axial tomography (CAT) and sonograms to the simplest chest **radiograph**. As a limited practitioner, a PCT obtains some of the basic x-ray images (radiographs) while using a standard radiographic unit.

Basic Radiographic Unit

All basic radiographic units (x-ray machines) work in essentially the same way and have three common components: the x-ray tube and controls, the examination table and controls, and the operator console.

X-RAY TUBE AND CONTROLS

The x-ray tube is a glass vacuum tube containing high-voltage electric components. For protection against the potential hazards of unlimited x-ray exposure, the x-ray tube is supported and covered by a cylindrical housing that is lined with lead (Fig. 16–1). Only a small portion of the x-ray beam is permitted to pass from the interior of the x-ray tube and ultimately to the patient. Once the x-rays have exited the tube housing, the x-ray beam can be further shaped and restricted by lead shutters called **collimators.** The collimator is generally equipped with a collimator light that shows the position, size, and shape of the x-ray beam before making an exposure (Fig. 16–2). A **centering light** allows the x-ray beam to be directed to the center of the film cassette when it is placed in the **bucky tray** of the examination table (Fig. 16–3). This ensures that the x-ray image will be projected to that point and appear in the center of the film.

Other controls located at the x-ray tube allow the tube to be moved in certain directions. These **directional controls** allow the x-ray tube (and the x-ray beam) to be directed to specific anatomic points and at specific angulations (angles) in accordance with standard procedures for radiography. The controls are usually in the form of push-button electronic locks that are unlocked when depressed and locked in position when released. Most radiographic units have the following controls:

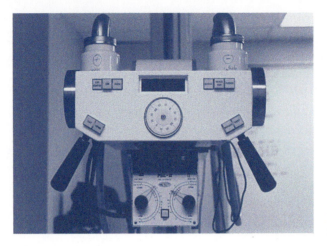

FIGURE 16–1   X-ray tube with covering and controls.

Longitudinal lock: allows movement of the tube along the length of the table
Transverse lock: allows movement of the tube across the table from side to side
Detente lock: locks the tube transversely to the exact center of the bucky tray
Vertical lock: allows movement of the tube straight up and down
Swivel lock: allows the tube to be swung left or right around the vertical axis
Angulation lock: allows the tube to be angled up and down the length of
   the table

EXAMINATION TABLE AND CONTROLS

The examination table is normally located in the center of the examination room. It provides a work surface that allows the patient to assume a comfortable position, whether lying on top of the table or seated next to it. Radiographs of the upper and lower extremities can be taken simply by placing the film cassette on the table and placing the specified anatomy directly on top of the cassette, as shown in Figure 16–4.

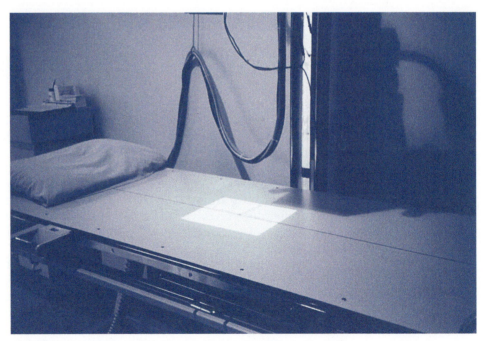

FIGURE 16–2   Collimator light focused on examination table.

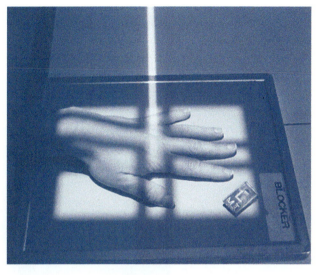

FIGURE 16–3 Collimator centering light.

Larger regions of the body measuring more than 10 cm in thickness require the use of a **grid** to enhance the visibility of the radiograph. For larger body regions, such as the abdomen or the vertebral column, the examination table has a cassette holder, sometimes called a bucky tray, that slides out from under the table's surface to accept a film cassette (Fig. 16–5). The cassette is locked in the center of the tray. The cassette can then be centered on the examination table by pushing the bucky tray all the way underneath. Although the cassette is hidden from view, the x-ray tube can then be directed to the center of the film cassette by using the detente lock (transversely) and the centering light (longitudinally).

In addition to the bucky tray located beneath the surface of the examination table, most radiography examination rooms also have a wall-mounted vertical cassette holder or upright bucky for use when performing chest x-rays. This cassette holder also contains a tray or slot to hold a cassette in place and a vertical lock to adjust the film height to the level of the patient's chest. The x-ray tube can sometimes be centered by using a detente lock. It can also be centered by sight by using the collimator light and the markings outlining the film size on the surface of the vertical cassette holder (Fig. 16–6).

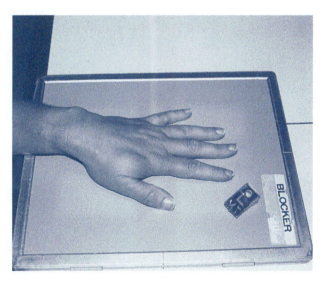

FIGURE 16–4 Positioning of an extremity.

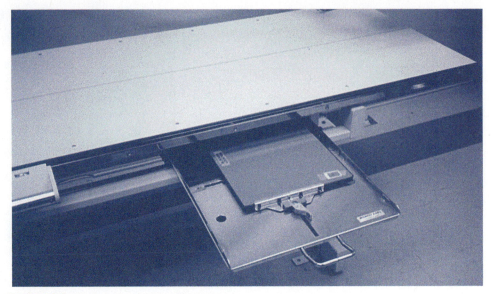

FIGURE 16–5   Bucky tray containing film cassette.

OPERATOR CONSOLE

The operator console is the panel at which the x-ray exposures are made. It also allows the radiographer to select the technical factors (exposure settings) that will determine the appearance of the radiograph. Most standard radiographic units have the following controls (Fig. 16–7):

Main or on/off switch	Supplies electric current to the radiographic unit and turns the unit on and off
Exposure switch	Usually a two-stage switch that allows the x-ray tube to prepare for an exposure; it produces the x-rays
mA selector	Allows the selection of electric current (milliamperage) to the x-ray tube and controls the density (overall blackness) of the radiograph
Exposure time	Controls the length of time that x-rays are produced by the tube and the density of the radiograph

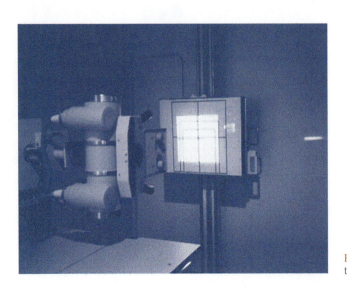

FIGURE 16–6   Wall-mounted vertical cassette holder.

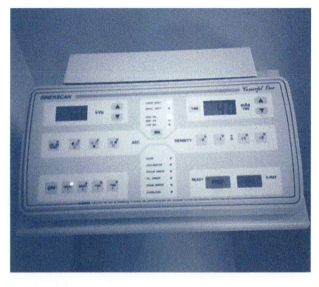

FIGURE 16–7   Radiographic control unit.

kVp or kV selector	Controls the penetrability of the x-ray beam in the patient's body and the level of contrast ("black and white" or "grayish" appearance) of the radiograph
Focal spot size selector	Controls the size of the area where x-rays are produced in the x-ray tube and the sharpness and clarity of fine details in the radiograph
Photocell selector	Used with automatic exposure control (**AEC**) and allows the exposure to be measured from a specific body region
Density selector	Used with AEC to control the density of the radiograph

Accessory Equipment

In addition to the radiographic unit itself, there are other accessories essential for the production of a radiograph.

RADIOGRAPHIC FILM

The radiograph is produced on a sheet of ***radiographic film***, which is manufactured in various standard sizes to accommodate different body regions. Because radiographic film is sensitive to both visible light and x-rays, it must always be protected from exposure until ready to be used. This is accomplished in two ways. First, boxes of unexposed film are usually stored in a lightproof ***film bin*** located in the darkroom, which is the area in which exposed films are chemically processed to form the familiar "black and white" appearance of a radiograph. Second, individual sheets of unexposed radiographic film are placed inside a lightproof container called a ***cassette***.

RADIOGRAPHIC FILM CASSETTES

Like radiographic film, radiographic film cassettes are manufactured in various standard sizes and are designed to accept a single sheet of radiographic film of matching size. The cassette is usually opened in a booklike fashion by releasing a pair of locking levers found on the back of the cassette. Inside the cassette are two **intensifying**

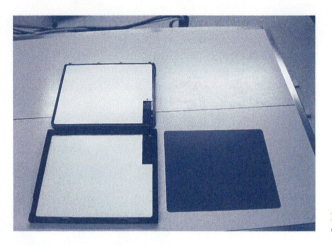

FIGURE 16–8   Radiographic film cassette and film.

screens that are designed to press on both sides of the radiographic film when a film is inserted and the cassette closed (Fig. 16–8).

When an unexposed film is placed in the cassette under darkroom conditions (in the absence of white light), the film can then be carried out into the examination room to be used for performing a radiograph. When the x-ray exposure is made, x-rays pass through the cassette and cause the intensifying screens to glow. The dim light produced by the intensifying screens exposes the film and forms the radiograph.

It is important to remember that:

1 The cassette has a front (or tube) side and a back side. The tube side must always face the x-ray tube during exposure.

2 The cassette has a small rectangular lead (Pb) blocker in one corner of the cassette that is protected from x-rays and remains unexposed. This area is used to provide the patient's name, number, date, and other useful information that is printed on the film using an identification flasher and flashcard. Anatomy of interest should never be placed over the lead blocker of the cassette.

3 Exposure to room light will destroy the radiograph. Cassettes containing film must never be opened in normal room light.

Technical Factors

The goal of selecting **technical factors** for a particular body region is to produce a visible image that contains sufficient density, contrast, and recorded detail to provide the unaided eye with a maximum of diagnostic information. This means that the region of the body under examination should be penetrated with an x-ray beam of sufficient quantity and energy to produce a clearly recognizable radiographic image that can be easily interpreted by a physician. In this unit we confine our discussion to chest radiography, although the basic principles of technical factor selection apply to other regions of the body as well.

RADIOGRAPHIC DENSITY AND MILLIAMPERE-SECONDS

The underlying principle of radiography is that x-radiation turns x-ray film black. The quality of blackness in the radiograph is termed *radiographic density*. When the x-ray beam passes through the chest, the air-filled lung fields absorb very little radiation, whereas the dense skeletal features absorb considerably more. As a result, the typical chest radiograph appears as black or dark gray lung fields with the white or light gray skeletal features superimposed. The heart, breasts, and other soft tissue structures appear to be a midrange or medium gray in appearance. Radiographic density is influenced by many factors, but it is controlled by **milliampere-seconds (mA-s).**

Milliampere-seconds represents the quantity of x-radiation produced by the exposure and can be easily calculated by multiplying milliamperage (mA) by the time of exposure (mA $\times$ second[s] = mA-s). For example, to calculate the quantity of radiation produced by technical factors set at 300 mA and 0.02 second, multiply milliamperage by exposure time (300 mA $\times$ 0.02 second = 6 mA-s).

Being able to calculate the milliampere-seconds used during an exposure is important, because occasionally it is necessary to compensate for a radiograph that exhibits excessive density (too dark) or insufficient density (too light). The clinical rule of thumb for correcting problems with radiographic density is as follows:

1 If a radiographic image appears too light, double the milliampere-seconds.
2 If a radiographic image appears too dark, reduce the milliampere-seconds by one half.

The changes to milliampere-seconds suggested by the clinical rule of thumb may be accomplished by changing either milliamperage or exposure time (in seconds), or both. In most cases, however, the necessary changes in milliampere-seconds are more easily accomplished by changing the exposure time only. Consider the following examples:

EXAMPLE 1: You have selected 300 mA at 0.02 second for a ***posteroanterior (PA)*** projection of the chest. When the film is processed, however, the radiograph appears too dark. To make the film visibly lighter, it is necessary to decrease the milliampere-seconds by reducing the exposure time to 0.01 second: 300 mA $\times$ 0.01 second = 3 mA-s.

EXAMPLE 2: You have selected 300 mA at 0.02 second for a PA projection of the chest. When the film is processed, however, the radiograph appears too light. To make the film visibly darker, it is necessary to increase the milliampere-seconds by doubling the exposure time to 0.04 second: 300 mA $\times$ 0.04 second = 12 mA-s.

KILOVOLTAGE

Kilovoltage (kVp, kV, or keV) is the technical factor that controls the penetrability of the x-ray beam as it passes through the patient's body. Generally speaking, higher levels of kilovoltage are used to penetrate thicker body regions, and lower levels of kilovoltage are used for thinner body regions. Kilovoltage also controls another aspect of image quality called ***radiographic contrast***. As kilovoltage is increased, the radiographic image becomes lower in contrast, that is to say, more featureless and grayer in appearance. As kilovoltage is decreased, the radiographic image becomes higher in contrast, or more black and white in appearance.

A complicating factor of kilovoltage selection is that whenever kilovoltage is increased or decreased, radiographic density also increases or decreases. Kilovoltage should be selected and fixed at a level sufficient to penetrate the thorax and provide sufficient contrast to easily distinguish the anatomic features of the heart and lungs.

Although kilovoltage influences radiographic density, it should remain fixed, depending on the body region being examined. Kilovoltage should not be used as a method of controlling radiographic density.

As a general rule, chest radiographs obtained without the use of a grid (using a cassette only) should be performed at a lower kilovoltage level than are radiographs obtained with a grid.

AUTOMATIC EXPOSURE CONTROL

Another method of setting the technical factors for chest radiography is accomplished through the use of AEC. In this case, the milliampere-seconds are regulated by a set of photocells located between the surface of the vertical cassette holder and the x-ray cassette/film. Although specific function depends on the manufacturer's specification for the radiographic unit, the radiographer usually needs to set milliamperage, kilovoltage, **photocell array**, and photocell density only. The radiographic unit automatically senses the correct amount of radiation for the optimum chest radiograph by regulating the exposure time.

PHOTOCELL ARRAY

The photocells of a standard radiographic unit are located between the surface of the vertical cassette holder (upright bucky) and the tray or slot that holds the x-ray film cassette. The three photocells are arranged in an inverted triangular pattern on a 14- by 17-inch field. The outline of the 14- by 17-inch field and the photocell pattern are often printed directly on the surface of the vertical cassette holder as a guide. Once the x-ray tube, cassette, and patient are properly positioned, the photocells can be independently activated at the operator console, depending on the position of the patient. When the exposure is made, the photocells will terminate the exposure after sufficient radiation has penetrated the patient to provide optimum radiographic density.

It is important to note that, when in the AEC mode, the only correction for errors in radiographic density caused by incorrect photocell selection is to use the correct photocell(s) on the repeat radiograph. Changing the milliampere-seconds at the console has no effect on the image when the photocells are activated.

PHOTOCELL DENSITY

Some adjustments to density can be made in the AEC mode by adjusting the relative density controls at the operator console. International symbols predominate the identification of these buttons (e.g., thin, medium, and heavy human figures or rectangles or fractions such as 1/2, 1, and 1 1/2). However, the radiographic unit should be calibrated to deliver optimum radiographic density when the selector is set at the middle, or normal, density setting. Chest radiographs should routinely be performed at the normal density setting.

X-ray Exposure

The x-ray exposure is made by first depressing the "rotor" or "prepare" button and waiting for the ready light to appear on the operator console. The exposure is then made by simultaneously depressing the "expose" button and holding it down until the "x-ray" light or audible signal terminates (usually a brief fraction of a second).

Radiographic Processing and Darkroom Procedures

Once the patient has been positioned and the x-ray exposure has been made, the film inside the cassette must be removed from the cassette and processed. That is to say, the film must be immersed in a sequence of chemical solutions for the radiograph to become visible. Because the exposed x-ray film is still very sensitive to light, this chemical process must take place in nearly total darkness, referred to as safelight conditions. Although many hospitals have advanced automated processing units that are self-contained and do not require a separate darkroom, most small healthcare facilities that provide radiology service are equipped with a small, light-tight working area designed for processing x-ray films.

DARKROOM

The darkroom is a lightproof working area usually located near the examination room and designed for unloading film from cassettes, placing the film inside the automatic film processor, and loading the empty cassette with fresh, unexposed film. As shown in Figure 16–9, the typical darkroom does not require excessive floor space but usually has the following basic features:

Water supply line	Automatic film processors are located partially inside the darkroom and require a constant water supply for the washing of processed films.
Lightproof construction	X-ray film is highly sensitive to light and will darken or "fog" if exposed to barely detectable levels of normal room light; the edges of the doorway, ceiling, and wall are especially susceptible to light leaks and must be sealed against light.
Working surface	A level countertop that provides an area to open cassettes and place films into the automatic film processor is needed.
Film bin	A lightproof cabinet for the storage of unexposed film in various sizes is used.
Safelight	Depending on the type of x-ray film being used, a dim light in the red spectrum can be used to illuminate the working surface when handling film; a 15-watt fluorescent bulb using a Kodak GBX filter is usually recommended.
Pass box	This is a double-door cabinet between the fully lighted working area and the darkroom. A pass box is usually installed in the wall at chest level and is used for passing cassettes to the darkroom without exposing the darkroom to light. When one side of the pass box is

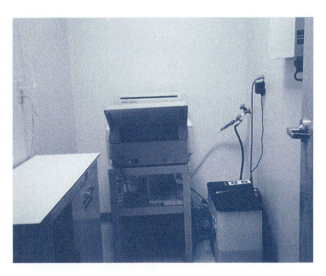

FIGURE 16–9 Typical darkroom.

opened, it automatically locks the door on the other side and prevents light from accidentally leaking into the darkroom.

AUTOMATIC FILM PROCESSOR

The automatic film processor is a device that performs the chemical processing of the exposed radiographic film (Fig. 16–10A and B). When a radiograph is produced, the film inside the cassette is exposed to a specific pattern of light from the intensifying screens that represents the body region being x-rayed. This pattern of light produces invisible chemical changes in the sensitive layer of the x-ray film. For a radiograph to be visualized as a black-and-white image, the areas of the film that have been exposed to light turn black, whereas those areas that have not been exposed turn white, or clear. This process is accomplished by placing the exposed film on a feed tray in the darkroom and transporting the film on a system of rollers through a series of chemical solutions contained inside the automatic film processor. Specifically, the process is as follows:

Developing	A brown-yellow alkaline solution containing reducing agents turns exposed x-ray film emulsion black, and unexposed film remains unaffected by the developer solution.
Fixing	A clear acidic solution containing a clearing agent dissolves unexposed x-ray film emulsion, giving it a white appearance on the view box, and film blackened by the developer solution remains unaffected.

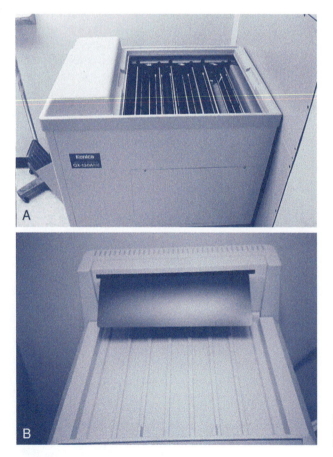

FIGURE 16–10 Automatic film processor. *A,* Inside view. *B,* Developed film leaving processor.

Washing	Circulating water removes the fixer solution from the surface of the film.
Drying	Circulating hot air from a blower removes water from the surface of the film.

FILM PROCESSING PROCEDURES

Film processing is a procedure that must be accomplished in a controlled environment. The three most important aspects of this environment are:

1 Maintaining *safelight conditions* and the prevention of light leaks
2 Maintaining consistent *developer solution temperature*
3 Maintaining consistent *developer solution*

Maintaining safelight conditions means that radiographic film is never removed from the film bin or the film cassette unless normal room lighting has been turned off and the door to the darkroom has been closed. Even the smallest light leak can result in *film fog*, a serious problem that appears on the radiograph as an increase in radiographic density (either black or gray in appearance) over the entire surface (or sometimes only a portion) of the film, making details of the radiographic image very difficult to see. Film fog can even appear under a properly filtered safelight if the film is left exposed on the working surface more than 1 to 2 minutes, or if the film is held more than 3 feet from the safelight fixture. This is easily avoided by promptly processing films as soon as they are removed from the cassette and by closing the film bin immediately after removing a film from it.

Because the temperature of developer solution has a significant effect on the radiographic density and contrast of the processed image, the temperature should be strictly maintained by an internal thermostat to within ± 1/2°F. Unless otherwise specified by the manufacturer, the temperature of the processing solutions should be maintained at 92°F.

When radiographic films are sent through the processing unit, a small amount of the developer and fixer solution is absorbed by the film. This means that over time these solutions become weaker and weaker. Automatic film processors are equipped with two small replenisher pumps that pump a few ounces of fresh developer and fixer solution from a reservoir tank into the processing tanks each time a film is processed. Unless otherwise specified by the manufacturer, the developer should be replenished at the rate of 60 mL per 14 inches of film, and the fixer should be replenished at the rate of 90 mL per 14 inches of film.

STEPS FOR RADIOGRAPHIC FILM PROCESSING

1 After exposing a film cassette, be certain that the correct identification flashcard is used to apply (or "flash") the patient's name and date of examination directly on the film. Refer to the manufacturer's instructions, because this may be done inside the examination room only if a daylight identification system is being used.
2 Before opening the door to the darkroom, be certain that other personnel are not working inside with unprocessed films that might be accidentally exposed. Enter the darkroom and place the cassette tube side down on the working surface. Close the door.
3 Turn off the room lights and turn on only the red filtered safelight. Release the dual locks on the rear of the cassette and remove the single sheet of radiographic film without bending or creasing it. If a darkroom identification system is in use, the film must be "flashed" with the identification card at this time.

4 Turn toward the feed tray of the processing unit and lay the film flat on the tray without advancing it. Slide the film laterally to one side of the tray to be certain that the film is aligned and in contact with the vertical edge of the tray.

5 Slide the film forward until the rollers begin to take up the film and the film can be felt moving into the processor. Avoid attempting to pull the film back out once this process has begun.

6 Open the film bin and remove a single sheet of film, taking care not to bend or crease it, and close the film bin.

7 Place the fresh sheet of unexposed film into the bottom of the cassette, termed "loading" the cassette. Be certain that the film lies flat and does not overlap the edge of the cassette. Close the cassette and secure the dual locks on the rear of the cassette. It is necessary to wait until the radiographic film has cleared the feed tray and has traveled into the processor before the door can be safely opened and the room lights turned on. Most automatic film processors are equipped with a small bell or buzzer to indicate when it is safe to return to normal room lighting.

8 Return the loaded and unexposed film cassette to the proper storage area until it is to be used again.

TROUBLESHOOTING

Occasionally, some difficulties with a processing system may arise. Most problems can be solved by establishing a regular system of cleaning and preventive maintenance. Depending on the number of films being processed, this type of service should be per-

TABLE 16–1   **Processing System Troubleshooting**

Problem	Probable Cause	Solution(s)
Dark films	Developer temperature too high	Check technical factors. Check thermostat. (Lower temperature to 92°F.)
Light films	Developer temperature too low	Check technical factors. Check thermostat. (Raise temperature to 92°F.) Wait for processor to warm up before processing films.
	Developer replenishment too low	Check replenishment pump. (Raise replenishment pump setting to 60–90 mL per 14 inches of film.) Check level of developer solution in reservoir tank and replace with fresh developer, if necessary.
Partially exposed films	Unlocked or damaged cassette	Identify cassette and check that locks are secure. (Replace cassette if damaged.)
	Films left inside room during performance of exposures	Remove extra cassettes from exposure examination room when exposures are being made.
	Light leak in darkroom	Seal all visible light leaks, be certain that film has cleared feed tray before opening door or turning on room lights, and keep film bin closed in normal room light.
Dirty films	Dirty rollers in processor	Remove racks from processor; wash, scrub, and rinse the rollers in the developer and fixer, and wash racks to remove surface "scum."
Black crescent pattern	Rough handling of film	Handle film with care.
Small white flecks	Dirty intensifying screens in cassette	Clean intensifying screens with cotton gauze and screen cleaning solution. (Allow to dry before reloading with fresh film.)

formed every 2 to 4 weeks. Table 16–1 lists the most common problems, causes, and solutions encountered with processing systems.

Radiation Protection

Studies of human populations exposed to high doses of radiation, including x-rays, have shown that exposure to radiation may be harmful to the body. Effects from low doses of x-radiation are less clear because information regarding low levels of radiation is limited. Therefore, the use of low doses of ionizing radiation for medical diagnosis can carry both risks and benefits. Each time a radiographic examination is ordered, the physician must consider the diagnostic value versus the potential biologic effects on the body. Once the examination is ordered, it is the radiographer's responsibility to perform the examination following the guidelines of the current radiation protection philosophy.

The goal of the radiographer is to control the level of radiation exposure so that it is kept to a level as low as reasonably achievable (**ALARA**). ALARA is an acronym based on the concept that exposure to radiation may be harmful and exposures should be kept as low as possible. Methods for achieving the ALARA concept for both the patient and the PCT are discussed in the following sections.

PATIENT PROTECTION

Effective Communication

As in all aspects of patient care, effective communication is a vital component to the successful completion of a radiographic examination. Procedures must be thoroughly explained if a patient is expected to cooperate. Generally, patients arriving for examinations are anxious and concerned about the unknown. It is the limited radiographer's responsibility to answer all appropriate questions concerning the examination to help ease the patient's anxiety. If a patient refuses an examination, it is the radiographer's obligation to seek out a supervisor or physician and discuss the situation and consequences.

Specific breathing instructions and body positions are critical to most radiographic examinations. Patients who are not fluent in English may have difficulty understanding instructions, which may result in a repeat examination. A repeat radiograph is a radiograph that must be done again because of human or mechanical problems. When an examination is repeated, a patient absorbs unnecessary radiation. Because x-rays may be harmful to the body, it is important to keep the number of repeat films to a minimum. Effective communication and patient understanding will help meet this goal. It may be necessary to locate an interpreter who can adequately communicate instructions to the patient. All female patients of childbearing age should be asked if they might be pregnant, and the date of the last menstrual period should be charted.

During the initial interview with patients, the PCT often has to gain important information that may affect the examination. A radiographic examination during the first 3 months of a pregnancy could be harmful to the fetus, and it is the responsibility of the radiographer to question and determine the status of the patient. If a woman is pregnant, it will be her physician's decision whether to continue with the radiographic examination. *A radiographer must always consult a physician before starting an examination on a pregnant woman.* Most hospitals post signs in many languages alerting patients to the potential dangers of having a radiologic examination while pregnant.

A trauma situation requires the localization of a possible injury. Effectively communicating with your patient will allow you to be certain about the location of an injury. It is important to understand how the injury occurred and how painful it might be to move the injured body part to different positions for the radiographic examination.

Pregnant Patients

A pregnant patient may be required to have a radiographic examination during her pregnancy. It is the physician's responsibility to determine whether the need for x-ray examination outweighs the potential risk from harmful radiation. If the physician concludes that a radiograph is essential, the radiographer must proceed following all the rules of the ALARA philosophy on radiation protection. In addition, a pregnant patient must be given a gonadal shield for the front and back of the abdominal area.

Collimation

A collimator is a device attached to the x-ray tube housing that controls the size and shape of the radiographic beam as it enters the patient's body. The proper use of a collimator limits the area of the body exposed to the x-ray beam. The radiographic beam should always be limited to the area of clinical interest. This results in reduction of the radiation dose to the patient and increases the quality of the radiographic image.

A collimator consists of two sets of lead shutters, one vertical and one horizontal, that are controlled by the radiographer. The collimator also contains a light field that mirrors the radiographic exposure area. When the shutter is correctly positioned, a picture frame effect should be visible around the parameter of the radiographic cassette. The light image that is displayed on the film cassette should demonstrate a 1-inch border on all sides. The following rules apply to collimation:

1 All radiographic examinations require the use of a collimator.
2 It is the radiographer's responsibility to collimate to the area of clinical interest.
3 Proper collimation reduces the patient dose.
4 A collimated border should be demonstrated on the final radiograph.

Figure 16–11 demonstrates the proper collimation for a PA and **lateral** chest examination. A 14- by 17-inch cassette is required for one projection of the chest examination. In Figure 16–11A the collimator is adjusted so the light field is smaller than the cassette. When the patient is positioned against the cassette (Fig. 16–11B and C), the collimator restricts the radiographic beam to the portion of the chest that is the area of clinical interest.

Gonadal Shielding

In addition to collimation, **gonadal shielding** is another method of minimizing patient exposure. It is important to remember that collimation and shielding complement each other and result in a lower radiation dose to the patient.

A gonad shield is a piece of lead vinyl material placed between the x-ray beam and the patient's testes or ovaries. Figure 16–12 illustrates two types of gonad shields. A contact or flat shield is the most effective in radiation protection. The flat shield is placed on the lower abdomen in female patients and over the reproductive organs in male patients. Gonadal shielding is *required* on all examinations in which the x-ray beam enters the body 0.5 cm or less from the reproductive organs. Examples of areas that require gonadal shielding are the abdomen, vertebral column, pelvis, and femur. In some instances, a shield may compromise the visualization of specified anatomy and cannot be used.

Additional criteria for the use of gonadal shielding include the following:

1 *Gonadal shielding must always be used on children.* Children are more sensitive to the effects of radiation than are adults; therefore, radiographers must be extremely cautious to protect the reproductive organs of children. *Shields should be provided in all pediatric radiographic examinations.*
2 *A gonad shield must be provided for patients of reproductive age.* A lead shield must be provided for any person of potential reproductive age. Gen-

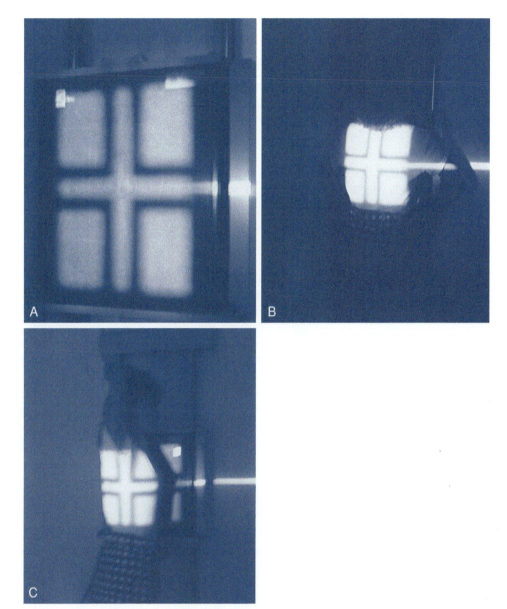

FIGURE 16–11   Collimation of a radiograph. *A,* Initial adjustment of collimator light. *B,* PA collimation. *C,* Lateral collimation.

erally, men have a longer reproductive period than do women. Many facilities have chosen to provide gonadal shielding for all patients to eliminate any questions concerning a patient's reproductive age. Consumers today are much more aware of radiation safety. The use of a gonadal shield on all examinations may alleviate a patient's anxiety concerning the potential hazards caused by radiation exposure.

Technical Factors

The exposure factors of milliamperage, kilovoltage, and exposure time not only affect the image on the radiograph, as discussed previously, but also determine the amount of radiation a patient receives. To reduce the patient's dose of radiation, an exposure technique using high kilovoltage and low milliampere-seconds is preferred.

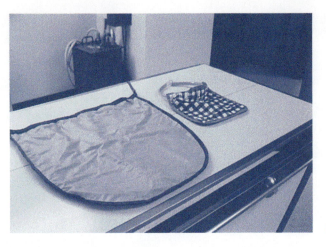

FIGURE 16–12   Gonadal shields.

PERSONNEL PROTECTION

PCTs working in areas with routine exposure to radiation must take precautions so they are not exposed to unnecessary radiation. Limited radiographers are exposed to the same potential hazards from radiation as are patients. Practitioners are exposed on a routine basis, however, and therefore the following preventive methods must be followed:

1   While an exposure is taking place, a radiographer should be located in the control booth and not in the x-ray room. The control booth is a small room adjacent to the radiography room that houses the x-ray generator and control panel (Fig. 16–13).

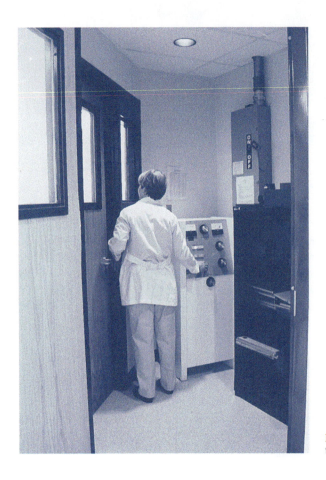

FIGURE 16–13   Radiographer in control booth.

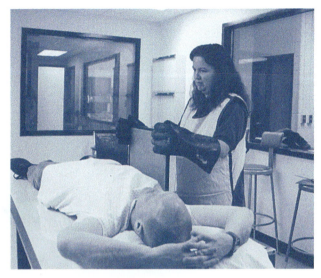

FIGURE 16–14   Protection for radiographer remaining in room during exposure.

The walls are constructed with impregnated lead that absorbs radiation and prevents the radiographer from being exposed to x-rays. The control booth also consists of a clear lead plastic barrier that allows for unobstructed visibility of the patient and communication of specific instructions.

2   A radiographer *should not* hold a patient, such as an uncooperative child, for a radiographic examination. To obtain the correct positioning, it may be necessary to resort to immobilization devices that will keep a child steady while the radiographic exposure takes place. If there are no restraining devices available, a nonradiographer may be asked to assist the child during the examination. A person who remains in the radiography room during an exposure must be given a full lead apron and gloves (Fig. 16–14). Similar to the lead in gonad shields or lead-impregnated walls, these aprons prevent individuals from absorbing radiation.

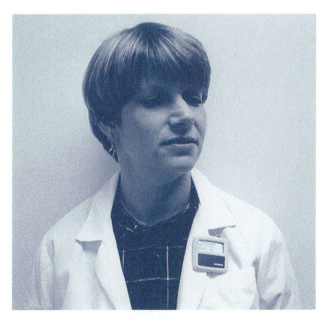

FIGURE 16–15   Radiographer wearing personnel monitoring device.

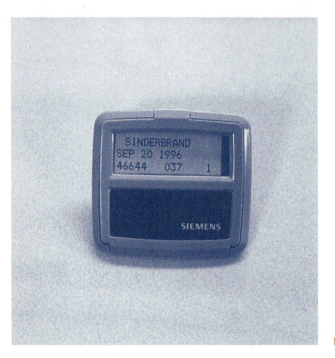

FIGURE 16–16   Film badge.

Monitoring Devices

Standards developed by the federal government limit persons working in diagnostic x-ray to receive only a certain quantity of radiation exposure annually. A radiography personnel monitoring device can determine the quantity of radiation an operator has absorbed. A monitoring device should be worn at the level of the waist or preferably at the chest near the collar to measure thyroid and eye exposure (Fig. 16–15) and should be worn at all times when performing radiographic procedures.

A **film badge** is the most common monitoring device used in radiology. It consists of a piece of radiation dosimetry film, similar to dental film, and a plastic holder (Fig. 16–16). The film is sensitive to radiation and when a radiographer is exposed to x-radiation the film is also exposed. After film processing and development, the density of the image is proportional to the exposure dose or the amount of radiation absorbed by the radiographer.

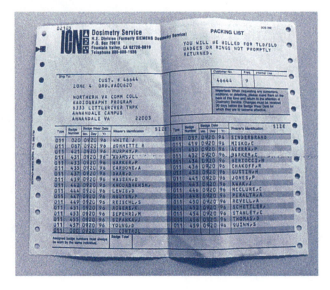

FIGURE 16–17   Monthly exposure report.

The film badge is sensitive to heat, humidity, and sunlight and should be kept in a safe area at the workplace and not transported back and forth from home. The film in a film badge must be changed on a monthly basis and sent back to the healthcare agency. A monitoring company reads the films and returns a copy of exposure doses (Fig. 16–17) that becomes part of an employee's permanent record. It is the responsibility of the employer to maintain exposure records on all employees.

Radiographic Procedures

As a member of the healthcare team, a limited radiographer or PCT is responsible for the successful completion of the radiographic examination and the well-being of the patient. A radiographer must adhere to a strict set of moral principles (acceptable conduct toward patients and other members of the healthcare team). The American Society of Radiologic Technologists has adopted a professional Code of Ethics that describes appropriate attitudes and behaviors for personnel working in the field of radiology.

GENERAL GUIDELINES

1 Always review the radiography request form to obtain information concerning the examination ordered and the patient. A patient's medical history can provide important information relating to the radiographic examination. Be certain to explain the procedure clearly to your patient. Answer any appropriate questions, and refer the patient to his or her physician for any unanswered questions.

2 A radiograph is a permanent record that belongs to the institution at which the examination was performed. Therefore, the radiograph must remain on file at the hospital or the physician's office. A radiograph can be released on loan to another physician or to the patient, who may wish to take it to another physician for a consultation. The radiograph must be returned to the original institution. A patient receives a bill for the interpretation of the film, not the actual radiograph.

3 A radiograph must have two forms of visible identification:
   • An identification marker that includes the patient name, date, ID number, and physician or institution. This information is written on a special card transferred photographically to the radiograph and appears on the radiograph after processing. This is a legal requirement for proper identification of an x-ray. When a chest radiograph is performed, the information blocker should be placed in the upper right-hand corner.
   • Right (R) and left (L) lead markers to accurately identify the orientation of radiographic films relative to the position of the patient's body. The markers should also contain a small set of initials or numbers that identify the radiographer who performed the examination (Fig. 16–18). If the radiograph is of an extremity, the lead marker will indicate which extremity is being radiographed (Fig. 16–19). Remember, *radiographs are considered legal medical records and should always be accurately marked and identified and treated with confidentiality.*

4 A radiograph is placed on the view box for review as if the patient were in anatomic position. More simply, the radiographer would be facing the radiograph (or the patient) with the patient's right on the radiographer's left. A radiograph with a left marker is placed on the view box so the left marker is facing the right side of the viewer's body.

5 Two projections are the minimum required to evaluate any anatomic structure. A chest examination requires a standing PA projection with the patient's chest

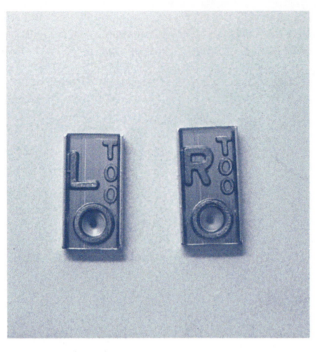

FIGURE 16–18   Lead markers.

placed against the cassette. The second required position is a side position or a lateral (**lat**). When a chest radiograph is being performed, the left side of the patient's body is placed against the cassette.

CHEST RADIOGRAPHY

The purpose of the chest radiograph is to evaluate the lung fields and bony anatomy surrounding the lungs. A chest radiograph must be performed with the patient erect, if possible, to demonstrate the length of the lung field, which is required to diagnose many pathological conditions, such as pneumonia, bronchitis, tuberculosis, and cancer.

Equipment Preparation

The following equipment setup should be completed prior to positioning the patient:

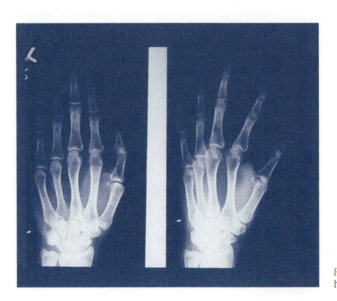

FIGURE 16–19   Radiograph of left hand.

1 Cassettes (two 14- by 17-inch cassettes). One cassette should be placed in the operator's booth to protect it from exposure. The second cassette should be placed in the erect film holder. For small- or medium-sized persons, the cassette should be placed lengthwise (14 by 17 inches). In this position the film blocker appears in the upper right corner of the cassette. For large persons, the cassette must be turned to a horizontal position. The film is then sized at 17 by 14 inches, and the left marker is taped on the upper left corner of the film.

2 Position of the x-ray tube. The x-ray tube must be directed to the upright or wall cassette holder. The distance from the x-ray to the cassette (source-to-image-receptor distance [**SID**]) should be 72 inches. The x-ray tube must be centered to the cassette longitudinally (up and down) and transversely (side to side). This is accomplished when the height of the cassette is adjusted for the individual patient.

3 Automatic exposure requirements. When positioning for a PA projection of the chest, only the two outer photocells should be activated. Using the center cell for a PA projection of the chest will result in a radiograph that is too dark. When positioning for a lateral projection of the chest, only the center photocell should be activated. Using the two outer cells for a lateral projection of the chest will result in a radiograph that is too light.

The kilovoltage should be set at 120 kVp for PA and lateral projections with a grid. Films without a grid (cassette) require 80 kVp for the PA and 90 kVp for the lateral projections.

Patient Instruction

The patient should be given a hospital gown and instructed to remove all clothing, including undergarments, above the waist. Necklaces, long earrings, and metal clips or barrettes should be removed, and valuables should be brought into the x-ray room.

The following steps are necessary to produce a radiograph:

PA Projection

1 The patient should be directed to place his or her chest against the erect film holder. Adjust the height of the film holder so the top of the cassette is approximately 1 1/2 inches above the shoulder.

2 Ask the patient to step aside for a moment and adjust the x-ray tube so it is centered to the cassette or erect film holder. The crosshair or center point of the collimator light should be centered to the middle of the cassette.

3 Adjust the patient so the frontal surface of the chest is centered to the cassette. The vertebral column should be in the middle of the cassette and the chest should be centered evenly between the borders of the cassette. Ask the patient to place equal weight on both feet. Extend the patient's chin above the cassette, and place the patient's hands on his or her hips and roll the shoulders forward (Fig. 16–20). Use a half-apron gonad shield.

4 Direct the central ray of the x-ray tube to the seventh thoracic vertebra, which is often at the level of the inferior (lower) angle of the scapula, as shown in Figure 16–11*B*.

5 Collimate to the borders of the skin.

6 Inform the patient that you are going into the radiographic exposure room. (Explain suspended inspiration to the patient [Take in a deep breath and hold it]). Inspiration lengthens the lung field to demonstrate lung anatomy.

7 Enter the radiographic exposure room and ask the patient to take in a deep breath and hold it.

8 Take the exposure.

9 Instruct the patient to resume breathing.

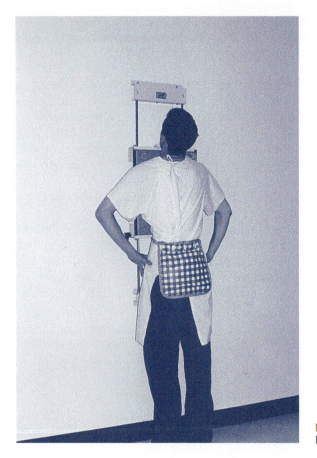

FIGURE 16–20   Patient positioned for PA chest film.

10 Remove the cassette after exposure and place it in the operator's booth. Place the other cassette in the holder for the next projection.

Lateral Projection

1 A lateral is generally performed with the left side of the body against the cassette unless there is specific pathology on the right side of the chest.

2 The patient should be directed to place his or her chest against the erect cassette holder. Adjust the height of the film holder so the top of the cassette is approximately 1 1/2 inches above the patient's shoulder.

3 Ask the patient to step aside for a moment and adjust the x-ray tube so it is centered to the cassette or erect film holder. The crosshair or center point of the collimator light should be centered to the middle of the cassette.

4 Place the patient's left side against the cassette holder. Raise the arms up over the head and have the patient grasp his or her elbows. Adjust the patient's position so that the body is centered to the cassette. Ask the patient to place equal weight on both feet and check for body rotation. Tape a left marker about 2 inches anterior to the front of the chest. Use a half-apron gonad shield as shown in Figure 16–21.

5 Direct the central ray of the x-ray tube to enter just inferior to the right axilla (approximately 2 inches below the right armpit), as shown in Figure 16–11C.

6 Collimate to the borders of the skin.

7 Inform the patient that you are going into the radiographic exposure room. (Explain suspended inspiration to the patient [Take in a deep breath and hold it]). Inspiration lengthens the lung field to demonstrate lung anatomy.

8 Enter the radiographic exposure room and ask the patient to take in a deep breath and hold it.

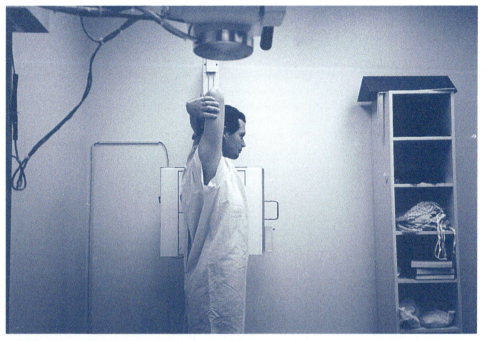

FIGURE 16–21   Patient positioned for lateral chest film.

9 Take the exposure.
10 Instruct the patient to resume breathing.
11 Remove the cassette after exposure and place it in the operator's booth.

CHEST ANATOMY

The following structures must be identified on a chest radiograph:

1 The entire length of the right and left lungs, including the following structures, as shown in Figure 16–22*A* and *B*.

- Apex—the most superior portion of the lung field, located above the **clavicles**

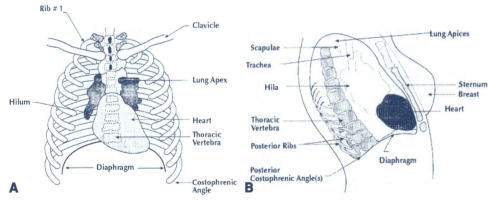

FIGURE 16–22   Structures visible in radiographs. *A*, PA chest exposure. *B*, Lateral chest exposure.

- Base—the most inferior portion of the lung field
- Axilla—the lateral-most portion of the lung field
- Diaphragm—a dome-shaped muscle that separates the chest and abdominal cavities
- Hilum—an area of the lung where blood vessels, nerves, bronchi, and lymph nodes enter the lung
- Costophrenic angle—the angle at the bottom of the lung field where the lungs meet the diaphragm

2 The **mediastinum** is the anatomic area between the two lung fields. The heart, trachea, and esophagus are located in the mediastinum. The heart, aorta, and trachea are easily identifiable on a chest radiograph.

3 The bony structures visualized on a chest radiograph include two clavicles, **sternum**, thoracic vertebrae (visualized behind the mediastinum), and rib cage.

CRITERIA FOR EVALUATION OF CHEST RADIOGRAPHS

The following structures should be visible on chest radiographs to indicate correct positioning, breathing instructions, and exposure settings:

PA Projection

1 Rotation of the chest could indicate a distortion of the heart or a pathology. It is critical that no rotation appear on the film. Rotation on the film is demonstrated by the ends of the clavicle meeting the sternum in the midline of the body. This articulation is known as the **sternoclavicular articulation**, which must be symmetrical on both sides of the chest (Fig. 16–23A and B). Rotation of the clavicle away from the sternum indicates that the patient's body is rotated to the left or right.

2 A minimum of 10 rib pairs above the diaphragm must be identifiable on the PA radiograph. The demonstration of the rib pairs is dependent on the correct breathing instructions being given to the patient. When a patient inhales, the di-

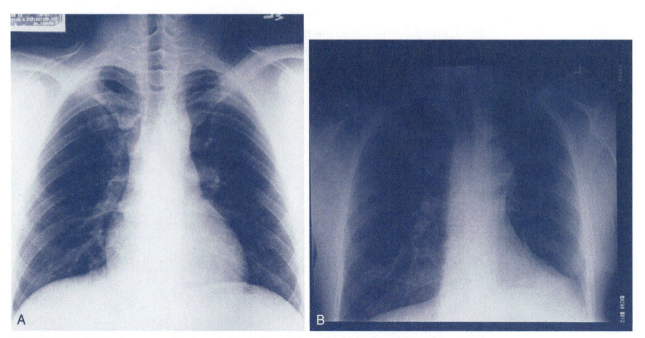

FIGURE 16–23   PA chest exposure showing rotation. *A,* Correct sternoclavicular articulation. *B,* Incorrect sternoclavicular articulation.

aphragm lowers to demonstrate more rib pairs. So, the instructions should state "Take in a deep breath and hold it." In Figure 16–24A, notice the length of the lung field on a cassette taken after inspiration, on which 10 rib pairs are demonstrated, and in Figure 16–24B, with the film taken after expiration, on which about 8 rib pairs are demonstrated.

3 The **scapulae** should be lateral to the lung field. Proper positioning of the hands and rolling the shoulders forward will place the scapulae to the lateral border of the chest. This allows the radiologist to receive more information concerning the chest anatomy.

4 The apices of the lung field will be cut off the film if the anatomy is placed too close to the top border of the cassette. This problem is avoided by making certain the top of the cassette is approximately 1 1/2 inches above the shoulder.

5 The *costophrenic angles* of both lung fields must be demonstrated. This is accomplished by making certain the entire chest fits on the cassette and the lungs are centered to the cassette.

6 When adequate kVp is used, the thoracic spine is visible through the heart. Inadequate kilovoltage will result in a bright white area in the mediastinum because of insufficient density.

Lateral Projection

Detecting rotation on the lateral projection is equally important. Identification of rotation is determined by looking at the posterior ribs behind the vertebral column. A correctly positioned lateral demonstrates superimposition of the posterior ribs (Fig. 16–25). Inaccurate positioning results in ribs that are demonstrated posterior to the vertebral column. Correct positioning results when the shoulders and pelvis are checked for true lateral positioning.

In summary, limited radiographers must incorporate patient care skills and technical abilities to produce quality radiographs. The following steps are the keys to a successful radiographic examination:

1 Effective communication
2 Good patient care skills
3 Radiation protection

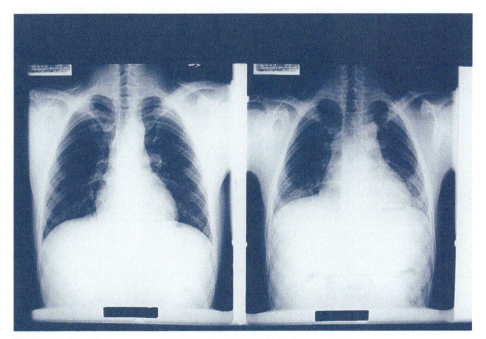

FIGURE 16–24   Chest exposures. *Left*, After inspiration. *Right*, After expiration.

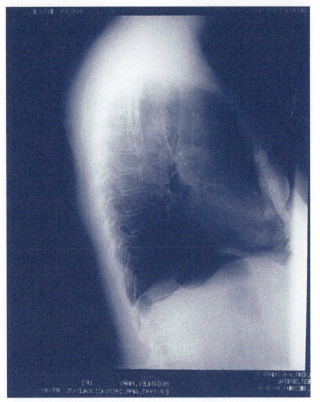

FIGURE 16–25 Radiograph showing correct lateral positioning.

4 Correct use of radiographic equipment
5 Correct selection of technical factors
6 Radiographic positioning
7 Evaluation of radiographic images

BIBLIOGRAPHY

Ballinger, P: Merrill's Atlas of Radiographic Positions and Radiologic Procedures, Volume I, ed. 8. CV Mosby, St. Louis, 1991.

Bontrager, K: Radiographic Positioning and Techniques, Student Edition. Bontrager Publishers, Peoria, AZ, 1994.

Campeau, F, and Phelps, MJ: Limited Radiography. Delmar Publishers, Albany, NY, 1993.

Statkiewicz-Sherer, MA, Visconti, PJ, and Ritenour, ER: Radiation Protection in Medical Radiography, ed. 2. CV Mosby, St. Louis, 1993.

STUDY QUESTIONS

1. List six directional controls that allow x-ray tube movement.

   a. _____

   b. _____

   c. _____

   d. _____

   e. _____

   f. _____

2. List the eight controls that are generally located on an operator's console.

   a. _____

   b. _____

   c. _____

   d. _____

   e. _____

   f. _____

   g. _____

   h. _____

3. Place the following steps in the film processing technique in the correct order by numbering them 1 though 9:

   a. _____ Open the film bin, remove a single sheet of film, and close the film bin.

   b. _____ Slide the film forward until the rollers take up the film.

   c. _____ Open the cassette and remove the film.

   d. _____ Turn on the room lights when the processor rings or buzzes.

   e. _____ Align the film with the vertical edge of the feed tray.

   f. _____ Place the cassette tube side down on the working surface.

   g. _____ Place the loaded cassette in an area for unexposed films.

   h. _____ Turn off the room lights.

   i. _____ Identify the film using a daylight identification system.

4. What is the most likely cause of processed films that are too dark?

   _____

5. Calculate the following:

   a. 100 mA $\times$ 0.5 second = _____ mA-s

   b. 200 mA $\times$ 0.2 second = _____ mA-s

   c. 100 mA $\times$ 1 second = _____ mA-s

6. How do technical factors differ with the use of a grid during an examination?

_____

7. Identify the photocells used for the following projections of the chest:

   a. PA _____

   b. Lateral _____

8. Explain the function of the following in the processing procedure:

   a. Developer _____

   b. Fixer _____

   c. Washer _____

   d. Dryer _____

9. Identify four methods of patient protection.

   a. _____

   b. _____

   c. _____

   d. _____

10. List four rules of collimation.

    a. _____

    b. _____

    c. _____

    d. _____

11. How does radiation protection for a pregnant patient differ from routine patient protection?

    _____

    _____

12. List the criteria used for gonadal shielding.

    _____

    _____

13. Why is it important to protect radiographic film from light?

    _____

    _____

14. Discuss a good location for a film badge when you are not in the radiology department.

    _____

15. State two forms of identification that must be visible on all radiographs.

    a. _____

    b. _____

16. A patient arrives for a chest examination. The patient is very broad and will not fit on the standard orientation of film (14 by 17 inches). What options do you have in performing this examination?

_____

_____

17. As a limited radiographer, you are evaluating a PA projection of a chest to determine whether it is a quality image. Upon viewing the radiograph you notice the apices have been cut off the radiograph by poor positioning. How can you correct for this error?

_____

_____

18. A PA chest radiograph is obtained using 200 mA at 0.03 second at 80 kVp. If the resulting radiograph appears too dark, what new level of milliampere-seconds should be used to correct the excessive density?

_____

_____

19. Match the following structures with the appropriate description:

a. _____ Base   1. The most superior portion of the lung field

b. _____ Apex   2. The most inferior portion of the lung field

c. _____ Hilum   3. Angle between the diaphragm and the lungs

d. _____ Costophrenic angle 4. Lateral-most portion of the lung field

e. _____ Axilla   5. Area of the lung where blood vessels and lymph nodes enter the lung

20. List six criteria for evaluation of a PA projection of the chest.

a. _____

b. _____

c. _____

d. _____

e. _____

f. _____

EVALUATION OF SETTING TECHNIQUE AND MAKING AN EXPOSURE

■ ▬▬▬▬▬▬▬▬▬▬▬▬▬▬▬▬▬▬▬▬▬▬▬▬▬

RATING SYSTEM   2 = Satisfactory   1 = Needs improvement   0 = Incorrect/did not perform

_____ **1.** Measures patient and/or correctly determines technical factors from chart

_____ **2.** Selects appropriate milliampere (mA) setting

_____ **3.** Selects appropriate kilovoltage (kVp) setting

_____ **4.** Selects appropriate exposure time (seconds) setting

_____ **5.** Sets the proper SID, if necessary

_____ **6.** Selects the correct photocell array for PA chest radiograph

_____ **7.** Selects the correct photocell array for lateral chest radiograph

_____ **8.** Provides the correct verbal commands and breathing instructions

_____ **9.** Depresses rotor (or prepares) button and waits for the "ready" indicator

_____ **10.** Depresses the expose button at the proper moment without releasing the rotor

_____ **11.** Releases the rotor and expose buttons only after the exposure is completed

_____ **12.** If resulting film is too light, correctly adjusts technical factors for repeat film

_____ **13.** If resulting film is too dark, correctly adjusts technical factors for repeat film

Total points _____

Maximum points = 26

COMMENTS

EVALUATION OF RADIOGRAPHIC FILM PROCESSING PROCEDURE

RATING SYSTEM   2 = Satisfactory   1 = Needs improvement   0 = Incorrect/did not perform

_____ **1.** Properly "flashes" or imprints radiograph with correct patient information

_____ **2.** Checks darkroom occupancy before opening door to enter darkroom

_____ **3.** Places cassette tube side down on working surface of darkroom

_____ **4.** Turns off normal room lighting and turns on appropriate safelight

_____ **5.** Opens cassette and carefully removes film without bending or creasing

_____ **6.** Aligns film on the processor feed tray without prematurely advancing film

_____ **7.** Slides film forward until processor rollers take up the film

_____ **8.** Opens film bin and removes a single sheet of film

_____ **9.** Closes the film bin immediately after removing film

_____ **10.** Places unexposed film in the bottom of cassette without overlapping the edge

_____ **11.** Closes and securely locks the cassette

_____ **12.** Waits for the film in the feed tray to enter the processor before opening door

_____ **13.** Places the loaded cassette in appropriate area reserved for unexposed film

Total points _____

Maximum points = 26

COMMENTS

EVALUATION OF POSTEROANTERIOR CHEST RADIOGRAPH PERFORMANCE

RATING SYSTEM   2 = Satisfactory   1 = Needs improvement   0 = Incorrect/did not perform

_____ 1. Greets patient and explains procedure

_____ 2. Examines requisition form

_____ 3. Asks patient to state full name

_____ 4. Directs patient to dressing room and gives proper disrobing instructions

_____ 5. Directs patient to remove earrings and necklaces and bring valuables into the radiography room

_____ 6. Questions female patients concerning the possibility of pregnancy

_____ 7. Selects correct-size cassette with proper film screen system

_____ 8. Places the cassette properly in the erect cassette holder

_____ 9. Places a left lead marker in the upper left-hand corner of the cassette

_____ 10. Manipulates x-ray tube so it is directed at the erect film holder

_____ 11. Sets SID to 72 inches

_____ 12. Centers x-ray tube transversely to cassette

_____ 13. Places patient's chest against cassette

_____ 14. Adjusts height of cassette so the top border is approximately 1 1/2 inches above the patient's shoulder

_____ 15. Asks patient to step aside and centers x-ray tube longitudinally to cassette (Collimator crosshairs should be centered to the midpoint of the cassette.)

_____ 16. Places patient's chest against properly adjusted cassette

_____ 17. Centers the median sagittal plane of the patient to the midline of the cassette

_____ 18. Adjusts patient's chin so it is sitting in the chin holder

_____ 19. Places patient's hands on hips and rolls shoulders forward into cassette

_____ 20. Directs the central ray to the seventh thoracic vertebra (approximately inferior angle of the scapula)

_____ 21. Collimates to demonstrate four borders of collimation

_____ 22. Places gonad shield around patient's waist

_____ 23. Sets correct exposure technique

_____ 24. Gives proper breathing instructions

_____ 25. Removes cassette from radiography room to darkroom

_____ 26. Properly marks film with patient identification

_____ **27.** Develops x-ray film

_____ **28.** Reviews resultant radiograph

Total points _____

Maximum points = 56

COMMENTS

EVALUATION OF LATERAL CHEST RADIOGRAPH PERFORMANCE

RATING SYSTEM   2 = Satisfactory   1 = Needs improvement   0 = Incorrect/did not perform

_____ **1.** Greets patient and explains procedure

_____ **2.** Examines requisition form

_____ **3.** Asks patient to state full name

_____ **4.** Directs patient to dressing room and gives proper disrobing instructions

_____ **5.** Directs patient to remove earrings and necklaces and bring valuables into the radiography room

_____ **6.** Questions female patients concerning the possibility of pregnancy

_____ **7.** Selects correct-sized cassette with proper film screen system

_____ **8.** Places the cassette properly in the erect cassette holder

_____ **9.** Manipulates x-ray tube so it is directed at the erect film holder

_____ **10.** Sets SID to 72 inches

_____ **11.** Centers x-ray tube transversely to cassette

_____ **12.** Places patient's chest against cassette

_____ **13.** Adjusts height of cassette so the top border is approximately 1 1/2 inches above the patient's shoulder

_____ **14.** Asks patient to step aside and centers x-ray tube longitudinally to cassette (Collimator crosshairs should be centered to the midpoint of the cassette.)

_____ **15.** Places the patient so his or her left side is against the cassette

_____ **16.** Places a left lead marker anterior to the chest on the cassette

_____ **17.** Adjusts patient so the chest is centered to the cassette

_____ **18.** Has patient raise arms above head and grasp his or her elbows

_____ **19.** Directs the central ray to enter axilla at the level of the seventh thoracic vertebra (approximately inferior angle of the scapula)

_____ **20.** Collimates to demonstrate four borders of collimation

_____ **21.** Places gonad shield around patient's waist

_____ **22.** Sets correct exposure technique

_____ **23.** Gives proper breathing instructions

_____ **24.** Removes cassette from radiography room to darkroom

_____ **25.** Properly marks film with patient identification

_____ **26.** Develops film

_____ **27.** Reviews resultant radiograph

Total points _____

Maximum points = 54

COMMENTS

APPENDIX

BASIC TERMINOLOGY

Medical terminology is derived primarily from the classic Greek and Latin languages. However, it is not necessary to master either of these languages to obtain a solid background in basic medical terminology. Medical terms consist of combinations of three major word parts: prefixes, roots, and suffixes. The same prefixes and suffixes are frequently used with different roots; therefore, knowledge of the commonly used prefixes, roots, and suffixes can provide the basic communication skills necessary for successful job performance.

Prefixes and Suffixes

Prefixes are letters or syllables added to the beginning of a root to alter its meaning. Likewise, suffixes are letters or syllables added to the end of a root to alter its meaning. In medical terminology, suffixes often indicate a condition or a type of procedure.

The most commonly used prefixes and suffixes are presented in this appendix. It will be necessary to memorize these common prefixes and suffixes. This will be easier if you relate them to terms that are already familiar to you.

> **EXAMPLE:** In medical terminology, the prefix "post-" means "after," just as it does in the term "postgraduate."
> The suffix "-ectomy" means "surgical removal," and the term "tonsillectomy" is a familiar word to most people.

COMMONLY USED PREFIXES

Prefix	Meaning
a-, an-	no, not, without
ab-	away from
ad-	toward
ambi-	both
ana-	up
anti-, contra-	against
auto-	self
bi-	two
brady-	slow
cata-	down
centi-	hundred
chromo-	color

Prefix	Meaning
circum, peri-	around
co-, con-	together, with
dia-	through, complete
dys-	difficult, painful
ecto-, exo-, extra-	outside
endo-, intra-	inside, within
epi-	on, over
ex-	out, away from
hetero-	different
homo-	same
hydro-	water
hyper-	increased
hypo-	decreased
infra-, sub-	below
inter-	between
iso-	equal
macro-	large
mal-	bad, ill
mega-	great
meta-	beyond
micro-	small
milli-	one-thousandth
mono-, uni-	one
multi-, poly-	many
neo-	new
oligo-	little, scanty
pan-	all
para-	beside, abnormal
post-, retro-	after
pre-, ante-	before, in front
primi-	first
pseudo-	false
semi-	half
supra-, super-	above
sym-	together
tachy-	fast
trans-	across
tri-	three

COMMONLY USED SUFFIXES

Suffix	Meaning
-ac, -al, -ar, -ary, ic	pertaining to
-ad	toward
-agon	assemble, gather together
-algesia	excessive sensitivity to pain
-algia, dynia	pain
-arche	beginning
-ase	enzyme
-asthenia	lack of strength
-blast	immature cell
-capnia	carbon dioxide

-centesis	surgical puncture
-cidal	pertaining to death
-clast	break
-coccus	spherical
-crine	secrete
-cyte	cell
-cytosis	abnormal condition of cells
-ectasis	distention
-ectomy	surgical removal
-emesis	vomit
-emia	pertaining to blood
-esthesia	nervous sensation
-genesis	formation
-globin, -globulin	protein
-gram	written record
-graphy	method of recording
-gravida	pregnancy
-ion	process
-ism	condition of
-ist	specialist
-itis	inflammation
-kinesia	movement
-lepsy	seizure
-lith	stone
-logist	one who studies
-logy	study of
-lysis, -rrhexis	rupture
-malacia	softening
-megaly	enlargement
-meter	instrument to measure
-metry	measurement
-oid	like, similar to
-oma	tumor
-opia	eye, vision
-ose	sugar
-osis, iasis	abnormal condition
-ostomy	surgical opening
-paresis	weakness
-pathy	disease
-penia	decrease in cell numbers
-pepsia	digestion
-pexy	fixation
-phagia	eating, swallowing
-philia	increase in cell numbers
-phobia	fear
-phonia	voice
-phylaxis	protection
-physis	growth
-plasty	surgical repair
-plegia	paralysis
-pnea	breathing
-prandial	meal
-ptysis	bursting out
-rrhea	discharge
-scope	instrument for viewing
-scopy	visual examination
-spasm, -stalsis	contraction

Suffix	Meaning
-stasis	controlling, standing still
-stenosis	narrowing
-stomy	new opening
-tension	pressure
-therapy	treatment
-tome	instrument for cutting
-tomy	incision
-toxic	poison
-tripsy	crushing
-trophy	development
-tropin	stimulation
-uria	pertaining to urine

Roots/Combining Forms

Roots are the main part of a word and may be combined with prefixes, suffixes, or other roots. The combining form of a root contains a vowel, usually an "o," which is used to facilitate pronunciation when the root is combined with a word part that does not begin with a vowel.

> **EXAMPLE:** The root word for "heart" is "cardi"
> The combining form is "cardi/o"
> The study of the heart is "cardiology"

Roots frequently refer to body components. Therefore, common roots are listed with their corresponding body system in this appendix.

Body System	Root/Combining Form	Meaning
Anatomy	antero/o	front, before
	dist/o	distant
	dors/o	back
	kary/o	nucleus
	later/o	side
	medi/o	middle
	poster/o	back, behind
	proxim/o	near
	viscer/o	internal organs
Integumentary	albin/o	white
	carcin/o	cancer
	cutane/o, dermat/o	skin
	erythemat/o	redness
	hidr/o	sweat
	hist/o	tissue
	hydr/o	water
	kerat/o	hard tissue
	melan/o	black
	onych/o	nail
	seb/o	sebum, oily secretion
	squam/o	scalelike

	trich/o	hair
	xanth/o	yellow
Skeletal	arthr/o	joint
	axill/o	armpit
	caud/o	tail
	chrondr/o	cartilage
	cost/o	ribs
	dactyl/o	finger or toe
	fibul/o	fibula
	humer/o	humerus
	mandibul/o	lower jawbone
	maxill/o	jawbone
	myel/o	bone marrow
	orth/o	straight
	oste/o	bone
	patell/o	kneecap
	rheumat/o	watery flow
	sacr/o	sacrum
	scapul/o	shoulder blade
	spondyl/o	vertebrae
	synov/i	synovial membrane
Muscular	fibr/o	fibrous connective tissue
	my/o, muscul/o	muscle
Nervous	cephal/o	head
	cerebell/o	cerebellum
	cerebr/o	cerebrum
	crani/o	skull
	encephal/o	brain
	gli/o	glue
	meningi/o	meninges
	neur/o	nerve
Respiratory	alveol/o	alveolus, air sac
	cyan/o	blue
	nas/o, rhin/o	nose
	olfact/o	sense of smell
	pector/o, thorac/o	chest
	pleur/o	pleura
	pneum/o	air, lung
	pulmon/o	lung
	spir/o	breathe
	steth/o	chest
	trache/o	trachea, windpipe
Digestive	adip/o, lip/o, steat/o	fat
	amyl/o	starch
	bil/i, chol/o	bile, gall
	bucc/o	cheek
	celi/o, lapar/o	abdomen
	cholecyst/o	gallbladder
	choledoch/o	common bile duct
	cirrh/o	yellow
	col/o	colon
	dent/i, odont/o	tooth
	enter/o	intestine
	gastr/o	stomach

Body System	Root/Combining Form	Meaning
	gingiv/o	gums
	gloss/o, lingu/o	tongue
	gluc/o, glyc/o	glucose
	hepat/o	liver
	icter/o	jaundice
	lith/o	stone
	or/o, stomat/o	mouth
	proct/o	rectum
	sigmoid/o	sigmoid colon
Urinary	cyst/o	urinary bladder
	glomerul/o	glomerulus
	micturit/o	urination
	nephr/o, ren/o	kidney
	noct/i	night
	olig/o	scanty
	pyel/o	renal
	ur/o, urin/o	urine
Endocrine	aden/o	gland
	andr/o	male
	cortic/o	cortex
	crin/o	secrete
	kal/o	potassium
	natr/o	sodium
	somat/o	body
	ster/o	solid structure
	thyr/o	thyroid gland
Reproductive	amni/o	amnion
	balan/o	glans penis
	colp/o	vagina
	episi/o	vulva
	gonad/o	sex glands
	gynec/o	female
	hyster/o	uterus, womb
	lact/o	milk
	mamm/o, mast/o	breast
	men/o	menses, menstruation
	nat/o	birth
	oopho/o, ovul/o	ovary
	orch/o	testes
	ovari/o	ovary
	salping/o	fallopian tubes
	spermat/o	spermatozoa
	test/o	testicle
Circulatory	angi/o	vessel
	ather/o	fatty substance
	brachi/o	arm
	cardi/o, coron/o	heart
	cyt/o	cell
	electr/o	electricity
	erythr/o	red
	leuk/o	white
	scler/o	hardening
	ser/o	serum

	sphygm/o	pulse
	thromb/o	clot
	vas/o	pertaining to blood vessels
Lymphatic	immun/o	protection
	lymphaden/o	lymph node
	splen/o	spleen
	tox/o	poison
General	agglutin/o	clumping
	ambul/o	to walk
	anis/o	unequal
	audi/o	to hear
	aur/o, ot/o	ear
	bacill/o	rod
	bi/o	life
	coagul/o	clotting
	contag/i	unclean
	esthesi/o	feeling
	febr/o	fever
	gen/o	formation
	ger/o	old age
	hem/o, hemat/o	blood
	isch/o	to hold back
	kil/o	thousand
	macr/o	large
	morph/o	form
	myc/o	fungus
	myring/o	eardrum
	necr/o	death
	nos/o	pertaining to disease
	ocul/o, ophthalm/o	eye
	onc/o	tumor
	opt/o	vision
	path/o	disease
	ped/i	children
	pharmac/o	drug
	phleb/o	vein
	prandi/o	meal
	psych/o	mind
	pur/o, py/o	pus
	quadri/o	four
	radi/o	x-ray, radiant energy

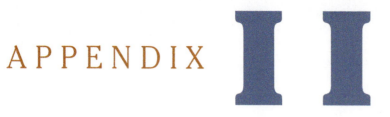

ABBREVIATIONS

Abbreviations	Definitions
Ab	Antibody
ABGs	Arterial blood gases
ABO	Blood groups
ACD	Acid citrate dextrose
ACT	Activated clotting time
ACTH	Adrenocorticotropic hormone
ADH	Antidiuretic hormone
AEC	Automatic exposure control
AFB	Acid-fast bacilli (tuberculosis)
Ag	Antigen
AIDS	Acquired immunodeficiency syndrome
ALARA	As low as reasonably achievable
ALP	Alkaline phosphatase
ALS	Amyotrophic lateral sclerosis
ALT (SGPT)	Alanine aminotransferase
ANA	Antinuclear antibody
ANS	Autonomic nervous system
APTT (PTT)	Activated partial thromboplastin time
ARD	Antimicrobial removal device
ASO	Antistreptolysin O
AST (SGOT)	Aspartate aminotransferase
AV	Atrioventricular
BaE	Barium enema
BM	Bowel movement
BP	Blood pressure
BSI	Body substance isolation
BT	Bleeding time
BUN	Blood urea nitrogen
Bx	Biopsy
C & S	Culture and sensitivity
Ca	Calcium
CAD	Coronary artery disease
CAP	College of American Pathologists
CAT (CT) scan	Computerized axial tomography
CBC	Complete blood count
cc	Cubic centimeter
CCU	Cardiac care unit
CDC	Centers for Disease Control and Prevention

CEA	Carcinoembryonic antigen
CEU	Continuing education unit
CHF	Congestive heart failure
CK-BB, MB, and MM	Creatine kinase isoenzymes
CK (CPK)	Creatine kinase
Cl	Chloride
CLIA '88	Clinical Laboratory Improvement Act of 1988
CLS	Clinical laboratory scientist (MT)
CLT	Clinical laboratory technician (MLT)
cm	Centimeter
CNA	Certified nursing assistant
CNS	Central nervous system
CO$_2$	Carbon dioxide
COLA	Commission on Office Laboratory Accreditation
COPD	Chronic obstructive pulmonary disease
CPR	Cardiopulmonary resuscitation
CPU	Central processing unit
CQI	Continuous quality improvement
CRP	C-reactive protein
CSF	Cerebrospinal fluid
CTS	Carpal tunnel syndrome
CVA	Cerebrovascular accident
CVC	Central venous catheter
CVS	Chorionic villus sampling
Cx	Cervix
DAT	Direct antihuman globulin test
DI	Diabetes insipidus
DIC	Disseminated intravascular coagulation
DM	Diabetes mellitus
DOB	Date of birth
Dx	Diagnosis
ECG (EKG)	Electrocardiogram
EDTA	Ethylenediaminetetraacetic acid
EEG	Electroencephalogram
EMG	Electromyography
ENT	Ear, nose, and throat specialty
ER	Emergency room
ERV	Expiratory reserve volume
ESR	Erythrocyte sedimentation rate
FANA	Fluorescent antinuclear antibody
FBS	Fasting blood sugar
FDA	Food and Drug Administration
FDPs	Fibrin degradation products
FEV$_1$	Forced expiratory volume in one second
FiO$_2$	Fraction of inspired oxygen
FMS	Fibromyalgia syndrome
FRC	Functional residual capacity
FSH	Follicle-stimulating hormone
FTA-ABS	Fluorescent treponemal antibody–absorbed
FUO	Fever of unknown origin
FVC	Forced vital capacity
Fx	Fracture
GGT	Gamma glutamyltransferase
GH	Growth hormone

Abbreviations	Definitions
GI	Gastrointestinal
GTT	Glucose tolerance test
GU	Genitourinary
GYN	Gynecology
H & H	Hemoglobin and hematocrit
HBsAg	Hepatitis B surface antigen
HBV	Hepatitis B virus
HCG	Human chorionic gonadotropin
Hct	Hematocrit
HDL	High-density lipoprotein
HDN	Hemolytic disease of the newborn
Hgb	Hemoglobin
HIV	Human immunodeficiency virus
HMO	Health maintenance organization
Hx	History
IC	Inspiratory capacity
ICU	Intensive care unit
Ig	Immunoglobulin
IM	Infectious mononucleosis
IM	Intramuscular
I & O	Intake and output
IRDS	Infant respiratory distress syndrome
IRV	Inspiratory reserve volume
IV	Intravenous
JCAHO	Joint Commission on Accreditation of Healthcare Organizations
K	Potassium
kg	Kilogram
KOH	Potassium hydroxide
kVp	Kilovolts-peak
L & D	Labor and delivery
lat	Lateral
LD (LDH)	Lactic dehydrogenase
LDL	Low-density lipoprotein
LH	Luteinizing hormone
Li	Lithium
LLQ	Left lower quadrant
LP	Lumbar puncture
LPN	Licensed practical nurse
LUQ	Left upper quadrant
Lytes	Electrolytes
mA-s	Milliampere-seconds
MD	Muscular dystrophy
MDI	Metered-dose inhaler
mg	Milligram
Mg	Magnesium
MI	Myocardial infarction
μL	Microliter
mL	Milliliter
MLT	Medical laboratory technician (CLT)
mm	Millimeter

mm Hg	Millimeters of mercury
MRI	Magnetic resonance imaging
MS	Multiple sclerosis
MSDS	Material Safety Data Sheets
MSH	Melanocyte-stimulating hormone
MT	Medical technologist (CLS)
mV	Millivolt
Na	Sodium
NFPA	National Fire Protection Association
NPO	Nothing by mouth
NSR	Normal sinus rhythm
O$_2$	Oxygen
O & P	Ova and parasites
OB	Obstetrics
OR	Operating room
OSHA	Occupational Safety and Health Administration
OT	Occupational therapy
P	Phosphorus
PA	Posteroanterior
PaO$_2$	Partial pressure of oxygen in arterial blood
Pap	Papanicolaou stain for cervical cancer
PAP	Prostatic acid phosphatase
PCT	Patient care technician
PEFR	Peak expiratory flow rate
PF3	Platelet factor 3
PFT	Pulmonary function test
PID	Pelvic inflammatory disease
PKU	Phenylketonuria
Plt	Platelet
PMS	Premenstrual syndrome
PNS	Peripheral nervous system
POCT	Point-of-care testing
POL	Physician's office laboratory
pp	Postprandial
PPD	Purified protein derivative
PPE	Personal protective equipment
PRL	Prolactin
PRN	Allowable as needed
PSA	Prostate-specific antigen
psi	Pounds per square inch
PST	Plasma separator tube
PT	Physical therapy
PT	Prothrombin time
PTH	Parathyroid hormone
PVC	Premature ventricular contraction
q	Every
QA	Quality assurance
QC	Quality control
qh	Every hour
qid	Four times a day
QNS	Quantity nonsufficient
R/O	Rule out
RA	Rheumatoid arthritis
RAM	Random access memory

Abbreviations	Definitions
RBC	Red blood cell
Retic	Reticulocyte
RF	Rheumatoid factor
Rh	The D (Rhesus) antigen on red blood cells
RLQ	Right lower quadrant
RN	Registered nurse
ROM	Read-only memory
RPR	Rapid plasma reagin
RUQ	Right upper quadrant
RV	Residual volume
Rx	Treatment (prescription)
SA	Sinoatrial
SB	Sinus bradycardia
SID	Source-to-image-receptor distance
SLE	Systemic lupus erythematosus
SOB	Shortness of breath
SpO_2	Oxygen-hemoglobin saturation
SPS	Sodium polyanetholesulfonate
SST	Serum separator tube
ST	Sinus tachycardia
stat	Immediately
STD	Sexually transmitted disease
SVN	Small-volume nebulizer
T & C	Type and crossmatch
t-PA	Tissue plasminogen activator
TB	Tuberculosis
TDM	Therapeutic drug monitoring
TIBC	Total iron-binding capacity
TLC	Total lung capacity
TP	Total protein
TPN	Total parenteral nutrition
TPR	Temperature, pulse, and respirations
TQM	Total quality management
TSH	Thyroid-stimulating hormone
TSS	Toxic shock syndrome
T_3	Triiodothyronine
T_4	Thyroxine
UA	Routine urinalysis
URI	Upper respiratory infection
UTI	Urinary tract infection
UV	Ultraviolet
VC	Vital capacity
VDRL	Venereal Disease Research Laboratory
V_t	Tidal volume
WBC	White blood cell

GLOSSARY

Terms	Definitions
Adrenocorticotropic hormone	Hormone produced by the anterior pituitary gland to stimulate secretion of adrenal cortex hormones
Aerosol	Fine suspension of particles in air
Aldosterone	Hormone produced by the adrenal cortex to regulate electrolyte and water balance
Alveoli	Air sacs in the lungs in which the exchange of O_2 and CO_2 occurs
Amphiarthrosis	Slightly movable joint
Amylase	Pancreatic enzyme to digest starch
Androgen	Male hormone produced by the adrenal cortex to maintain secondary sex characteristics
Angioplasty	Reconstruction of a blood vessel
Anterior (ventral)	Pertaining to the front of the body
Antidiuretic hormone	Hormone produced by the posterior pituitary gland to stimulate retention of water by the kidney
Antiglycolytic agent	Substance that prevents the breakdown of glucose
Aortic semilunar valve	Structure that prevents backflow of blood from the aorta to the left ventricle
Apex	Rounded tip of the heart
Apical pulse	Heartbeat taken at the fifth intercostal space (apex of the heart)
Appendix	Small organ that extends from the cecum
Arachnoid membrane	Middle layer of the meninges
Arteriospasm	Spontaneous constriction of an artery
Atria	The two upper chambers of the heart
Atrial fibrillation	Rapid, random contractions of the atria
Atrioventricular node	Heart pacer cell area capable of generating impulses at the rate of 40 to 60 per minute
Atrioventricular valve	Structure that prevents backflow of blood from the right ventricle to the right atrium
Auscultation	Listening with a stethoscope
Autoantibody	Antibody formed against a self-antigen
Autonomic nervous system	System regulating the body's involuntary system functions by carrying impulses from the brain and spinal cord to the muscles, glands, and internal organs
Axillary	Pertaining to the armpit
Basilic vein	Vein located on the underside of the arm
Benign	Noncancerous

Terms

Bevel
Bicuspid valve

Bilirubin
Bowman's caps

Brachial artery
Brain stem

Bronchi
Bronchioles
Buccal
Bulbourethral

Bundle of His

Calcitonin

Cannula
Carcinogenic
Cardiac cathete
Cardiologist
Carpals
Cecum
Celite
Cephalic vein
Cerebellum

Cerebrospinal
Cerebrum

Certification

Chorionic gona
Circumflex arte

Clavicle
Coccyx

Collagen
Collecting duct

Computerized
   tomography
Congenital
Conjugated
Constipation
Contracture
Cortisol

Coumadin
Cranium
Cubic centimet
Cuvette

Terms	Definitions
Foley catheter	Retention urinary catheter held in place by inflation of a balloon
Follicle-stimulating hormone	Hormone produced by the anterior pituitary gland to stimulate estrogen secretion and egg production by the ovaries and sperm production by the testes
Fowler's position	The head of the bed is elevated to 90 degrees
Functional residual capacity	Amount of gas left in the lungs after a normal exhalation
Gastrin	Hormone secreted by the gastric mucosa to stimulate gastric acid secretion
Gauge	Unit of measure assigned to the diameter of a needle bore
Genitalia	Reproductive organs
Geriatric	Pertaining to old age
Glomerulus	Collection of capillaries enclosed by the Bowman's capsule where filtration occurs
Glucagon	Hormone produced by the pancreas to stimulate conversion of glycogen to glucose
Glucosuria	Glucose in the urine
Grid	Thin, waferlike barrier placed between the patient and the radiographic cassette to absorb scattered radiation
Growth hormone	Hormone produced by the anterior pituitary gland to stimulate growth of the bones and tissues
Hemodialysis	Technique to remove waste products from the blood when the kidneys are not functioning
Hemoglobinometer	Instrument that measures the concentration of hemoglobin in a solution
Hemolysis	Destruction of red blood cells
Hemolytic disease of the newborn	Blood group or type incompatibility between mother and fetus that can cause hemolysis of the fetus's red blood cells
Heparin	Anticoagulant monitored by the activated partial thromboplastin time
Human chorionic gonadotropin	Hormone produced by the placenta during pregnancy to stimulate the ovaries to produce estrogen and progesterone
Humerus	Long bone of the upper arm
Hypoglycemia	Decreased blood glucose
Hypothalamus	Part of the brain that regulates body temperature and the secretions of the pituitary gland
Hypothyroidism	Reduced thyroid function
Hypoventilation	Below-normal level of ventilation that increases the partial pressure of carbon dioxide
Hypoxemia	Less than normal partial pressure of oxygen in the arterial blood
Ileum	Last part of the small intestine
Immune	Resistant to certain diseases
Infection	Multiplication of microorganisms in body tissues
Inferior	Pertaining to a position below another structure
Inspiratory reserve volume	The amount of gas that can be inhaled above that of a normal inhalation
Insulin	Hormone produced by the pancreas to promote the utilization of glucose by the body

Intensifying screens	Internal sides of a radiographic film cassette
Intercostal	Between the ribs
Interneuron	Nerve cell entirely within the central nervous system
Internodal pathways	Area of the heart that conducts impulses from the SA node to the AV node
Interstitial fluid	Fluid located in the spaces between cells
Ischemia	Deficiency of blood to a body area
Jaundice	Yellow appearance
Jejunum	Second part of the small intestine
Kilovoltage	Electric potential of one thousand volts
Labia	Outer folds of the vagina
Larynx	Organ between the pharynx and the trachea containing the vocal cords
Left anterior descending artery	Branch of the left coronary artery that supplies the anterior of the heart
Left bundle branch	Division of the bundle of His transmitting impulses to the Purkinje system
Licensure	Authorization by an agency to practice a profession
Lipase	Pancreatic enzyme to digest fats
Loop of Henle	Part of the renal tubule between the proximal convoluted tubule and the distal convoluted tubule
Lot	Group of products manufactured at the same time under the same conditions
Lumbar puncture	Procedure used to remove cerebrospinal fluid from between the vertebrae of the lower spine
Lumen	Cavity of an organ or a tube, such as a blood vessel or a needle
Luteinizing hormone	Hormone produced by the anterior pituitary gland to stimulate ovulation
Lymphokines	Chemicals released by activated T cells that attract macrophages
Macrophage	Cell derived from monocytes capable of phagocytosis of pathogens, damaged cells, and old red blood cells
Magnetic resonance imaging	Procedure producing body images in three planes using a magnetic field
Malignant	Cancerous
Manometer	Instrument used to measure pressure
Median cubital vein	Vein located in the center of the antecubital area
Mediastinum	The space between the lungs
Medulla oblongata	Part of the brain that regulates heart rate, respiration, and blood pressure
Melanocyte-stimulating hormone	Hormone produced by the anterior pituitary gland to stimulate pigmentation of the skin
Melatonin	Hormone produced by the pineal gland that regulates the body's internal clock
Metabolism/Metabolic	Chemical changes taking place in the body/pertaining to
Metacarpals	Bones of the hands
Metastasis	Spread of cancer from a primary site to another site
Metatarsals	Bones of the feet
Milliampere-seconds	Radiologic unit of measurement that determines the amount of x-ray energy produced
Milliliter	One thousandth of a liter
Mitosis	Cell division
Mitral valve	Valve between the left atrium and the left ventricle of the heart

Terms	Definitions
Myocardium	Muscle layer of the heart
Necrosis	Death of cells
Norepinephrine (noradrenalin)	Hormone produced by the adrenal medulla to constrict blood vessels and increase blood pressure
Occult	Hidden (not visible)
Olfactory receptors	Sensory receptors in the nasal cavity that provide the sense of smell
Oncology	Branch of medicine specializing in tumors
Oral	Pertaining to the mouth
Osteoblast	Bone-producing cell
Osteoclast	Bone-destroying cell
Osteomyelitis	Inflammation of the bone
Ostomy	Surgical opening for the elimination of waste
Ovaries	Female gonads that produce ova
Ovulation	Release of ovum from the ovary
Oxytocin	Hormone produced by the posterior pituitary gland to stimulate contraction of the uterus at delivery and release of milk into the breast ducts
Pacemaker cells	Cells that determine the rhythm of the heart
Palpation	Examination by touch
Parathyroid hormone	Hormone produced by the parathyroid gland to regulate calcium levels in the blood
Pathogen	Microorganism capable of producing disease
Pathology	Branch of medicine specializing in the study of disease
Pathophysiology	Disease affecting a body function
Perfusion	Passage of blood or other fluids through the vascular system
Pericardium	Membrane surrounding the heart
Perineum	Region between the anus and the female urethra or male scrotum
Peritoneum	Membrane lining the abdominal cavity
Phagocytosis	Ingestion of bacteria or other foreign particles by a cell
Pharynx	Tubelike structure located behind the nose that is a passageway for air and food
Phenylalanine	Naturally occurring amino acid
Phlebitis	Inflammation of a vein
Phlebotomy	Puncture or incision into a vein to obtain blood
Photocell array	The activation of the cells in a radiographic unit that determines the necessary amount of exposure to radiation
Photometer	Instrument that measures light intensity
Pia mater	Innermost layer of the meninges
Plasma cell	Cell derived from an activated B cell that produces antibodies to a specific antigen
Platelet	Blood-clotting cell
Polycythemia	Markedly increased red blood cells
Polyuria	Marked increase in the urine flow
Pons	Part of the brain stem that influences respiration
Porphyrins	Intermediate compounds in the formation of heme
Posterior (dorsal)	Pertaining to the back of the body
Postprandial	After eating
Prenatal	Before birth

Procedure manual	Detailed documentation of procedures and methods used in performing tests
Progesterone	Female hormone produced by the adrenal cortex and the ovaries to promote conditions suitable for pregnancy
Prognosis	Forecast of a disease course or outcome
Prolactin	Hormone produced by the anterior pituitary gland to stimulate breast development and milk secretion
Prostate gland	Gland that surrounds the first inch of the male urethra and secretes an alkaline fluid to maintain sperm motility
Prothrombin	Protein converted to thrombin in the coagulation process
Proximal convoluted tubule	Part of the renal tubule between the Bowman's capsule and the loop of Henle
Pulmonary semilunar valve	Structure that prevents backflow of blood from the pulmonary arteries to the right ventricle
Pulse	Measurement of pressure when blood is forced out of the heart as the ventricles contract
Purkinje fibers	Cardiac muscle fibers that conduct electricity
Purkinje system	Cardiac electric system capable of generating impulses at a rate of 20 to 40 per minute
Radial artery	Artery located on the thumb side of the wrist
Radioisotope	Substance that emits radiant energy
Radius	Large bone of the lower arm located on the lateral or thumb side
Rectum/Rectal	End part of the colon/pertaining to
Reducing valve	Device used to lower the pressure of a gas leaving a container
Regulator	Combination of a reducing valve and a flowmeter on high pressure medical gas cylinders
Renin	Hormone produced by the kidney to increase blood pressure
Residual volume	Amount of gas remaining in the lungs after a maximum exhalation
Reticulocyte	Developing red blood cell
Reverse Trendelenburg's position	The head of the bed is raised and the foot of the bed is lowered
Right bundle branch	Division of the bundle of His transmitting impulses from the SA node to the Purkinje system
Right lymphatic duct	Collects the lymph from the right upper quadrant to return it to the blood
Rotor head	Movable part of a centrifuge
Sacrum	Five fused sacral vertebrae at the base of the spine
Scapula	Flat bone forming the back of the shoulder (shoulder blade)
Scrotum	Sac that contains the male testes
Sebum	Oily secretion of the sebaceous gland
Semi-Fowler's position	The head of the bed is raised 45 degrees and the foot, 15 degrees
Seminal vesicles	Glands that secrete an alkaline fluid that becomes part of semen
Septicemia	Pathogenic microorganisms in the blood
Septum	Partition between the right and left sides of the heart
Shock	Sudden decrease in blood flow interfering with heart and tissue function

Terms	Definitions
Sinoatrial node	Mass of pacer cells considered the dominant pacemaker of the heart
Sphygmomanometer	Instrument that measures blood pressure
Sputum	Expectorated matter from the lungs
Sternoclavicular articulation	Joint that connects the collarbone with the breast bone at the location of the first rib
Sternum	Breastbone (alternate site for the collection of bone marrow specimens)
Stethoscope	Instrument used to listen for body sounds
Stratum corneum	Outermost layer of the epidermis consisting of dead cells filled with keratin
Stratum germinativum	Innermost layer of the epidermis in which cell division occurs
Sublingual	Under the tongue
Superficial	On the surface
Superior	Pertaining to a position above another structure
Synarthrosis	Immovable joint
Systole	Contraction phase of the heartbeat
Tarsals	Bones of the ankles
Technical factors	Control determining the appearance of an x-ray
Testes	Male gonads that produce sperm
Testosterone	Hormone produced by the testes and responsible for the development of male sexual characteristics
Thalamus	Part of the brain that regulates subconscious sensations
Thixotropic gel	Substance that undergoes a temporary change in viscosity during centrifugation
Thoracic	Pertaining to the chest
Thoracic duct	Collects the lymph from the lower body and left upper quadrant to return it to the blood
Thrombin	Enzyme that converts fibrinogen to fibrin
Thrombolytic	Clot destroying
Thrombophlebitis	Inflammation of a vein producing clots
Thymosin	Hormone produced by the thymus gland for the maturation of T cells
Thyroid-stimulating hormone	Hormone produced by the anterior pituitary gland to stimulate secretion of thyroid hormones
Thyroxine/ triiodothyronine	Hormones produced by the thyroid gland to stimulate energy metabolism of cells
Tibia	Largest bone of the lower leg
Tidal volume	Amount of gas exhaled after a normal inhalation
Tonicity	Active resistance to stretching in muscles (maintains posture)
Trachea	Organ that provides the opening between the larynx and the bronchi
Trendelenburg's position	The head of the bed is lowered and the foot is raised
Tricuspid valve	Valve between the right atrium and right ventricle
Trochanter roll	Support placed at the hip joint to prevent movement
Tunica adventitia	Outer layer of blood vessels composed of connective tissue
Tunica intima	Inner layer of blood vessels composed of endothelial cells
Tunica media	Middle layer of blood vessels composed of smooth muscle tissue

Tympanic membrane	Eardrum
Ulna	Long bone of the forearm opposite the thumb
Ultrasonography	Examination of deep body structures using high-frequency sound waves
Umbilicus	Pertaining to the navel
Ureters	Tubes that carry urine from the kidney to the bladder
Urethra	Organ that carries urine from the bladder to the outside of the body
Uterus	Female organ that forms a placenta to nourish a developing embryo
Valve	Structure in veins and the heart that closes an opening so that blood flows in only one direction
Variable performance system	Oxygen delivery system that does not provide a constant and consistent FiO_2
Vas deferens	Tube that carries sperm from the epididymides to the circulatory duct
Vector	Carrier that transfers an infective agent from one host to another
Ventral	Pertaining to the front of the body
Ventricle	One of two lower chambers of the heart
Ventricular fibrillation	Rapid movement of the ventricular muscle fibers without coordinated ventricle contraction
Ventricular tachycardia	Extremely rapid heartbeats generated within the ventricle
Visceral	Pertaining to organs within a body cavity

INDEX

An "f" following a page number indicates a figure; a "t" following a page number indicates a table.